Contents

RUNNING

BIOMECHANICS AND EXERCISE PHYSIOLOGY IN PRACTICE

Frans Bosch
Medical illustrator
National coach for jumping events in athletics
Athletics coach
Tilburg, The Netherlands

Ronald Klomp
Exercise physiologist
Sport psychologist
Olympic coach
Waalwijk, The Netherlands

Illustrations by Frans Bosch

Translation by Dee Wessels Boer-Stallman

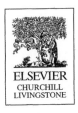

ELSEVIER
CHURCHILL
LIVINGSTONE

EDINBURGH   OXFORD   PHILADELPHIA   ST LOUIS   SYDNEY   TORONTO   2005

ELSEVIER
CHURCHILL
LIVINGSTONE

ISBN 0 443 07441 0

British Library Cataloguing in Publication Data
A catalogue record for this book is available from the British Library.

Library of Congress Cataloging in Publication Data
A catalog record for this book is available from the Library of Congress.

Note
Medical knowledge is constantly changing. As new information becomes available, changes in treatment, procedures, equipment and the use of drugs become necessary. The author/contributors and the publishers have taken great care to ensure that the information given in this text is accurate and up to date. However, readers are strongly advised to confirm that the information, especially with regard to drug usage, complies with the latest legislation and standards of practice.

your source for books, journals and multimedia in the health sciences
www.elsevierhealth.com

Transferred to digital print 2007

Printed and bound by CPI Antony Rowe, Eastbourne

The publisher's policy is to use paper manufactured from sustainable forests

Foreword

For 2 years I trained under the supervision of Ronald Klomp. With considerable experience behind me, I first thought that there were not too many new things that I could still be taught. In that I was greatly mistaken. Inspired as Ronald is, my coordination was almost immediately compared to that of a very young puppy we encountered on the sidewalk, which could barely stand on its own four feet and constantly toppled over. Naturally, I was insulted, but it could not be denied that Ronald was honest and indeed showed some insight. Those first months were tough and painful, and all those strange exercises drove me nearly crazy, although I saw their results.

Years before, during my very first training at an athletic club, I had arrived at the race track wearing tennis shoes. I had had no idea that this was not such a good idea. After scraping together some money in the following weeks I bought some real running shoes and I noticed the difference immediately. Although this opened my eyes, at the same time it showed my ignorance regarding running as a sport. Everyone can run can't they? You really don't need anything else to help? Many people still think this way. Some people will even ask themselves if so much can be written about the sport. Running always looks so easy. It may wear you out but it isn't that difficult is it? Indeed it is! There is much more involved than merely putting one foot in front of the other. People cannot run fast and perform well just by having talent and simply training a lot. Details are so very important here, and will decide whether you continue to enjoy running, whether your performance improves and whether you can protect your body from injury. Pleasure, as well as improvement, can be increased so much if someone reaches out to you with a helping hand. This book is about these details. It charts the territory between tedious incomprehensible theories and the actual practice of running.

According to the authors, this is the ultimate book about running. Such a claim creates expectations, but that is what Ronald and Frans are all about – convinced about what they are writing. They have walked a long road before writing this book. Ronald and Frans have both had years of experience working with top athletes, guiding athletes from their first step to a high level of performance. They have been part of and have counseled each phase in an athlete's development. They have attended international athletic tournaments, and spent many hours during warm-ups observing top athletes preparing themselves to compete. They have watched how an athlete moves and seen which techniques are correct for the most efficient way to run. Based on this experience, they have written this book.

Read it and run!

Ellen van Langen
Summer 2001

Introduction

During a symposium on middle- and long-distance running held in 1983, Peter Coe, the father and trainer of Sebastian Coe (at that time holder of the world record for the 800 m, 1500 m and English mile), spoke the following introductory words:

Coaching is an art. Although it is science based, it is still an art.

This book about running, which has since come into existence after an encounter between 'artist' Frans Bosch and 'scientist' Ronald Klomp, bears the same characteristic. Intuition, observation, experience and speculation have been brought together on a scientific basis, resulting in a practical book with a scientific background.

Starting with a general knowledge of anatomy and physiology, one progresses towards the application of specific ways of training, directed at improving running performance in the broadest sense of the word. It is concerned with the running performance of recreational as well as top runners, of patients in physiotherapy, of sportsmen and school-aged youths. Using the information presented in this book, trainers as well as physiotherapists and physical education teachers can gain better insight into running, which might, at first glance, appear so simple. Moreover, this book presents many ways to influence adequately the running performance of a specific target group.

The chapters have been arranged taking into account both the reader's areas of interest and their level of knowledge. For example, if the reader is highly knowledgeable about anatomy and the physiology of exercise, then Chapters 1 and 2 can be skipped over and left to function as reference material. When the reader is particularly interested in the practical application of a particular form of training, he or she is advised to read Chapters 4–6. Here it should be noted that justification for many of the forms of exercise chosen can be found in the defined running model discussed in Chapter 3.

In Chapter 1, a number of anatomical and biomechanical principles important for understanding running are discussed. These basic data, together with more general information on anatomy and biomechanics, form the blocks with which the model for running is constructed.

In Chapter 2, the processes in the physiology of exercise that play an important role during running are presented. For example, attention is paid to how energy is generated and to how the cardiorespiratory system functions.

In Chapter 3, a model for running is described. Although relevant anatomical, biomechanical and physiological data are integrated into this model as much as possible, one can speak only of a model, not of a certain and proved system. The question remains whether science will ever be able to document completely the total pattern of running with proven facts. The description chiefly concentrates on running at a high and constant speed. The role of reactivity, the avoidance of interfering rotations, and movements during the floating and stance phases are described in detail, with both text and illustrations.

In Chapter 4, the general principles of training are presented. Thorough attention is given to adaptation as a consequence of training. Finally, the means that can be applied during training are derived.

In Chapter 5, running instruction is discussed. Here the relationship between physical condition, the sensory system and coordination is shown. The principles of overload, specificity and transfer of training are explained in relation to instructing running technique. Exercises to practice teaching technique are aimed at the basic components of the running technique, the total motion of running, and the start and acceleration.

In Chapter 6, strength andstrength training are discussed. The manifestations of strength are described and analyzed according to their applicability within the training process. Furthermore, adaptation resulting from strength training is discussed, with strong emphasis on the relationship between strength and coordination. In the second half of this chapter, the relationship between the various muscles and muscle groups, which are specialized for a particular type of work, and forms of strength training in which such specialization is used is shown. Subsequently, forms of strength training best suited for the most important groups of muscles are discussed, with reference to the underlying principle as well as to the exercises themselves. The established patterns by which individual muscles work together during strength training are shown and, finally, forms of strength training that are related to running are discussed.

Frans Bosch and Ronald Klomp
Summer 2001

1
Anatomy of the locomotor apparatus and basic principles of motion

1.1   COORDINATION AND RUNNING: MECHANICS OR BIOMECHANICS?

Without auxiliary tools, one would only be able to study the mechanics of running by observing the body's outer surface. At a glance, one might see the upward and downward oscillation of the limbs. Such a segment can be thought of as a fixed unit with a certain unchanging mass, and its movement can be plotted graphically. For example, the thigh oscillates up and down while its velocity accelerates or slows. Using a video camera, one can record changes in the angular velocity of the hip joint during locomotion. Using information obtained during such observations, it is possible to draw a number of conclusions regarding the amount of energy required for the pendular motion of the oscillating leg. However, it will be more difficult to designate which muscles are providing the necessary power. When a muscle is located superficially near the outer surface, it can clearly be seen to contract. However, no sign of surface activity can be observed for other (more deeply lying) muscles. In order to chart muscle activity accurately, one needs to use technical tools such as electromyography (EMG). Although it is relatively easy to use EMG to record the activity of muscles situated close to the surface, recording the activity of the iliopsoas, for example, will prove quite difficult, if not impossible. If more accurate information is needed on the activity of a certain musculature (e.g. how a change in muscle length during prestretch is divided between the changes in length of the passive and contractile muscle segments), laboratory experiments must be set up in which dissected muscle can be studied as isolated tissue. However, the deeper one delves into the topic of muscle tissue by way of such interventions, the further one drifts away from the area of functional movement. One can make extremely exact observations (e.g. with respect to an isolated muscle fiber) without being able to draw significant conclusions about how muscles function in sports.

Technical descriptions of running all too frequently include what can be observed on the body's surface, but do not take into consideration what EMG studies and tested models for muscle activity can contribute. Such an approach completely anchors any analysis of running to the mere rise and fall of body segments, so that the analysis misses its mark, not with regard to small details, but on essential issues. For speed running, the end of the support phase is always seen as a very important moment for propulsion or thrust. American sprinters who hold their upper body erect, or even inclined slightly backward, and who fail to push off at the end of the stance phase until the stance leg is fully extended have been frequently judged as being technically weak. At first glance, the mechanics of running gives support to this opinion, because the direction of thrust is particularly favorable at the end of the support phase. Therefore, the end of thrust should be a very good time to exert a great deal of force. However, from EMG recordings of the hamstrings (a muscle group that can direct the force of thrust favorably) (see Section 1.6.1), one can deduce that these muscles are silent, having already stopped working by that time. Apparently there are other factors at play that help determine whether the end of support will be favorable for forward propulsion. Many of these factors lie 'hidden' within the body. For example, one such important factor is the lever arm of the hamstrings with respect to the hip joint, which is less favorable by the end of thrust.

The mechanics of running is therefore decided, to an important extent, by factors that cannot be observed on the body's surface. Understanding how a running technique is effective goes hand in hand with one's knowledge about the processes that take place within the body: i.e. how the lever arm of a muscle works upon a joint that must move, as well as how the lever arm can change; how energy can be stored before being released in forward thrust, from which more than half of the total energy needed is derived; how one muscle group can exert an eccentric moment on another muscle group during movement; or how, by tilting the pelvis forward, the dorsal muscles can exert an eccentric moment on the hamstrings, which makes them work better in terms of reactivity* thereafter (leveraged action of the pelvis). Therefore, many mechanisms are at work deep within the recesses of the body, and have a decisive effect on running. The prefix 'bio' in the word 'biomechanics' is thus essential to a good understanding of the concept of 'running technique'. Many aspects in the total pattern of movements involved in running are still unknown. Through evolution, locomotion has been designed to be energy efficient, but the price that must be paid is the complexity of the entire mechanical pattern of locomotion. Because of such efficiency, running is more complicated than other forms of movement (e.g. backflip, skating, swimming) that are further removed from man's natural state and, therefore, more difficult to learn. Opinions on running techniques are really more like models for movement than patterns that have actually been measured. Unraveling the secrets of running will prove more difficult than unraveling those of less natural forms of motion.

1.2 STRUCTURE AND WAYS IN WHICH JOINTS CAN MOVE

The range within which a joint can move depends to a large extent on what movement the structure of the joint allows in different directions. As well as being limited by its structure, the movement of a joint can also be limited by the range of a muscle. For functional movement, the degrees to which different joints move must be coordinated accurately if they are to work well together. Analyzing what happens in a single joint during running will only prove worthwhile if that movement is also considered in relation to movement in the other joints. Descriptive analysis of a running technique should integrate the movements occurring in all the joints.

Note on translation Two of the more widely used technical words in the Dutch original of this book are the noun 'reactiviteit' and the associated adjective 'reactief', which have been translated here as 'reactivity' and 'reactive'. In English, 'reaction' almost always implies a neurally mediated response. However, in this book 'reactivity' refers instead to the almost instantaneous resistance to stretch of muscle cross-bridges already active at the time the stretch is imposed. So the response to the imposed load is not an active, neurally mediated process, but a passive reflection of the muscle's properties at the instant concerned. Of course, these properties depend critically on the neural activation operating on the muscle, as well as on its length, at the moment of the stretch. This neural activation *prepares* the muscle for its 'reaction', and is sustained essentially constant throughout it – the reaction is not *caused by changes* in the activation. Thus it is important for readers to bear in mind that the 'reactivity' referred to is that of a muscle actively braced and so stiffened against impact, *not* one that is relaxed and easily extended. A full explanation of the phenomenon is given in Section 1.4.2.

1.2.1 Hip, back, and pelvis

The hip joint is a functional, spherical joint that has six degrees of freedom for movement:

- forward flexion (maximum 120° possible)
- backward flexion (maximum 13°)
- adduction (maximum 20°)
- abduction (maximum 40–60°)
- medial rotation (maximum 13–40°)
- lateral rotation (maximum 36–60°).

There is greater freedom of movement for abduction, medial rotation, and lateral rotation when the hip is bent rather than extended. The hip is considered to be extended when the femur is positioned so that the axis of the knee joint is in the frontal plane. The femur is a torqued bone and, when in this position, its head is turned to the front, creating an angle averaging 12° with the frontal plane. The range of movement in this position is less for lateral rotation (36°), medial rotation (13°), and abduction (40°). Forward flexion allows a greater range of movement in the intended direction. For abduction and adduction, the optimum angle is about 60°, while for medial and lateral rotation it is about 90°.

During the first strides of a sprint after leaving the starting block, forward flexion in the hip is about 90° at the moment when the foot is placed on the ground surface. As speed increases, the hip is less bent at foot placement and, once constant speed has been achieved, there is only slight forward flexion at foot strike. During the first strides after the start, a sprinter will evert his foot as he places it on the ground (lateral rotation and abduction in the hip, and lateral rotation in the lower leg). This is possible due to greater freedom of movement in the hip joint when the hip is bent. Why sprinters do this is not known. The reason might be the fact that, during the start, the hip and knee are extended quite far by the end of the support phase, so that strong medial rotation has developed in the hip. Setting the leg down in a position of lateral rotation will limit the degree of medial rotation during push-off. The athlete will not need to push himself to reach the upper boundary for medial rota-

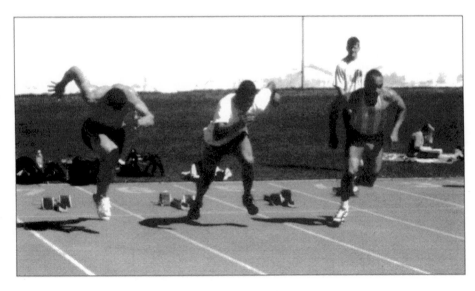

Figure 1.1 Degree of movement during the start

During the start, at the moment of foot placement (right-hand runner), the hip and knee are bent, giving the joints a great degree of freedom to move. The hip is laterally rotated and abducted; the lower leg is rotated laterally. The foot is turned outward (eversion) at ground contact. At the end of the support phase (center and left runners), the hip and lower leg revert from a lateral rotation to the neutral position. At the end of push-off, the heel points directly toward the rear. This typical sequence of movements is observed for most athletes during the start.

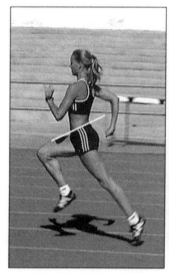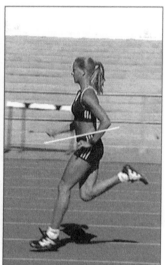

Figure 1.2   Forward pelvic tilt
Ligaments lying in front of the hip joint allow only up to 13° backward flexion. The pelvis tilts forward, increasing the range in which the foot can be moved backward. Muscles responsible for forward pelvic tilt are important during running.

tion (36°). It is also possible that outward rotation of the stance leg will allow more force to be exerted for acceleration. Once the athlete has attained speed, lateral rotation in the hip can be omitted. During the support phase, the foot will now be able to point in the direction in which the athlete is running (i.e. the line of progression). Moreover, there are many athletes who, even when running at speed, also rotate the hip outward before foot placement. When running at speed, some athletes (e.g. Ato Boldon) who compete at international level will use a different position for each leg during foot placement: e.g. foot strike without more lateral rotation in the hip (the foot pointing directly forward) and foot strike with the leg strongly laterally rotated (with the foot everted) (Lohman 1977, Tittel 1990, Rozendal & Huijing 1996).

Freedom of movement for medial rotation, lateral rotation, and adduction is so slight in an extended position because important and very strong ligaments (the iliofemoral, pubofemoral, and ischiofemoral) lying in front of the hip joint resist any greater degree of movement. In particular, limiting backward flexion to 13ffl has important consequences for the total pattern of movement seen for running. This means that being able to move the stance leg toward the rear, up until the foot leaves the ground, is partly brought about by tilting the pelvis forward. Pelvic tilt should hold a place of importance in any theoretical discussion of the technique of running.

All the ways in which the hip joint can move are called upon during running. During the support phase, medial rotation, abduction, and backward flexion take place, while forward flexion, lateral rotation, and adduction develop during the swing phase.

Movements made by the hip joint can also be translated into movement of the pelvis. After all, tilting the pelvis forward will cause the hip joint to move, which equals forward flexion in the thigh. Tilting the pelvis backward corresponds to backward flexion in the hip joint. When standing on one leg, moving the contralateral free hip in various directions causes the hip joint to move in different ways: i.e. rotating the free hip forward causes medial rotation, moving it backward causes lateral rotation, lifting it causes abduction, and dropping it causes adduction in the hip joint. Whether it is the leg or pelvis that changes its position when the hip moves

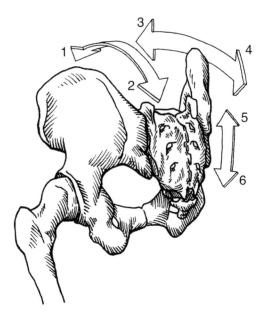

Figure 1.3   Ways in which the pelvis can move when standing on one leg
Forward (1) and backward (2) pelvic tilt are identical to forward flexion and backward flexion in the hip joint. Forward (3), backward (4), upward (5), and downward (6) movement of the free hip are identical to medial rotation, lateral rotation, and abduction and adduction in the hip joint, respectively.

depends on the situation in which the motion is carried out. In an open-chain movement (in the hip of the swing leg), using sufficient force to tighten abduction-producing muscles causes the leg to be lifted laterally; in a closed-chain movement (in the hip of the stance leg), the free side of the pelvis undulates upward. For a good understanding of running, it is important that both these possible results of hip joint movement (i.e. movement of the leg and of the pelvis) be included in the analysis. In the methodology of training an athlete to run, it is useful to approach movement in the hip joint from both perspectives: how the leg moves (at the knee, fast pendular

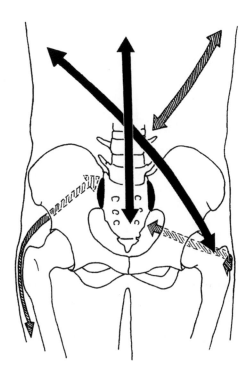

Figure 1.4   Passage of muscles within the area around the pelvis
Many muscles around the hip run diagonally in the body. The sacroiliac joint is bridged, and thus affected, by many such muscles.

motion of the leg, etc.) and how the pelvis moves (use of dorsal, abdominal, and small gluteal muscles, etc.).

The pelvis articulates not only with the thigh, but also with the spinal column, by way of the sacroiliac joint. Much is still unknown about the exact function of this joint. The sacroiliac joint can only move within a very small range (2–4° rotation), but despite its limited mobility it still has a certain function. Because the pelvis works like a lever with large lever arms, even a small degree of movement can have a large effect on the total locomotor system. In addition to its motor function, the sacroiliac joint also has an important sensory function, because many muscle groups (e.g. the gluteus maximus, oblique and transverse abdominal muscles, hamstrings, iliopsoas, and latissimus dorsi) exert force on it from different directions. The sacroiliac joint lies at the meeting point of various force trajectories. As far as running is concerned, the sacroiliac joint only draws attention to itself when complaints arise. Oblique muscles (i.e. the gluteus maximus and oblique abdominal muscles), which are very important for running, also affect how well the sacroiliac joint will function. Training these muscles professionally can therefore help prevent the development of problems in the sacroiliac joint (Snijders et al 1995).

Flexion, extension, lateral flexion, and axial rotation (i.e. torsion around the longitudinal axis) can all take place in the spinal column. The degree of movement is dic-

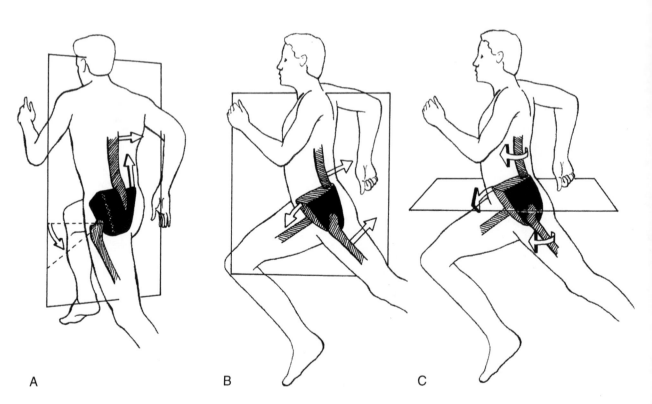

A   B   C

Figure 1.5   Coordination between degrees of movement during the support phase
(A) Frontal plane: abduction in the hip joint (the free side of the pelvis is lifted), lateral flexion in the spinal column.
(B) Sagittal plane: backward flexion in the hip joint, pelvis tilted forward, spinal column extended.
(C) Transverse plane: medial rotation in the hip joint (the free side of the pelvis is bent forward), torsion in the spinal column.

tated to a large extent by the position of the joint surfaces to which the vertebrae are connected. In particular, flexion, extension, and lateral flexion can occur in the spine. Rotation, or torsion, is generally seen at a thoracic level. Moreover, lateral flexion is always accompanied by some rotation, and vice versa. For running, flexion and extension (especially lumbar) and rotation (especially thoracic) are important.

Movements in the hip, pelvis, and spinal column are closely interrelated during running. In the sagittal plane, backward flexion in the hip of the stance leg, forward pelvic drop, and extension in the spinal column all occur simultaneously during push-off. In the transverse plane, there is medial rotation in the hip of the stance leg, while the contralateral free side of the pelvis moves toward the front and the spinal column rotates in the opposite direction. In the frontal plane there is abduction in the stance leg and lateral flexion in the spinal column, while the contralateral free side of the pelvis undulates upward. The relationship between the degree of movement in the hip joint and the movements in the pelvis and spinal column provides a complete picture, in which the pelvis functions as a lever when the body moves. Because of their attachment to the pelvis, muscles can have a very large levered arm with regard to the hip joint or spinal column. First, using their large lever arm, muscles can affect the joint that they span (e.g. abdominal muscles with regard to the spinal column, and gluteus maximus, rectus femoris, and the hamstrings with regard to the hip joint). In addition, due to the specific structure of the pelvis, its musculature (e.g. the dorsal and abdominal muscles, which can affect the hip joint by rotating the pelvis forward and backward) can have an influence on joints that the muscles do not span. In this way the pelvis is responsible for the transfer of force from the upper body to the legs, or from the left to right side of the body. For example, when standing on the right leg, if the erector spinae contracts strongly on the contralateral side, the left side of the pelvis will be raised, resulting in abduction in the right hip. When the left leg is lifted toward the front while standing, the hamstrings of the contralateral leg can increase the degree of movement possible by pulling the pelvis backward. This aspect of the pelvis, which can function as a lever, is central to further discussion of the technique of running.

1.2.2 Knee

The most important degree of movement in the knee occurs during the swing phase. In this phase the position of the knee changes from nearly straight at the end of the support phase, to quite bent at the middle of the swing phase, to slightly bent during the next foot placement. The maximum degree of flexion found during speed running varies greatly between athletes. Some runners bend the knee so far that the heel nearly touches the buttocks, while other runners bend the knee to just 90°. During the support phase (especially when running fast), the angle made by the knee is able to change much less.

Due to the structure of the femoral epicondyle, which looks like a snail shell when viewed from the side, the ligaments are tightened as the knee straightens. In addition to this tension, the differences in structure between the lateral and longer medial femoral condyls are responsible for holding the knee stable (i.e. there is no movement in the transverse and frontal planes) and for protecting the joint adequately when the knee is in an extended position. Thus when an athlete running at high speed sets his foot down in an everted position, he is able to do this not by moving his knee within the transverse plane, but rather by developing strong lateral rotation in the hip.

When the knee is bent, it can also produce movements other than flexion and extension. The lower leg can rotate medially and laterally so that the tibial tuberosity shifts medially or laterally, respectively. During functional movement, medial (maximum 30° when the knee is bent 90°) and lateral rotation (maximum 45° when the knee is bent 90°) in the knee are always accompanied by inversion and eversion of the foot.

In addition to these rotations, when the knee is bent and then straightened, the tibia will slide relative to the femur. The knee joint is quite a complex mechanism, because it allows many possibilities for movement. The menisci play an important role in guiding these sliding, rotating, and rolling motions, during which they undergo distortion and their positions shift. To prevent injury to the knee, one must coordinate quite precisely the various possible movements. When the knee is bent and the lower leg or shank laterally rotated (e.g. when squatting), the form of the medial meniscus is strongly distorted and its position will have shifted quite far. Subsequently, when the leg is straight, medial rotation must be carried out in the lower leg, to ensure that the medial meniscus is returned correctly to its original position. If such medial rotation does not take place, the meniscus can become damaged (Snijders et al 1995, Rozendal & Huijing 1996).

As already stated, sprinters evert their feet during their first steps after leaving the starting block. The heel is inverted as the foot touches the ground. When the knee is bent, there will be lateral rotation in the lower leg. As the foot pushes off, the heel is subsequently everted again, so that the lower leg rotates medially. One aim, for example, of this medial rotation is to return the meniscus to its original position. The same type of rotation across the ball of the foot during push-off can be observed in tennis players, who initiate a quick sprint after the opponent has hit an unexpected dropshot. Skaters, on the other hand, cannot rotate on the blades of their skates, and consequently must avoid everting the heel during push-off. They cannot make use of the possibility for lateral rotation in the lower leg because, thereafter, it will be impossible to develop medial rotation, which is needed during push-off. In order to direct sufficient force of thrust toward the rear during the start, the foot must still be everted as it is placed on the surface. To solve this problem, a skater will begin by rotating the hip strongly laterally so that the knee is pointing further outward during the first part of the start than is customary for a runner.

1.2.3 Ankle and foot

The foot is an especially complicated structure, with 12 bones, 14 phalanges, and 108 ligaments. The ways in which the foot can move, and in particular the relationship between its segments, are so complex that the best approach to understanding its function is to use a greatly simplified model.

One should first differentiate between the upper and lower tarsal joints. In the upper tarsal joint the distal ends of the tibia and fibula articulate with the upper plane of the talus joint. Although the joint is hinged, it can also make important rolling and sliding movements. To do this, its rotational axis is not rigid, but rather adapts as the foot changes position. Roughly explained, the axis runs mediolaterally at the level of the medial malleolus. Both dorsiflexion and plantar flexion are possible in the upper tarsal joint. Due to its structure, the upper tarsal joint is most stable during dorsiflexion.

In the lower tarsal joint, the talus (a bone to which no muscles attach) articulates with the navicular bone and the calcaneus. The axis of this joint also shifts during movement, running approximately laterally upward from behind, through the heel

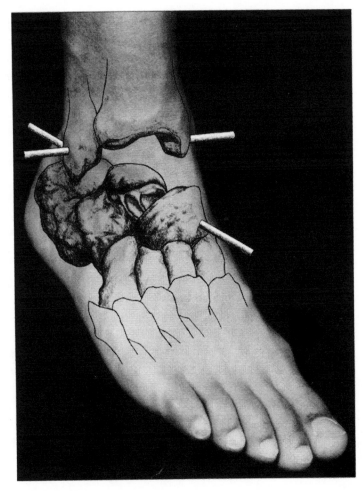

Figure 1.6 Axes of the upper and lower tarsal joints
Bones surrounding the ankle, excluding the talus, are illustrated.

bone, and then medially upward toward the front through the navicular bone. When the foot is dangling freely, there is 5° eversion (i.e. pronation + abduction + dorsi-flexion) and 20° inversion (i.e. supination + adduction + plantar flexion) around the axis (Snijders et al 1995, Rozendal & Huijing 1996).

The arches of the foot are not rigid structures and can actually change form. If the medial arch is raised and lowered while standing on the ball of the foot, this will not only cause a certain degree of movement in the lower tarsal joint, but it will also change the positions of all the other joints in the tarsal bone and mid-foot. All the rotations and distortions in the tarsal bone and arches of the foot can be described as supination and pronation. The motion of flattening the arch of the foot is called pronation, while that of making it hollow is called supination.

The ways in which all the joints of the foot can move together ensure that the foot can adapt optimally to the conditions in which it must function during running. Different demands are constantly being made on the foot's ability to distort its shape to suit various ground surfaces, different running speeds, and changes in velocity.

During foot strike, it can clearly be observed that the tarsal joints, tarsus, and arches of the foot are quite flexible. Due to its ability to transform its shape, the foot can adapt well to the demands made on it by the ground surface, body posture, etc. Flattening of the arch of the foot by about 1 cm during foot strike will be absorbed by the very strong ligaments and the action of its muscles. The energy that is absorbed here does not disappear as frictional heat, but rather is stored in elastic tissues until it can be released during the following push-off (McNiell Alexander 1987, Snijders et al 1995). Thereafter, during the support phase, the foot becomes less flexible. The upper tarsal joint assumes the position of dorsiflexion, in which it is most stable but its flexibility is most limited. As the plantar aponeurosis (a very strong structure on the underside of the foot) tightens, its flexibility is further limited. This strong fascia transverses beneath the foot from the calcaneal tubercule toward the area of the metatarsophalangeal joints. Together with the application of muscle strength, the plantar aponeurosis works to stop the structure of the foot arches from flattening. As soon as the metatarsophalangeal joints begin to bend (toward the end of support), the plantar aponeurosis tightens and the arches of the foot become quite taut. Because the foot has become more rigid by the end of the support phase, force can be unloaded much better to the ground. The cycle in which the foot first distorts in order to store energy and then becomes more rigid in order to unload energy, takes less time during high-speed running than during slow running. In order to complete this cycle rapidly, an athlete must remember to generate a great deal of prestretch and tension in the tendons around the ankle, even before the foot touches ground. Therefore, tension must already be present in the lower-leg muscles before foot placement. These muscles can only tighten optimally when the position of the ankle is neutral. Controlling the cycle in which the form of the foot is first transformed and then energy is transferred to the ground is therefore closely related to controlling the position of the upper tarsal joint.

The shape of the tarsus and foot arches is also affected by how the lower leg moves. If the lower leg rotates medially while standing, the arches of the foot will flatten (pronation). During lateral rotation, the foot arches will hollow (supination).

Figure 1.7 Ways in which the foot can move

Movements in the foot should be considered together. On the left, the lower leg rotates medially (the tibial tuberosity serves as an orientation point and turns medially). Medial rotation causes the tarsal bone to turn inward and downward from its neutral position, thus flattening the foot. Pronation in the lower leg flattens the foot and is caused mainly when the forefoot moves with regard to the tarsal bone (black arrows). The tarsal joints (white arrows) move only slightly. On the right, the lower leg rotates laterally. Lateral rotation causes the tarsal bone to turn upward and outward from its neutral position, thus rounding out the arch of the foot. This distortion of the entire foot is called supination, and is caused mainly by movement in the tarsal joints (black arrows). The forefoot (white arrows) moves only slightly.

When the foot can hang freely, pronation accompanies eversion and supination inversion.

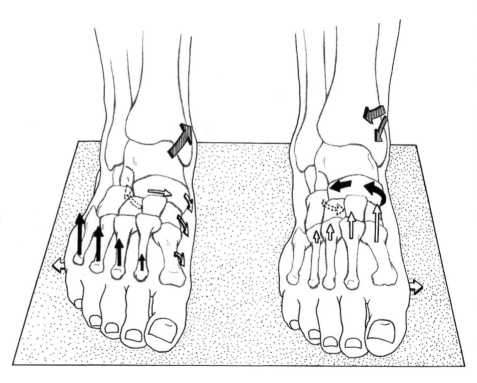

If the foot is off rather than on the ground, lateral rotation in the lower leg will be accompanied by eversion in the foot (Rozendal & Huijing 1996).

In summary, movement in the foot is a combination of movements in the lower leg, upper and lower tarsal joints, foot arches, and tarsus, each of which strongly affects the other.

1.3 GENERATION OF POWER AT MUSCLE LEVEL

The way in which all the muscles involved in running can generate power determines how speed can be increased and maintained. Speed will remain constant if there is exactly enough power to overcome opposing forces (e.g. air shear and contact friction) and to compensate for the loss of internal energy as parts of the body constantly accelerate and slow down. Speed will increase when there is more than enough power available to compensate for the energy wasted by antagonistic forces. In this section, attention is given to the delivery of power (P) at muscle level, which is determined by the amount of force generated (F) and the speed of muscle contraction (v): $P = Fv$.

The morphology of a muscle has a great effect on the force and speed of muscle contraction, independent of biochemical or physiological factors. To gain insight into the role played by muscle morphology during a functional movement such as running, it is necessary first to study the structure and function of muscle tissue on a microscopic level. Starting at the level of the sarcomere, the discussion below progresses to the level of the muscle–tendon–bone complex, passing through a number of intermediate steps. At each level it is possible to identify which factors determine force and speed and, finally, to what extent these factors can be applied when setting up a strength-training program for runners, for example.

1.3.1 Force and speed at sarcomere level

Skeletal muscle is composed of muscle fibers grouped together in small bundles. A muscle fiber is an elongated cell, 10–80 μm in diameter, with many nuclei. The muscle fiber, which is surrounded by a membrane called the sarcolemma, contains sarcoplasm, which is the fluid component of the muscle cell. The sarcoplasm contains myofibrils, in addition to dissolved amino acids, minerals, various organelles, glycogen, and fats. These strings of contractile protein are stretched along the entire length of the muscle fiber. One muscle fiber can contain from many hundreds to several thousand myofibrils. In turn, a myofibril is built up of sarcomeres, which are considered to be the smallest basic functional unit of skeletal muscle. Three categories of protein can be found in a sarcomere:

(1) proteins directly involved in the process of contraction taking place within the sarcomere
(2) proteins regulating such processes (Jones & Round 1990, Huijbregts & Clarijs 1995, Brooks et al 1996)
(3) proteins serving to maintain the spatial structure within a muscle cell (Huijbregts & Clarijs 1995).

In this section attention is focused on the types of protein listed under (1) and (2). More information about the third category of proteins can be found in textbooks of physiology (Wilmore & Costill 1994, Brooks et al 1996, Fox et al 1996).

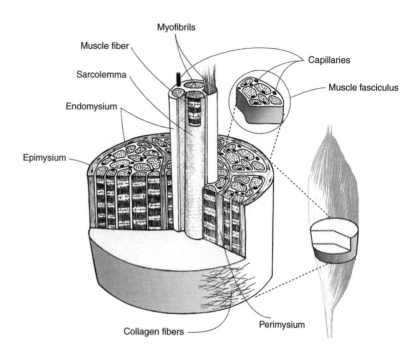

Figure 1.8 Schematic illustration of a muscle segment
A segment of muscle showing the pathways for muscle fibers and layers of connective tissues (endomysium, perimysium, and epimysium). A small bundle of fibers belonging to one muscle fasciculus is shown.

Contractile proteins

The most import proteins involved in muscle contraction in a sarcomere are myosin and actin. Typically, some 1500 myosin and 3000 actin filaments are arranged side by side in the cross-section of a myofibril. These numbers are somewhat misleading because, based on mass, two-thirds of muscle protein consists of myosin (Wilmore & Costill 1994). Myosin is the chief constituent of thick myofilaments and actin is the chief constituent of thin myofilaments. To gain insight into the generation of force and speed of contraction, it is important to look more closely at the structure and function of thick and thin myofilaments.

Thick myofilaments
The myosin molecule consists of two equal-length intertwined chains with a globular head on one terminal end. A myosin chain is composed of a relatively lightweight tail segment (light meromyosin) and a relatively heavy head–neck segment (heavy meromyosin). In the head–neck segment, one can differentiate two components: S1 and S2. The S1 component, the actual myosin head, makes an angle of 90° in relation to the length of the myofibril, and at this angle is able to bind with actin. It is also the site where the enzyme myosin–ATPase is located. (The role of myosin–ATPase is outlined on pp. 15–16) S2 is the neck component, which forms a flexible elastic connection with S1. The elastic properties of the S2 component are part of the sliding-filament theory (Huxley & Huxley 1957) (see pp. 14–15). The various forms of muscle contraction can be considered and explained using this theory. When the S1 units are positioned with at right angles to the myofibril fibers at the start of a possible cross-binding with actin, the S1 and S2 components together are called 'cross-bridges'.

The thick filament consists of a braid intertwined from the tails of 200–300 myosin molecules. The cross-bridges are located on the terminal ends so that only the braided body of the tails is found in the mid-section. Therefore, in this region (10% of the total length) cross-bridges are unable to bind to the actin filament.

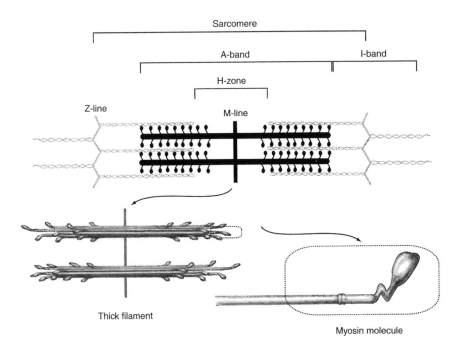

Figure 1.9 Two-dimensional organization of a sarcomere
A sarcomere runs between Z-lines. A thick myofilament, called myosin, is illustrated.

Thin myofilaments

The chief constituent of the thin myofilament is the globular protein actin (g-actin). Inside a sarcomere, actin is found only as string-like chains, so-called filamentous actin (f-actin). The thin myofilament is mainly composed of two intertwined f-actin chains. To visualize this structure clearly, imagine a pearl necklace in which g-actin represents a single pearl and f-actin the entire necklace.

Lying in the groove formed when two f-actin chains are twisted together is an elongated regulatory protein called tropomyosin. At regular intervals along the actin is another regulatory protein called the troponin complex, which is composed of the

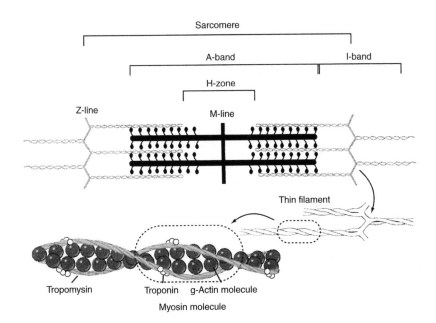

Figure 1.10 Two-dimensional organization of a sarcomere
A thin myofilament, called actin, is illustrated.

subunits troponin-C, troponin-I, and troponin-T. These regulatory proteins are involved in allowing the creation of bonds between actin and myosin filaments.

Actin filaments come together at one terminal end in the Z-disc (Zwischen membrane), where they bind to four actin filaments from the next half-sarcomere. The Z-discs are considered to be the boundaries of a sarcomere (Jones & Round 1990).

Sliding-filament theory

In the past, many models were devised that might be used to explain the phenomenon called 'muscle contraction'. The most frequently asked question was 'In what manner do actin and myosin filaments interact?'. In 1954, Huxley and Huxley made a number of remarkable discoveries, which eventually led to the sliding-filament theory. One proof for the sliding-filament theory was the stearic change in the structure of the sarcomeres involved in contraction. In addition, the basis for the theory was formed from experiments in which the force of isometric contractions was measured using muscle fibers set at various lengths. The latter is further elaborated on in Section 1.4.1, where the first-mentioned evidence for the sliding-filament theory (i.e. sarcomere structure) is discussed in depth.

Differences in size, density, and division of actin and myosin filaments are responsible for the characteristic transverse stripes, or striations, of a sarcomere that can be seen under the microscope (Martini 1998). A schematic model of the sarcomere structure shows the reasons for this phenomenon. Darker zones, called A-bands, alternate with lighter zones, called I-bands. The A-band contains myosin filaments as well as a zone where there is partial overlap with actin filaments. In this area of overlap light is able to pass through less easily, in contrast to I-bands where actin filaments are the main constituent. To complete the description, there is an area within the A-band where only myosin filaments are found (the H-zone).

The following changes in sarcomere structure can occur during muscle contraction:

- the H-zone and I-band shorten
- the zones where actin and myosin overlap increase in size
- the Z-discs come to lie closer together
- the width of the A-band remains unchanged.

The observations made by Huxley and Huxley (1954) concerning changes in sarcomere structure during contraction can only be explained if the thin filaments actually slide along the thick filaments toward the center of the sarcomere. In other words, the length of the actin and myosin filaments does not change. The way in which the actin and myosin filaments interact was discovered by experimenting with dissected contractile segments of muscle fiber. When an active muscle fiber shortens rapidly by 1% of the total fiber length, the force generated temporarily drops to zero before building up again. If the actin and myosin filaments were to assume the structure of a long spring during contraction, the force would only decline by 1% during this rapid 1% shortening of the total length of the muscle fiber. This discovery pointed to the existence of many short components generating force and working along a short trajectory, because slight shortening would completely remove stretch from these components (Jones & Round 1990). This short force-generating component is the S1 segment of the globular myosin head that clamps itself to a free binding site on the actin filament and subsequently topples over toward the H-zone, pulling the actin filament toward the center of the sarcomere. The entire cross-bridge cycle is discussed below.

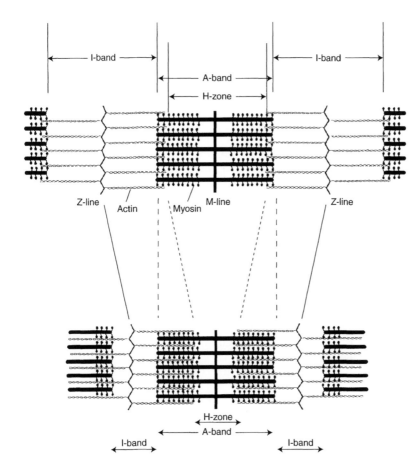

Figure 1.11 Section of a sarcomere shortened by contraction
The lengths of the myosin and actin filaments do not change. The filaments slide over each other (sliding filaments), whereby the A-band keeps its length and the H-zone and I-band shorten.

Cross-bridge cycle

A cross-bridge cycle consists of a number of successive steps, starting from the moment that a myosin head binds to actin until the moment that the bond has been broken and the process must repeat itself (Brooks et al 1996).

When a signal from the nervous system is strong enough to initiate muscle contraction, a number of processes begin within the muscle cell. First, the sarcoplasmic reticulum, where calcium ions are stored, is stimulated so that calcium ions are released into the sarcoplasm. The calcium ions bind to troponin-C, which is part of the troponin complex on actin. As a result, the troponin complex undergoes stearic alteration, by which the tropomyosin is pulled, as it were, a little farther into the groove of the actin filament. The result is that the binding sites on actin that had previously been masked by tropomyosin are now available for the globular myosin heads. Once myosin–ATPase has activated the myosin head by hydrolyzing ATP to ADP and P_i, which remains bound to the myosin head, then an actomyosin complex can be formed. This process can be compared to tightening the spring of a mouse trap. The myosin head is activated and swings in the direction of a binding site on actin, where it forms a weak bond with actin. The myosin head now forms an angle of 90° with the myosin filament. The release of P_i on the myosin head initiates the power stroke (i.e. the myosin head tumbles over, thus pulling actin towards the center of the sarcomere). At the end of the power stroke, ADP and P_i are released, and a strong bond (the 'rigor complex'), is formed between actin and myosin. ATP is needed to uncouple the rigor complex and produce relaxation.

If sufficient calcium ions remain on hand, through constant stimulation by the nervous system, the cross-bridge cycles will continue to repeat (frequency, say, 5/s). The myosin heads uncouple from actin, swing back to their initial positions, are reactivated by myosin–ATPase, and then bond at a new free binding site further along the actin filament. One might say that the actin filament is 'rowed' toward the center (the myosin heads acting as oars). When sufficient calcium ions are available, the cross-bridge cycles can continue repeating until the ends of the myosin filaments reach the Z-discs. When the time comes that muscle is being activated only slowly by the motor nerve bundles, or when activation has stopped completely, the concentration of calcium ions in the sarcoplasm decreases, because they are continuously being pumped back into the sarcoplasmic reticulum. The calcium ions bound to troponin-C are released and tropomyosin returns to its original position, so that the binding sites on actin are once again masked against interaction with a myosin head (Fox et al 1996).

Force of contraction and sarcomere structure

The maximum force generated by a sarcomere depends on the fiber length and the speed of shortening (Rozendal & Huijing 1996). The force that a single sarcomere can generate when static is a fixed value of 22–28 N/cm^2 cross-section. Moreover, there is no difference between slow and fast muscle fibers. The arrangement of sarcomeres, however, affects not only the force generated but also the speed of con-

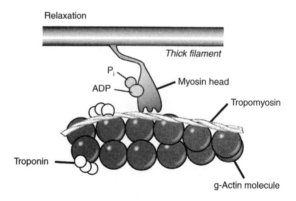

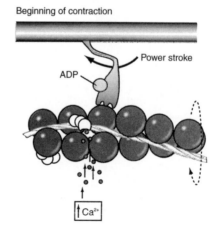

Figure 1.12 Formation of the actomyosin complex
The troponin complex undergoes a change in configuration when calcium ions bind to troponin-C within the troponin complex on actin. Binding sites on actin that were first hidden by tropomyosin are now freed for the myosin heads.

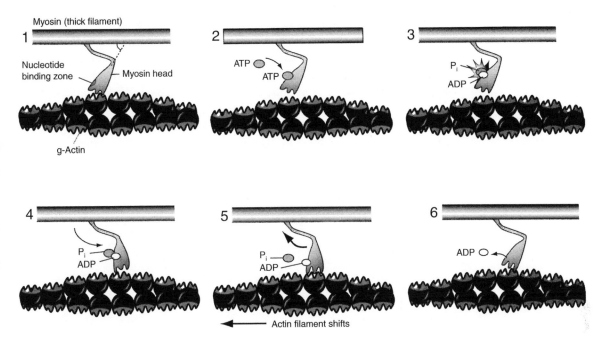

Figure 1.13   Molecular basis for muscle contraction
1 The rigor complex.
2 Unlinking the rigor complex with the help of ATP.
3 Activation of the myosin head by hydrolysis of ATP with the help of myosin-ATPase.
4 The beginning of a weak binding between a myosin head and actin.
5 Power stroke.
6 Development of the rigor complex at the end of the power stroke as ADP is released from the myosin head.

traction. The way in which the arrangement of sarcomeres within a muscle fiber exerts an influence is discussed in Section 1.3.2. Differences in the amount of force generated have been registered at the level of a single sarcomere, under isometric conditions using varying lengths of sarcomere. The relationship between force and sarcomere length is discussed in more detail in the following section.

Each sarcomere has a maximum speed of contraction that is chiefly determined by the specific activity of myosin–ATPase, which has a number of isoforms (small deviations in structure) that determine the speed of contraction. Slow and fast muscle fibers (see Section 1.3.2) can be categorized on the basis of certain isoforms of myosin–ATPase found on the myosin head. The speed at which a muscle shortens is inversely related to the force generated (this is discussed in detail in Section 1.4.1).

Force–length diagram
The experiments that led to the discovery of the force–length relationship in a sarcomere were carried out to measure its isometric activity. Both ends of a muscle-fiber segment were held fixed while an instrument for measuring force was attached to one end (Rozendal & Huijing 1996). After applying maximum stimulation, the force generated during the isometric contraction was measured. It was assumed that the various sarcomeres found in a muscle fiber were of uniform length. However, it appeared that the sarcomeres located at the terminal ends were shorter than those found in the center of the muscle fiber.

Assuming that the same force is generated for each cross-bridge interaction, the force generated by a sarcomere will depend on the number of possible cross-bridge interactions. In other words, the total force is dependent on the degree of overlap between actin and myosin filaments. Maximum force will develop if all the cross-bridges are able to bond to an actin binding site (i.e. the sarcomere has an optimum length when the overlap between actin and myosin filaments is maximum). The isometric force that a muscle fiber can produce when the length of its sarcomeres vary can be plotted on a force–length diagram.

The characteristic pattern found in a force–length diagram shows that force decreases when sarcomeres are shorter (Fig. 1.14, left) or longer (Fig. 1.14, right) than the optimum length. When they are longer than optimum there is less overlap between actin and myosin. Conversely, when sarcomeres are very short the myosin filaments come to butt against the Z-discs, so that further shortening becomes impossible. Just before such a situation has been reached, when the sarcomeres are still a bit longer, the actin filaments lying longitudinally to each other are already partly overlapping, and thus normal interaction between thick and thin filaments becomes impossible.

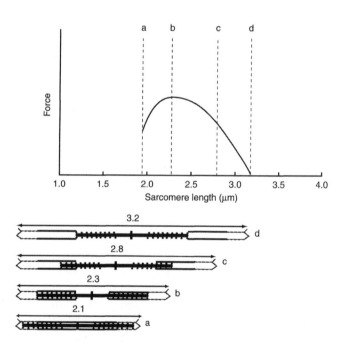

Figure 1.14 *Force–length relationship in a sarcomere*
The relationship between force and length in a sarcomere is explained by the degree of overlap between actin and myosin filaments.

Force–velocity diagram

As described above, the force generated by a sarcomere depends on the degree of overlap between actin and myosin filaments. In addition, the developing force depends on the speed at which the fiber is shortened and/or elongated. When a muscle has been stretched to its optimum length, but the length is not held fixed during stimulation, it is possible to measure the force generated at different speeds of contraction. It is found that there is an inverse relationship between the maximum force generated and the speed of contraction. At higher speeds of contraction the force generated decreases. When the muscle is stretched while activated, the force generated increases (Fig. 1.15, left-hand side) by as much as 50–100% of the isometric value. When constructing a graph to plot the power of a muscle fiber, each coordinate in the force–velocity diagram represents the product $P = Fv$. This power curve is discussed in Section 1.8.

An explanation for the relationship between force and speed of contraction can be found in cross-bridge kinetics; i.e. in the important role played in this process by the elastic S2 segment. Under isometric conditions, the globular myosin head can be compared to a rotating gear that grasps the active binding sites located on actin. The actin filament remains in place while the elastic S2 segment of the cross-bridge elongates. When the sarcomeres shorten, there are fewer cross-bridge interactions and the S2 segment has less time in which to stretch. When the speed of contraction is rapid, it is possible that the myosin head cannot release its hold in time, so that the movement of filaments sliding past each other is hindered by the crumpled S2 segment. As the speed of contraction increases, the number of interfering cross-bridges increases and there is a further decline in force.

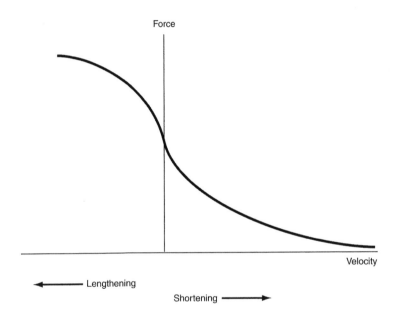

Figure 1.15 Force–velocity diagram

When a sarcomere elongates, the S2 segment becomes increasingly stretched, thus causing higher tension. Moreover, it is thought that the myosin head makes a rotation in the opposite direction, by which means it can come in contact with several free binding sites on actin during a single cross-bridge interaction. In this manner, more force can be generated during one cross-bridge cycle than when a sarcomere shortens.

1.3.2   Force and speed of contraction at muscle-fiber level

A muscle fiber is composed of myofibrils, which can be arranged in various ways. Here, attention is directed at how contractile material is arranged, and so the effect of elastic components is not taken into consideration. When the junctions of two sarcomeres are connected end to end in series, the total force that can be generated is equal to the force generated by one sarcomere. After all, the forces that are being exerted on the common Z-disc are in opposition and therefore do not contribute to the total force of contraction. The changes in length can be summed, so that the total is twice that for two sarcomeres connected in parallel (Rozendal & Huijing 1996). When several sarcomeres are connected end to end in series, those situated more toward the center can act as a strong connection at the moment when an isometric force is needed (Jones & Round 1990). As already stated, because the lengths of sarcomeres are not uniformly distributed along the muscle fiber, activating sarcomeres that have already reached their maximum overlap has an eccentric effect on other sarcomeres that have not yet attained their maximum overlap. In this situation, the total force generated is greater than if the sarcomere lengths were uniformly distributed (Huijbregts & Clarijs 1995). In particular, this situation can be said to occur when the muscle-fiber length is nearly maximum.

When two sarcomeres are connected in parallel, the situation is reversed: i.e. the change in length is equal to that of a single sarcomere, while the force generated is twice as large as that for two sarcomeres connected in series. Muscle strength is therefore proportional to the cross-section rather than to the length of the muscle. The characteristics of the force–length and force–velocity diagrams have been determined experimentally under conditions for maximum muscle-fiber stimulation (Rozendal & Huijing 1996). The degree of stimulation also determines how much force of contraction will be generated.

In vivo, muscle strength can be regulated in one of two ways. First, more muscle fibers can be called into action. Muscle fibers are organized in motor units. A single motor unit consists of a nerve cell and a motor nerve innervating a cluster of muscle fibers. Within a motor unit all the muscle fibers have identical biochemical and physiological properties (Brooks et al 1996). Slow-twitch (ST) motor units contain clusters of only 10–180 muscle fibers, while fast-twitch (FT) motor units contain clusters having as many as 300–800 muscle fibers. Motor units are recruited according to the 'size principle' (Henneman et al 1974), which means that the order of recruitment is closely related to the magnitude of stimulation originating in the nervous system. Each motor unit has a minimum stimulation threshold that must be exceeded if activation is to take place according to the 'all or nothing' principle. This stimulation

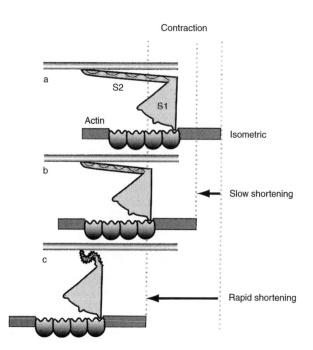

Figure 1.16 Types of contraction
Behavior of the elastic S2 segment of the cross-bridge during different types of contraction.

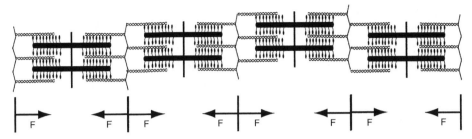

Sarcomeres in series

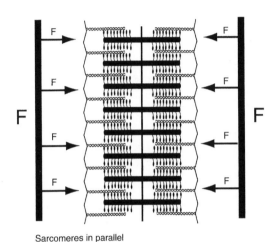

Sarcomeres in parallel

Figure 1.17 Generation of force by sarcomeres
Generation of force by serial and parallel joined sarcomeres.

threshold is strongly related to the size of the nerve cell body, which means that ST motor units, which have small cell bodies, are recruited before FT motor units, which generally have larger cell bodies and are called into action as stimulation increases. Selective recruitment of motor units is determined by the force of contraction demanded and not by the speed of movement (Gollnick et al 1974). The force that must be generated cannot be regulated simply by selectively recruiting motor units; the activities of various motor units must also be synchronized. However, it will never be possible to synchronize 100% of the motor units available in a muscle, because this would result in damage to muscle and tendon.

In addition to selective recruitment and eventual synchronization of motor units, muscle strength can also be varied by adapting the firing frequency, this being controlled from within the nervous system (rate coding). After a motor unit has been activated by way of a motor nerve, a single contraction occurs, followed by release of tension (relaxation) in the muscle fibers. If, before muscle relaxation is complete, another stimulus exceeding the stimulation threshold of the motor unit is applied, the forces produced by the two stimuli are summed. As the firing frequency increases, the force of contraction also increases.

1.3.3 Slow and fast muscle fibers

It has already been stated that both slow and fast muscle fibers are found in muscle. Fast muscle fibers can be further subdivided into types a, b, and c. In (English language) literature, slow and fast muscle fibers are classified as slow-twitch (ST) and fast-twitch (FT), or type-I and type-II, respectively. In spite of the fact that there

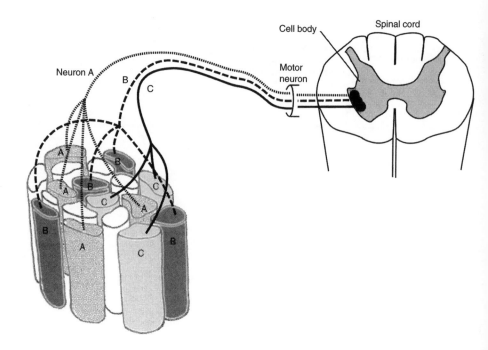

Figure 1.18 Motor units
Three motor units, each consisting of a cell body, motor neuron, and innervated muscle fibers.

are several classification systems available for differentiating various types of muscle tissue, in this book a classification has been chosen that is based on information obtained using histochemistry. This division shows a strong relationship to the classification based on contractile muscle properties. The similarities are sufficiently great that it is unnecessary to discuss both classifications explicitly. Using contractile muscle properties as the classification criterion, muscle fibers can be categorized as:

- slow
- fast, fatigue-resistant
- fast, readily fatigued.

Using histochemistry as the criterion for classification, muscle fibers can be categorized as:

- slow, oxidative (type I; ST)
- fast, oxidative, glycolytic (type IIa; FTa)
- fast, glycolytic (type IIb; FTb).

Slow, oxidative (ST) muscle fibers are suitable for long-duration low-intensity physical exercise. They are nearly unfatiguable and efficiently produce ATP aerobically from carbohydrates and fats (see Ch. 2). These muscle fibers are specialized to provide energy aerobically. The concentration of oxidative enzymes is higher in ST than in FT muscle fibers. Compared with FT muscle fibers, ST muscle fibers also have at their command more fat reserves, more mitochondria, and a more extensive capillarization. It is also notable that the Z-discs are thicker in ST than in FT fibers. The reason for this should probably be sought in the process of adaptation resulting from continuous physical exercise.

Muscle fibers categorized as fast, oxidative, glycolytic (FTa) are recruited during higher intensity exercise and, because they are supplied with oxidative and glycolytic enzymes, are capable of generating energy by both anaerobic and aerobic processes.

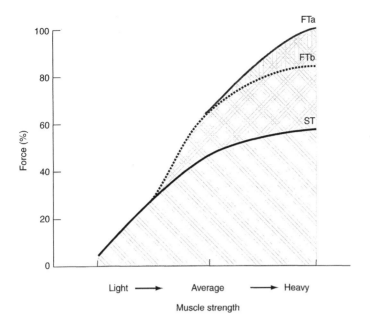

Figure 1.19 *Selective recruitment of motor units*
Motor units are selectively recruited according to the contractile force required. Slow-twitch (ST) motor units are recruited first, followed by fast-twitch (FTa and FTb) fibers when stimulation is intensified.

Of the three different types of muscle fibers, FTa fibers are more 'all round' in their performance. Like the slow, oxidative (ST) muscle fibers they have the ability to generate energy aerobically, and like the fast, glycolytic (FTb) muscle fibers they can generate energy anaerobically (see below). However, in both cases the FTa fibers are outperformed by the specialist fibers.

FTb fibers are the most difficult to recruit. Because of their high stimulation threshold, these fibers can only be activated when the contraction must be strong. The high concentration of glycolytic enzymes makes this type of muscle fiber especially suitable for generating energy anaerobically. However, the fibers become more easily fatigued.

The above-mentioned terms 'slow' and 'fast' twitch refer to the speed of a single contraction (twitch). Under isometric conditions, FT muscle fibers achieve their maximum force of contraction during a single twitch more rapidly than do ST fibers. The reason for this can be found in the differences between the isoforms of myosin–ATPase on the myosin head. FT fibers have an isoform characterized by a high myosin–ATPase activity, while ST fibers have an isoform characterized by a lower myosin-APTase activity. In addition, FT fibers are able to relax more rapidly, which has a direct effect on the firing frequencies at which motor units (composed of ST or FT muscle fibers) must stimulate them in order for the force of contraction to reach a maximum level. Because FT fibers need a shorter time to relax, a higher firing frequency is necessary in order for their force of contraction to reach a maximum level. As already stated, the order in which different motor units are recruited is determined by the differences in their stimulation thresholds. The firing frequency can then serve to make further subtle distinctions in terms of contractile force. The order of recruitment within FT muscle fibers is FTa first, then FTb. (FTc fibers are not considered here because they are only a small component of muscle tissue (<3%) and little is known about their properties.) In addition to having a higher speed of contraction, motor units composed of FT fibers can also provide a greater force of contraction, which can be explained by the presence of more FT muscle fibers. The force exerted by individual ST or FT muscle fibers does not vary greatly.

Muscles in untrained individuals have approximately equal amounts of ST and FT fibers. In long-distance runners, the ST/FT ratio favors ST fibers (90% of the muscle tissue in the calves of marathon runners able to compete at international level is ST fibers), while in elite sprinters the ratio favors FT fibers (nearly 80% of the muscle tissue in the calves of sprinters is FT fibers). Researchers have proposed the idea that it might be possible to determine an athlete's talent for running a specific distance by analyzing a muscle biopsy (the removal of a piece of muscle tissue using a hollow needle). However, such a method would have its limitations because a large number of performance-determining factors, such as coordination, muscle cross-section, and cardiovascular capacity, would not be taken into account. Moreover, with the use of increasingly refined techniques to differentiate types of muscle fiber, evidence is mounting that supports a continuum rather than three or four separate types of fiber. In particular, the activity of myosin–ATPase appears to range from low to high. Finally, the reasoning behind the idea that FT fibers provide speed, and thus good performance, during a sprint overlooks the important role played by reactivity, elasticity, prestretch, and the avoidance of rise delay (see Sections 1.4 and 1.5).

1.4 STRUCTURE AND DIFFERENTIATION OF MUSCLES, JOINT MOMENTS, AND PASSIVE-TISSUE FUNCTION

1.4.1 Different muscle structures

The morphology of the body's musculature is so diverse and remarkable that one is compelled to question why such differentiation exists. The most simple basic concept for muscle structure is the tendon–muscle belly–tendon complex connected in series. Each muscle in the human locomotor apparatus represents a unique variation of this basic concept. The angle that a muscle fiber makes with regard to its tendon, as well as the number and length of muscle fibers, can vary. This also holds true for the number, length, and structure of tendons, for the lever arm with regard to

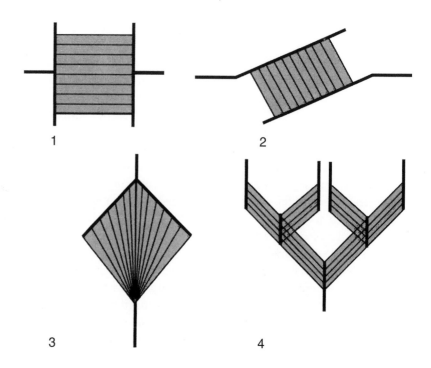

Figure 1.20   Different types of muscle structure
1 Parallel-fibered.
2 Unipennate.
3 Fusiform.
4 Multipennate.

the joint bridged, for passive tissues in and around a muscle, etc. Sometimes the variations are so pronounced that the basic concept can only be traced with difficulty.

Because of their differences in structure, not all muscles are suited to doing the same type of work. While one muscle may be able to contract concentrically over a large range with relatively little force (e.g. the sartorius), another muscle may be more suited to contract over a small range with greater force (e.g. the gluteus maximus), or for reactive muscle action. Before a muscle can work reactively, it must first be stretched by an external force. Due to stretch, energy is first stored in the elastic segments of the muscle before being subsequently released as the muscle shortens (e.g. the soleus). Such far-reaching specialization in muscle naturally has many consequences for functional movement. Muscles that are made to contract in a manner for which they have not actually been built cannot work efficiently. In order to analyze and to learn which techniques can be used correctly in sports, one must first understand both the structure and the specialization of different muscle groups (Rozendal & Huijing 1996).

Muscles that are part of the locomotor apparatus can be divided into three categories according to their structure:

- Parallel-fibered.
- Pennate:
  - unipennate (fibers ordered in one group)
  - bipennate (fibers ordered in two groups)
  - fusiform (fibers ordered like spindles)
  - multipennate (fibers ordered in multiple groups).
- Orbicular or sphincteric.

Pennate and fusiform muscles are characterized by the fact that their fibers make an angle with the muscle's line of action (i.e. the direction in which force is exerted). Muscles are labeled strongly pennate when the angle between the muscle fiber and line of action is large. In parallel-fibered muscles, the fibers run parallel to the line of action. In order to compare the 'properties' of pennate and parallel structures, the following comments must first be taken into consideration (Rozendal & Huijing 1996):

- There is a direct relationship between the force that a muscle can generate and its physiological cross-section (i.e. that section of muscle taken directly perpendicular to the length of the muscle fibers, which shows the maximum number of fibers that are connected in parallel). The larger the physiological cross-section of a muscle, the more isometric force it can produce.
- There is a direct relationship between the total length of sarcomeres connected in series and the speed at which the muscle can shorten. The longer the chain of sarcomeres, the faster the muscle will be able to shorten. For example, when 20 sarcomeres are connected end to end in series, if one sarcomere shortens by 1 unit within 1 s, the total length of contraction achieved will be 20 units. When 10 sarcomeres are connected in series, the total length shortened will be 10 units within the same timeframe.
- There is a direct relationship between the total length of sarcomeres connected in series and the range within which a muscle can exert a great deal of force. When 20 sarcomeres are connected in series, in order to shorten a fiber by a total of 10 units each fiber must contract by 0.5 units, while 10 sarcomeres connected in series have to shorten by 1 unit each to achieve the same effect. Because force

is related to fiber length (see Section 1.3.1), in contrast to a short chain, a long chain will be able to sustain a more constant force while shortening by 10 units.

A muscle that must simultaneously be able to generate a great deal of force, to contract rapidly, and to provide force over a long range will thus require not only a large physiological cross-section but also many muscle sarcomeres connected in series (i.e. a muscle with a large mass or volume, such as the gluteus maximus). Nearly all the muscles in the body have one specialization: they are built either for their physiological cross-section or for their length. We can partly deduce what type of work a muscle can perform by looking at its structure. Parallel-fibered and pennate structures are expressions of muscle specialization.

Parallel-fibered muscle

When the muscle structure is parallel-fibered, shortening the fibers will cause the largest possible decrease in total muscle length. Within a given mass, a parallel-fibered muscle can be short and thick or long and thin. In the first case, the muscle can pull harder, but will develop less speed and only work across a short range. When a muscle is long and thin, there are more sarcomeres lying in series, thus enabling the muscle to shorten more rapidly and exert force over a longer range. The maximum amount of force (related to its mass) that such a long parallel-fibered muscle can provide is slight. The sartorius, which like the rectus femoris bridges the knee and hip joints, and is approximately as long, is a muscle that satisfies this characteristic, albeit in a distinctive manner.

Figure 1.21 Two muscles of equal length
The left muscle is parallel-fibered (e.g. sartorius) and the right muscle has a pennate structure (e.g. rectus femoris). When the fibers in both types of muscle shorten equally (e.g. 10%), the parallel-fibered muscle shortens more than the pennate muscle. Parallel-fibered muscles are thus more suited to concentric and eccentric work and pennate muscles to isometric work.

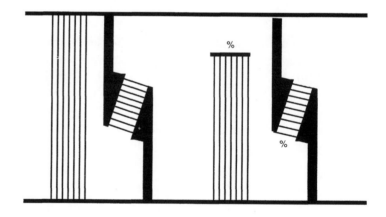

Pennate muscle

In a strongly pennate muscle, the specific structure demonstrates the following characteristics:

- A strongly pennate structure (i.e. a relatively large angle is formed between the length of the fiber and the line of action) makes a muscle suitable for attaining a large physiological cross-section, certainly when its origin and insertion are not located too close together and when the area of attachment to the bone is not too large. Because of its large physiological cross-section, such a muscle will generate a great deal of force in relation to relatively slight mass.
- The disadvantage of a pennate structure, however, is that not only the muscle fibers, but also the force generated, are at an angle to the muscle's line of action.

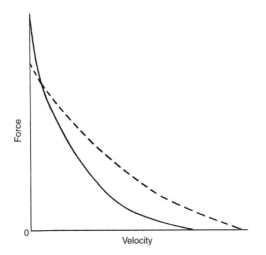

Figure 1.22 Force–velocity diagram
The force–velocity diagram for parallel-fibered (dotted line) and pennate (solid line) muscle. When both types of muscle have the same total mass, the pennate muscle will have the larger physiological cross-section and be able to exert the most force close to isometry. When the speed of contraction is more rapid, parallel-fibered muscle can continue delivering more force because it has longer chains of sarcomeres connected in series.

When the angle is 30°, only 87% of the force remains in a longitudinal direction (cos 30° = 0.87). As long as the pennate angle is less than 30°, the advantage of having a larger physiological cross-section per mass (and thus greater force) off-sets the disadvantage posed by the unfavorable direction of the force. A pennate structure is therefore favorable, up to an angle of 30°, for the magnitude of force that can be directed toward the line of action.

- A strongly pennate structure is less suitable for rapid shortening. There are two reasons for this. First, the total length of muscle fibers connected in series is limited, and the total change in length of fibers connected in series is small. Second, shortening the fibers through the angle that they make with the line of action has only a limited shortening effect on the total muscle. From this perspective, the mechanics of pennate muscle are extremely complicated. During contraction, the angles formed by muscle fiber, tendon, and the line of action change. Considering the aim of this book, delving deeper into the complexity of this material would serve no further purpose, nor would it help to clarify any consequences for locomotion in sports (see e.g. Rozendal & Huijing 1996).

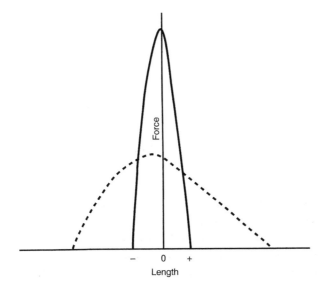

Figure 1.23 Force–length diagram for muscles
The 0-line is placed on the length of the fiber where the muscle can exert optimum force. In contrast to pennate muscle of a similar mass, parallel-fibered muscle (dotted line) can exert force over a longer range but not as much force within the optimum range. Muscles are specialized to perform certain types of work. Functional movement adheres as closely as possible to the specialized ability of a muscle.

- When its structure is strongly pennate, a muscle can only exert force across a small range. The reason for this again lies in the limited length of sarcomeres joined end to end and the angle formed by the fibers and the muscle's line of action.

The rectus femoris spans the hip and knee joints, is strongly pennate, and consequently is especially well suited to generating a great deal of force near isometry and close to the optimum length. This suitability for isometry is entirely in agreement with the biarticular nature of the muscle. Movement in one joint can be compensated for by movement in another joint, while the muscle remains close to its optimum length (Zuurbier & Huijing 1992, Rozendal & Huijing 1996).

In summary, it can be said that the structural characteristics of muscles differ, and therefore their suitability for the work that they must perform varies. Differences in suitability can be especially significant due to nothing more than the structure of the muscle itself. Pennate muscles, the fibers of which form a large angle with the line of action, are better able to do isometric work across a limited range. Parallel-fibered muscles, which have long chains of sarcomeres in series, are better able to make rapid shortening contractions involving relatively little force (related to the mass of the total muscle).

1.4.2 Passive tissues and their function

In the world of anatomy, passive tissues (tendons, fascias, aponeuroses, and connective tissue) belonging to the locomotor apparatus are attracting a lot of interest. In the past, these tissues were rather neglected, as can be seen from the marvelous prints, generally drawn from anatomical preparations, found in anatomical atlases. For didactic purposes it was attempted to achieve the greatest possible clarity in both the illustrations and the preparations (i.e. everything that impeded the clarity sought was simply removed). Usually much of the connective tissue was removed by dissection because it hindered the view of the muscle fibers themselves and blurred the boundaries between muscles. What remained were the muscle bellies and their terminal tendons. By omitting all sorts of passive tissue, the functionality of these tissues was repeatedly overlooked. Today, one realizes that connective tissue and fascias form important connections between the collaborating components of the locomotor apparatus. It is because of these tissues that the mechanics of motion within areas around joints is frequently different and more complex than was previously assumed. Moreover, attitudes towards anatomy are not only changing with respect to smaller structures, which can be easily overlooked (e.g. all sorts of connective tissue surrounding and between muscles), but also with respect to larger structures, such as the iliotibial tract, which are now being approached from a different perspective.

In the theory of running, the structures of passive tissues, especially their elastic properties, are gaining in importance. In particular, the concept of reactivity (i.e. the uptake of energy from forces working upon the body and the subsequent use of that energy to create movement) plays a large role in all movements seen in sports for which speed is crucial. In any case, how passive tissues work and how elasticity and muscle strength interact during functional movement have not yet been charted sufficiently. We certainly understand the concept of 'reactivity', but do not actually know enough about how it works. Nevertheless, during the practice of training, this phenomenon is frequently applied. Moreover, we have already formed a good and differentiated picture regarding which approaches will yield results and which will fail. In this respect, the use of reactivity during training is one step ahead of our understanding it in theory.

How passive tissues influence movement can be subdivided into two categories: the transfer of force and the delay of force.

Transfer of force

Passive tissues serve to transfer force from muscle fiber to bone. It will become clear that the more complex and more interwoven the passive system is, the more complicated is the transfer of force. In muscle, connective tissue can serve to enlarge the physiological cross-section by diverting the flow of force. It is not necessary for muscle fibers to be connected end to end in series if force can be diverted from one fiber by way of passive structures around another fiber. In this way, fibers that are situated longitudinally to each other can still be connected in parallel so that the physiological cross-section is enlarged. For example, the muscle bellies of the rectus abdominis lie head to toe, but function as if they were connected in parallel because they are attached to the sheath of the rectus. The force that the muscle can generate is more or less equal to the total sum of forces produced by the muscle bellies. When force is being transferred beyond the muscle, passive tissue not only serves to transfer it from muscle to bone, but also from one muscle to another. One important function of passive tissues is to integrate this flow during movement.

The passive tissues of the various abdominal muscles, for example, are strongly fused together so that the abdominal muscles can participate as one functional unit. From the perspective of function, the nature of their activity is more collective (modulating and maintaining body shape) than a matter of each muscle acting independently (to move the trunk in a predetermined direction).

The gluteus maximus is attached partly to the thigh and partly to the iliotibial tract, which spans the knee joint. Therefore, the force of this powerful muscle can work not only on the hip joint but also on the knee joint. This division of force is important when movement is taking place within a closed chain (i.e. jumping or running), whereby all the forces must work in a well-synchronized manner in relation to both joints (Snijders et al 1995, Rozendal & Huijing 1996, Bogduk 1997).

Delay of force (elasticity and isometry)

To some degree, passive tissues can all be stretched (i.e. they are elastic). Because of their elasticity, passive tissues have an important effect on how muscles change length and on the way in which force is built up. Tissue elasticity, together with the active functioning of muscle fibers, determines the way in which contractions progress. As a rule, Hill's model of the muscle is used to describe muscle contraction. In this model, the following elements can be differentiated (Ingen Schenau et al 1995, Jacobs et al 1996, Rozendal & Huijing 1996):

- contractile elements (muscle fibers) (CE)
- series-linked elastic components (to CE) (SEC)
- parallel-linked elastic components (to CE) (PEC).

Hill's model for the muscle is behavioral rather than anatomical. The exact location of SEC segments is of less interest with regard to how the model works. In addition to tendons and aponeuroses, elements that demonstrate SEC activity can also be located in muscle belly.

The elastic elements (SEC and PEC) can influence muscle action in one of two ways:

(1) SEC and PEC segments can store energy during stretch
(2) SEC segments affect changes in muscle-fiber length during stretching and shortening contractions.

With regard to (1), tendons, aponeuroses, fascias, SEC segments in muscle belly, etc., can all be stretched in order to store energy. Such stretch develops due to forces arising from contracting muscle fibers and from external resistance, the latter force being in opposition to that of the muscle fibers. The elastic properties of passive tissues can vary greatly. Most tissues are capable of storing large amounts of energy after being stretched somewhat from their resting state. Some tissues are supple and can be stretched quite far without storing much energy before reaching the range in which elongation will be accompanied by greater storage of energy. Other tissues are rigid and can store a great deal of energy after being stretched very little.

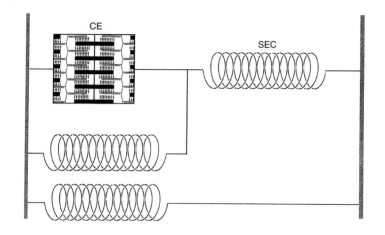

Figure 1.24 Hill's model for muscle CE, contracting element; PEC, parallel-linked elastic component; SEC, series-linked elastic component. In this scheme, PEC is divided into a segment connected in parallel only to CE and a segment connected in parallel to both CE and SEC. Both SEC and PEC segments can be divided further into different, individually distinguishable, segments. However, this is not necessary in order to understand how the complete model functions. SEC is represented as a coil to show that these segments have important elastic properties.

Figure 1.25 Storage of energy in elasticity When SEC segments are stretched, energy is stored in muscle tissue. The amount of energy stored per millimeter of stretch does not increase linearly. At the beginning of stretching, relatively little energy is stored. Thereafter, the structures become more rigid and loading capacity increases greatly per millimeter of stretch. When muscle reactivity must be extreme, such as during high-speed running, a muscle fiber should first be tensed (pretension means that muscle fiber must be tightened before absorbing an external force). There must be enough pretension in the muscle so that SEC segments can store the external energy load within the most suitable range of stretch and then release it. The plotted line ends abruptly once SEC segments have reached their maximum capacity for stretching. A larger external force will cause the muscle to rupture.

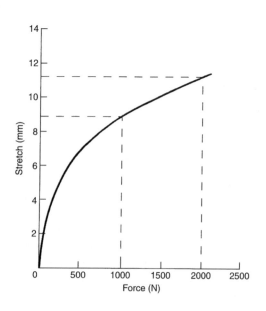

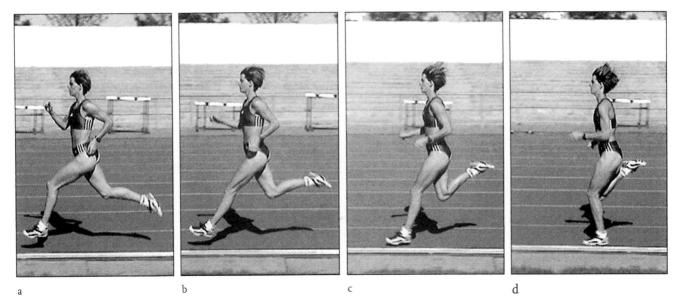

a   b   c   d

Figure 1.26a–d   Storage and return of energy
As the lower leg swings outward just before foot placement (a and b), the hamstrings tighten so that lengthening of the muscles occurs, as well as possibly some stretch in the SEC segments. Prestretch in the hamstrings is 'carried through' to the landing. During the floating phase, the body's center of mass is first displaced vertically upward before dropping again (c). During the landing, kinetic energy from the drop is also stored in elastic muscle segments (d). All the energy generated from the pendular oscillation of the leg and from the drop will be reused during the next push-off. Only a limited amount of positive work is needed because a significant amount of energy for push-off comes from muscle elasticity.

Segments connected end to end in series – particularly tendons and aponeuroses – have a greater effect than segments connected in parallel, which can only store energy after the muscle fibers have been stretched quite far.

Tendons and aponeuroses are not only important reservoirs for storing energy, but are also able to reconvert that energy during recoil into a shortening contraction. They can return up to 93% of the stored energy during recoil (Achilles tendon: McNiell Alexander 1987, 1988), while the remaining energy will be lost as frictional heat. There is only a limited amount of time possible between the storage and return of energy. If too much time is spent much of the energy will dissipate as heat (Aruin & Prilutskii 1985). For running this will not be a serious concern because the contact time with the ground is so brief that such a loss of energy will seldom occur and the return of energy can take place quite satisfactorily.

When a muscle is stretched by an external force (e.g. a hard foot strike during running) the SEC segment will be stretched. Such a stretch will be optimal if the CE does not stretch as well: indeed, because the muscle fibers work eccentrically, the muscle will lengthen at the expense of the amount of stretch of the SEC. The eccentric activity of muscle fibers counteracts energy storage in the SEC. Isometry (and eventually concentric activity, when external forces are low, and stretch, and therefore energy storage, is limited) and the preloading of elastic segments are mutually compatible processes (Ingen Schenau et al 1995). When seen in the context of running, this means that 'reactive' movement (i.e. the muscle action fueled by the return of stored (stretch) energy) is accompanied by relatively little spring as the landing energy is absorbed. In order for running to be energy efficient, a sufficiently

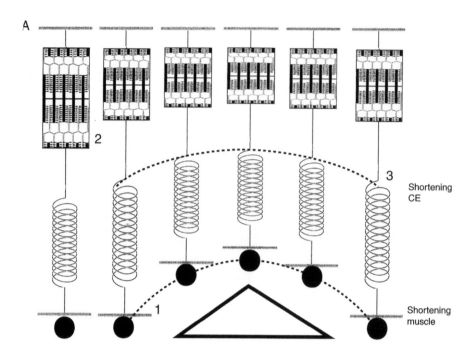

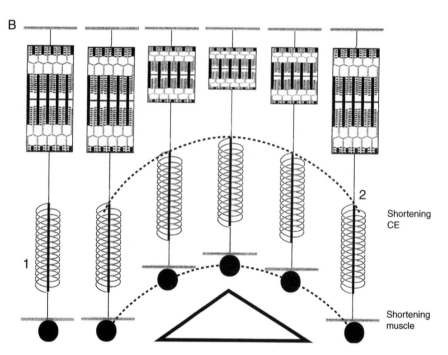

Figure 1.27A,B   Stretching SEC and shortening SE segments
(A) The force and speed of muscle contraction are not mutually compatible processes (see Section 1.3). When a weight is lifted quickly (A1), this problem is partly solved because the muscle fibers first shorten while the SEC segments are prestretched and preloaded (A2). When the weight then begins to move, SEC segments unload and shorten so that CE segments need to shorten less rapidly in order to move the external weight at a certain speed (A3). Using this mechanism (with which some of the movement is caused by stretching elastic segments), the body can partly bypass the very negative relationship between force and velocity. Such 'isometrization' of movement has an important role to play in the model which describes how to run (see also Ch. 3).
(B) If SEC segments lacked the potential for elasticity (B1), the shortening trajectory that CE segments would have to travel would equal the displacement of the object moved (B2).

hard foot placement is a prerequisite. During the swing phase, the link between isometry in the CE and preloading of the SEC will play a role. During the outward pendular action of the swing leg just before foot strike, for example, the hamstrings will be stretched (Chapman & Caldwell 1983). When CE elements are thereby working as isometrically (non-eccentrically) as possible, the elastic segments can be loaded almost optimally. (During slow running, the force exerted by the hamstrings on the tibia during the swing phase is nearly equal to the body's weight.) If a runner relaxes too much during the outward pendular swing of his leg, the loading of

SEC segments will be impeded by the eccentric action of the CE (the outward pendular action will not be slowed down sufficiently). The direction to always relax as much as possible when running, which many trainers give their athletes during practice, is therefore incorrect. Prestretch at the end of the swing phase is an important factor that is frequently underestimated.

It is extraordinarily difficult to quantify how much the SEC contributes and any estimate of this should only be made with great caution. One can estimate how much energy will be needed to accelerate and decrease the speed of different parts of the body during endurance running. One can then calculate how much oxygen a runner would have to take up per unit of time in order to produce the necessary energy via metabolic processes. In reality, it appears that only approximately half of the amount of oxygen required is actually taken up. This discovery indicates that elasticity plays an important role during functional movement (Cavagna et al 1964, Cavagna 1977).

With regard to (2), in addition to contributing to the energy needed, passive components connected in series are also responsible for a second important effect. In various situations, they can be held partly accountable for changes in muscle length (Ingen Schenau 1983, Ingen Schenau et al 1984, Bobbert et al 1992).

When a muscle is stretched by the action of external forces, the elongation of the muscle is partially absorbed by the SEC. When the muscle subsequently shortens during the reaction phase, less concentric response is required from the muscle fibers because of shortening taking place in the SEC. Due to stretch in the elastic tissues, muscle fibers are able to work at a lower speed of contraction, and thus with more force, after prestretch (reactive muscle action).

Even during contractions in which there are no external forces at work, the CE will also work first to stretch, or pre-load so to speak, the SEC. During the next shortening contraction, because the SEC relaxes, and therefore shortens, the CE will be able to work at a lower speed of contraction than would be deduced on the assumption that the total shortening was active. SEC segments serve to delay the force provided by the CE and to 'isometrize' its activity.

This reduction in the speed of contraction is important, because the force and speed of contraction are competing processes (see force–velocity diagram, Section 1.3.1). A muscle fiber that must provide a great deal of force will function best when made to contract slightly and slowly. The 'flexibility' of the SEC facilitates, so to speak, the activity of CE segments.

1.4.3   Rise delay, prestretch, and elasticity

There has been much discussion about the role played by elasticity in movement. It is beyond dispute that an elastic component is involved during muscle activity and that its role is important. However, how much this elasticity contributes is still unclear. Muscles frequently appear better able to perform after they have first been subject to a counter-movement force moment (i.e. if SEC segments have first been stretched) in contrast to having had no opposition (i.e. function without prestretch). To attribute this difference solely to the storage capacity of the SEC segments would be incorrect. Instead, yet another phenomenon plays an important role here, namely circumventing the rise of the force (Ingen Schenau et al 1984, Bobbert et al 1996).

Before a muscle can be made to contract, a concentric contraction must occur in order to bring the muscle to its primary length and to stretch the SEC segments to the right level of tension. The time taken for this shortening of contracting muscle fibers to a workable length is called the 'rise latency'. When there is little time for a muscle to act (e.g. during an explosive movement or when ground contact time is short during running), performance will be affected adversely by the rise latency. The muscle will not reach its optimum force output until the period of explosive contraction or the support phase. However, when a counteractive force moment (i.e. stretching SEC segments and contracting muscle fibers to a working length) provides prestretch, the rise latency will be shorter. The rise latency will be side-stepped so to speak. In this way, the muscle will be able to generate a high level of force from the beginning of the explosive movement or support phase. Therefore, the muscle can perform much better after prestretch.

The external forces that create the counteractive force moment within a muscle are not built up slowly during running, but rather peak within a very short time. During a sprint these peaks are larger and occur within a shorter time span than in slow running. In order to absorb such peaks without causing an eccentric response to occur in the muscle fiber (unfavorable for stretching SEC segments), there must be sufficient tension present in the muscle before external forces affect the body. This pretension (or 'rigidity') is of utmost importance for sprinters and should not be neglected by endurance athletes either.

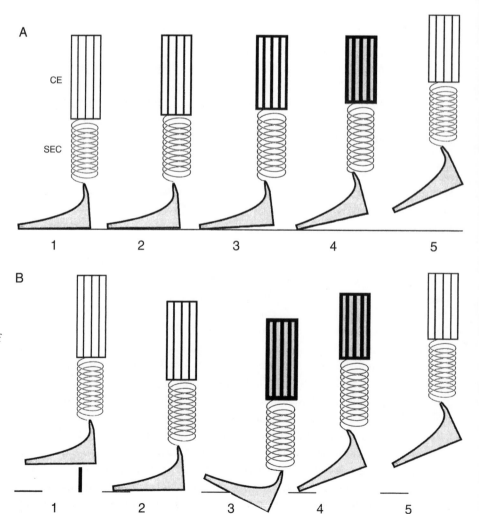

Figure 1.28 Problem of the rise latency
(A) Series A1–A5 shows a vertical push-off without prestretch. The SEC segments are stretched (2) as the force of contraction builds up in the CE segments. However, because the contraction is late in reaching its maximum level, the height of the jump will be restricted.
(B) Series B1–B5 shows a vertical reactive jump. From the drop (1), SEC segments are stretched (2). CE segments can readily build up force because prestretch guarantees that fibers need not shorten first (3). In this way, the rise delay can be avoided.

During reactive movement (e.g. during a technically well-executed plyometric jump across a hurdle), the following observations can be made:

- As the body drops directly before foot placement, while anticipating the reactive ground forces during the landing, there is a great deal of pretension in the muscles by which the SEC segments are already somewhat prestretched.
- During the landing, external forces work to stretch the SEC segments even further and to exert an antagonist moment on the CE segments without causing an eccentric movement in the muscle fibers.
- Very soon after the external forces have been absorbed, CE segments reach their maximum level of force, SEC segments unload their energy, and (eventually) yet another concentric contraction follows in the CE segments.
- The ground contact phase is quite short, the degree of movement in the joints is limited, and the body constantly tends toward an upright posture. The combination of elasticity in the SEC segments and of contractile segments working near isometry allows the muscle to work reactively, rapidly, and with a good deal of force. In contrast to athletes who are less proficient in the use of reactivity, those athletes who have been trained well in using it appear to run or perform bouncing jumps with less effort.

Because external forces, which create an antagonist moment, can 'solve' the problem of rise latency, one must question the premise that sprinters per se should have a high percentage of FT fibers. The reasoning that fast muscle fiber will provide speed, and thus good performance, in a sprint is not totally valid. ST fibers, which offer the possibility to avoid the rise latency, are also suited to reactive muscle work. This idea finds support in the fact that ST, in contrast to FT, fibers have stronger Z-discs and thus can absorb larger external forces. Moreover, because they not only turn on but also turn off more slowly, ST fibers are able to maintain muscle morphology, which is so important for sprinters (Ingen Schenau et al 1984, Jones & Round 1990, Bobbert et al 1996).

The soleus is a strongly specialized muscle, the structure of which has adapted optimally to its reactive function. The Achilles tendon is particularly long (about 37 cm), can store a great deal of energy, and can accommodate changes in muscle length well. The short muscle fibers of the strongly pennate soleus barely need to change in length during the concentric phase of the muscle. For the above-mentioned reasons, a pennate structure accompanied by the presence of many elastic structures is mutually compatible for muscle function.

Several points of particular interest

The terminology used for the type of muscle action described may be confusing. Terms such as plyometry and eccentric–concentric activity might imply that there is much movement in the contractile muscle segments and suggest the development of an eccentric movement in the muscle fibers. Instead, one can assume, for instance based on Hill's model, that reactivity is coupled to active segments working more or less isometrically. This assumption has also been confirmed during training practice. In the past, it emerged that training provided no extra effect when forms of exercise were used in which very large amounts of energy were applied to the muscle (e.g. during reactive jumping from extremely high drops (up to 1.5 m)). The eccentric activity that muscle fibers developed from such an overload was obviously poorly compatible with trying to improve the reactive properties of muscle.

Now, as a rule, it holds that the height of the drop, and thus the amount of energy absorbed, may not exceed what a muscle can cope with isometrically. Short ground contact is therefore required when training for reactive jumping. In addition, having a well-coordinated body is of the utmost importance. Working contractile segments should have no eccentric phase and must be exactly coordinated with regard to the way in which elastic tissues load or discharge and elongate or shorten.

Through practice it has become evident that reactive muscle action cannot be achieved equally well for every body posture used for jumping. The drop energy generated by a reactive jump can best be absorbed when the body's posture is nearly erect (i.e. hip and knee outstretched, with the ankle in a neutral position). When squatting (knee and hip bent, with the upper body slanting forward), it is quite difficult to absorb external forces adequately, to avoid the rise latency, and to take advantage of the benefits offered by reactivity. Choosing this position for reactive muscle work would thus appear improbable. Seen in this light, it is strange that frequent use is made of the so-called 'counter-movement jump' when taking measurements. During this type of jumping, one first squats and then pushes the body in a downward direction before pushing off vertically. The impact of the external forces and reactivity proceed 'softly', in contrast to a bouncing jump with the body extended. The impact of the external forces during the counter-movement is much lower than what the body would be able to absorb, and conversion into push-off proceeds much less abruptly than might be possible in really reactive jumps. The counter-movement jump can be compared to a leaky ball bouncing on a soft surface, whereas the bouncing jump with the body extended can be compared to a massive rubber ball bouncing on a hard surface. Thus, in fact, the counter-movement jump is an essentially non-functional movement, and therefore has little to say, with regard to reactivity, about the caliber of an athlete in sports (Bobbert et al 1996).

1.4.4 Moments in the joint

Neither the physiological cross-section nor whether a muscle's structure is pennate are the only factors that help determine how a muscle works during movement. The moment of a muscle with regard to the joint it must move is also of importance. When we want to include in our description of what affects functional movement (in addition to the structure of contractile and passive muscle segments) the location of a muscle with regard to the bone and/or joint that must be moved, we first need to clarify the term 'moment'.

Most movements made by muscles are rotations around an axis, usually located in a joint. However, during running, one nearly always aims to make a transition, such as a horizontal or vertical displacement of the body's center of gravity. The effect of a muscle's contractile force on a rotational movement depends not only on the magnitude of the force, but also on the distance between the line along which the generated force works and the rotational axis. This can easily be demonstrated using the example of a weightless board that is supported in such a way at point X located in the center of the board that rotation is possible. If identical weights are hung at each end of the board equidistant from point X, the board will remain balanced. However, if one of the weights is doubled, the other weight must be hung at twice the distance from point X to maintain balance. The shortest distance from the rotational axis X to the line along which a force works is called the lever arm of that force. The product of a force multiplied by a lever arm is the force moment with regard to the rotational axis X. If this calculation is then translated to a force moment of a muscle with regard to a rotational axis located in a joint, the force moment will be the

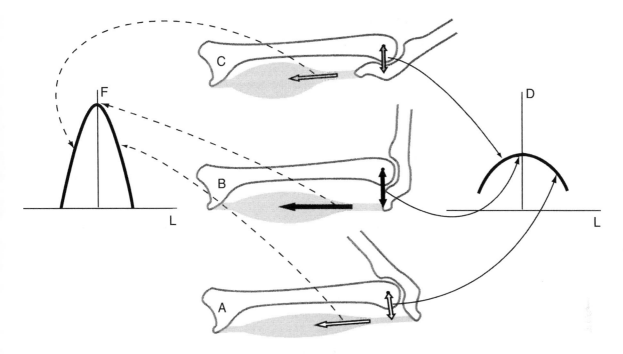

Figure 1.29   Relationship between the axis of rotation and the lever arm
When a joint changes position, it changes both the lever arm of the muscle, with regard to the joint, and the amount of force that the muscle can generate. Therefore, the amount of force that a muscle can exert, with regard to the joint depends not only on the force–length property of the muscle (left) but also on how its lever arm changes with regard to the joint (right).

product of the force component measured at a right angle to the bone multiplied by the shortest distance from the rotational axis to the muscle's insertion.

Because most muscles have relatively short moment arms with regard to the joints that they span (Ingen Schenau & Tousaint 1994), the muscle must be very strong even when the external force is relatively low.

Moreover, the perpendicular force component is dependent on the angular moment in the joint during movement. This is also true for the moment arm. Generally, the moment arm increases to its maximum from one extreme position before subsequently decreasing as it nears the other extreme position (Rozendal & Huijing 1996). The force moment of a muscle and its moment arm do not follow the same pattern because, based on the relationship between force and muscle length, the value representing muscle strength is variable along the trajectory in which it moves. This means that, during functional movement, there are multiple factors that can restrict the efficient use of a muscle.

The key to being able to run well lies in one's ability to integrate the efficiency of a muscle within the total pattern of functional movement. A muscle is like an instrument in a very large orchestra; it must meticulously follow the music score according to how it was composed so that beautiful music will be produced.

1.4.5   Important muscles for running

Erector spinae

The erector spinae group consists of a number of separately differentiated muscles, the fibers of which follow a particularly complicated pathway close to the spinal column. Caudally they are attached by means of a broad aponeurosis (fused with the thoracolumbal fascia) to the pelvic rim (iliac crista), to the sacral bone, and to the spinal processes of the lumbar vertebrae. The latissimus dorsi and posterior segments of the abdominal muscles also insert into the thoracolumbal fascia. It is particularly in the lumbar area that the muscle has many sheets of connective tissue running along complicated pathways. From where it originates, the erector spinae runs craniolaterally, subsequently crossing the thorax and becoming smaller, as it continues toward the cervical part (Bogduk 1997, Lohman 1977).

The most important function of the erector spinae group is to hold the body's trunk upright against the pull of gravity, an activity comparable to elongating the spinal column. At the start of a sprint, the upper body is leaning forward. This posture is achieved either by bending the spinal column quite far combined with a slight pelvic tilt forward, or by tilting the pelvis far to the front combined with little or no flexion in the spinal column. The advantage of starting with the back extended (slight flexion) is that the erector spinae is very active and can contribute to the impulse of push-off. When the spinal column is bent quite far, the action of the erector spinae declines. However, if the spinal column is completely bent, the function of the erector spinae will be completely taken over by tightly drawn dorsal ligaments. Starting a sprint with the back bent very round is thus more passive and less effective that when the back is straighter.

The same contraction by the erector spinae that is responsible for extending the spinal column can also cause the pelvis to tilt forward. When the hip joint is held rigid by muscle strength, this pelvic tilt will cause the ipsilateral leg to move backward. Even when the pelvis only tilts slightly forward the foot will be displaced quite a way toward the rear. Consequently, during running, the erector spinae acts to support backward thrust.

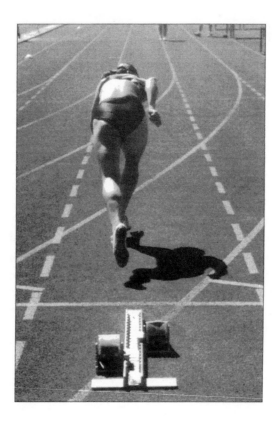

Figure 1.30   The function of the erector spinae
At the start of the race, the back is quite rounded and the pelvis tilted backward so that the dorsal muscles cannot work actively. The upper body will contribute only slightly during acceleration. The start appears to be passive.

Furthermore, through the action of the erector spinae, rotation as well as lateral flexion can be initiated or resisted. During rotation, movement in the spinal column as well as movement of the pelvis in the transverse plane form a functional unit. For axial rotations when the body is standing erect, the erector spinae and abdominal muscles will always work together. The lever arm of the abdominal muscles with regard to the spinal column is, moreover, much larger than that of the erector spinae group (Snijders et al 1995).

The role that the erector spinae plays during running is frequently underestimated. The force that it can contribute, via the pelvis, to thrust is substantial during running. The dorsal muscles of top sprinters are extraordinarily well developed, and their ability to coordinate the actions of these muscles optimally is quite important for a good performance.

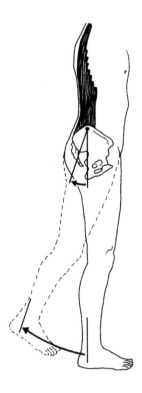

Figure 1.31   The function of the dorsal muscles
When the dorsal muscles are active, the pelvis can tilt forward. When the hip joint is held stationary, pelvic tilt will cause the leg to move toward the back. Any slight movement in the pelvis will result in a relatively large displacement of the foot. In this way, the dorsal muscles can help support push-off during running.

In the lumbar area, the erector spinae is attached not only to bones (pelvic rim, sacral bone, and spinal processes), but also to a strong aponeurosis. In this way, the physiological cross-section is greatly enlarged. Moreover, on a lumbar level, the erector spinae has many connective-tissue fascias running along complicated pathways. The muscle fibers that are attached to these connective tissues can transfer the force of contraction at these sites. Such forces are subsequently transferred by connective tissues to the sites where muscles attach. In this way, muscle fibers can lie longitudinally to each other without actually being connected in series. The physiological cross-section is enlarged, so to speak, by the presence of connective tissue. Thus the erector spinae is a group of muscles capable of providing an exceptional amount of force, although the possible pathway for and speed of contraction remain limited.

Iliopsoas and abdominal muscles

The iliopsoas is the most important and strongest muscle that can provide forward flexion. The structure of the muscle is parallel-fibered and it can provide force over a relatively large range. Because it is a large muscle, the iliopsoas has a large physiological cross-section. The origin of the iliacus segment can be found on the inner side of the pelvis, while that of the psoas major segment is at the front of the spinal column. The point of attachment for both segments is on the femur. In addition to backward flexion in the hip joint, the psoas major is also stressed eccentrically by extending the spinal column. In contrast, the iliopsoas can work to cause forward flexion in the hip joint and, when the abdominal muscles are inactive, will result in making the shape of the back hollow. When the abdominal muscles are also active, forward flexion in the hip joint is accompanied by flexion in the spinal column (Lohman 1977, Snijders et al 1995, Bogduk 1997).

The abdominal muscles have a small physiological cross-section, but a very large lever arm (with regard to the joints of the spinal column). The rectus abdominis segment lies anterior and between the thorax and trunk. The other segments are situated not only anterior to, but also laterally toward, the back, as far as the erector spinae group. The muscle fibers run vertically in the rectus abdominis and horizontally in the transversus abdominis. In the obliquus internus abdominis, the muscle fibers run obliquely, descending outward, while the fibers of the obliquus externus abdominis run perpendicular to it (i.e. moving down toward the interior). The muscle fibers are strongly interwoven with the various layers of fascia in the abdominal wall. With regard to their structure and function, the abdominal muscles are closely interrelated and thus form a functional unit. Because their fibers run perpendicular to each other, together they are well suited for maintaining the posture of the trunk in good form. This is generally more important for a body in motion than for the actual generation of motion itself.

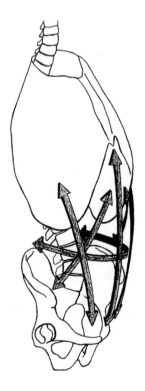

Figure 1.32 The interrelationship between abdominal muscles
Various abdominal muscles are strongly interwoven. These abdominal muscles can work in many directions, and thus function as a corset that can absorb external forces arriving from any direction.

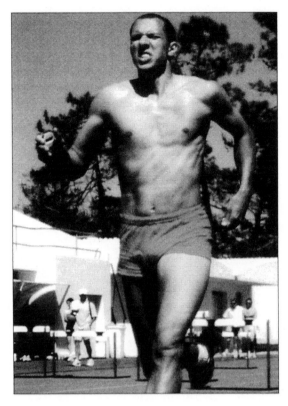

Figure 1.33 The corset activity of abdominal muscles during running
When the upper body is held upright, large external forces work on the abdominal muscles (because the stance leg trails behind). These muscles absorb the forces in repeatedly alternating diagonal lines.

During functional movement, the abdominal muscles always work together with other muscles (i.e. during flexion of the spinal column, with the iliopsoas; during axial rotation, with the erector spinae segments).

During strength training one frequently looks for forms of exercise in which an abdominal muscle can be tightened in isolation. Considering the dominant role that synergists play when the body is moving, this is understandable, but from the perspective of function, isolating the abdominal muscles during training (certainly for well-trained athletes) is of very limited use.

Moreover, the abdominal muscles do not work in isolation during running. In fact, at the end of thrust, these muscles are working reactively, especially when the upper body is held erect. Being able to handle a reactive load is therefore more important for abdominal muscles during running than being able to contract forcefully. During training, learning to work with external forces can only be taught if the abdominal muscles are able to work simultaneously with the iliopsoas. Athletes who are not able to keep their abdominal muscles in a correct form will tend to lean forward when running in order to avoid placing eccentric and/or reactive stress on these muscles.

The iliopsoas is a synergist of the abdominal muscles. During running, both muscle groups work closely together, and the concentric activity of the iliopsoas (as is the case for all muscles) is controlled by interpreting sensory information derived, for example, from registering prestretch in the muscles. There is much to be said for the idea that such data are only partially derived by prestretching the iliopsoas. However, when backward flexion in the leg is maximal, there can only be a great deal of stretch in the psoas major if there is hyperextension in the spinal column at the same time. Backward flexion in the hip is restrained by ligaments. Moreover, because of its long parallel-fibered structure, the iliopsoas can easily be stretched quite far.

Taken together, these data plausibly suggest that prestretching the iliopsoas is not enough to ensure precise control. At the end of support, prestretch in the abdominal muscles will provide extra valuable information so that mobilization of the knee can be well timed. The structure of the abdominal muscles (i.e. the strong interrelationship between the structure of their fibers and connective tissues, and the pathways along which the fibers run in all directions) makes them suitable for receiving impulses from the sensory system.

Gluteus maximus, tensor fasciae latae, and iliotibial tract

The gluteus maximus is the muscle that is capable of providing the strongest backward flexion in the hip. Moreover, it also allows lateral rotation in the hip. It is structured from coarse parallel-fibered bundles of muscle, which are bound together by many strong connective-tissue septa and which have a coarse innervation. The muscle is therefore specialized to contract very forcefully and is able to work over a large range. the gluteus maximus is considered to be the most important source of force during running. The muscle runs from the pelvis and sacral bone distally through to the upper third section of the femur, and has a very large lever arm with regard to the hip joint. It has its insertion mainly on the iliotibial tract. The tensor fasciae latae also inserts into this very strong thickening of the fascia lata. The iliotibial tract spans the knee and attaches to the lateral condyl of the tibia. In this way, the gluteus maximus works not only upon the hip but also upon the knee. Generally, the iliotibial tract is only accredited with having a stabilizing effect on the knee, but one must then question whether this is not an underestimate of the role that such a large, strong structure plays. The elastic capacity of the iliotibial tract is comparable to that of the Achilles tendon, and is influential during push-off in transferring force downward (comparable to the action of biarticular muscles).

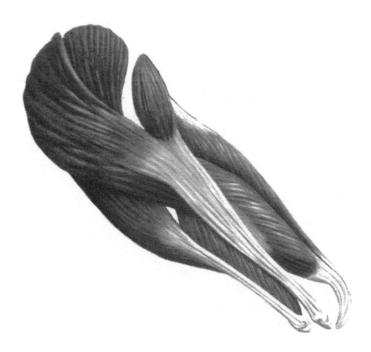

Figure 1.34   The gluteus maximus and tensor fascia latae
Anatomical illustration of the insertion of these muscles in the tibial tract.

The small gluteal muscles have their most important function when the body is standing on one leg, and therefore also during the support phase of running. They make it possible for the free side of the pelvis to undulate upwards and they also deliver a significant amount of the energy needed to displace the body's center of gravity vertically when running.

Hamstrings

The hamstrings are built up from the biceps femoris, the semimembranosus and the semitendinosus. The hamstrings arise from the ischial tuberosity of the pelvis, span the hip and knee joints, and attach medially (semimembranosus and semi-tendinosus) and laterally (biceps femoris) to the lower leg. Therefore the hamstrings are biarticular (with the exception of the short head of the biceps femoris). In recent years, our insight into the function of biarticular muscles has deepened and, certainly with regard to running, they are of major importance. Having a good understanding of the structure and function of these muscles is essential in order to analyze running.

The lever arm of the hamstrings with regard to the hip joint becomes significantly larger or smaller as the hip joint changes position. The lever arm with regard to the hip is much larger when the hip is bent (90° forward flexion) than when it is extended. In contrast, the lever arm of the hamstrings with regard to the knee remains more or less constant as the angle of the knee changes. Consequently, when movement is functional and within a closed chain, the hamstrings will particularly be required to work in situations where there is forward flexion in the hip, while they will also need to be active as the knee makes a large number of different angles.

Because the hamstrings are biarticular, their work is related to the range of movement in two joints. When a muscle is monoarticular, there is a simple relationship between the amount of force that the working muscle exerts and its effect upon the joint. If there is enough force to overcome the resistance, the muscle will work concentrically. If these forces are equal, the muscle will work isometrically. If there is insufficient force, the muscle will work eccentrically. For biarticular muscles, there is no such linear relationship between the amount of force and their effect on a joint. In addition, there is no direct relationship between muscle length and the position of one of the joints. As one of the joints moves, the muscle's origin is drawn closer to the insertion, while at the same time movement in the other joint shifts its origin away from the insertion. Movement occurs in both joints while the biarticular muscle remains the same length.

The concentric working of the hamstrings is also not linearly related to the degree of movement in either of the two joints. When the knee joint is held secure by other muscles, any concentric action of the hamstrings will result in backward flexion in the hip joint. In turn, if the hip joint is held secure, the knee will bend when this muscle works concentrically.

Because of the different ways in which the pelvis can move (forward and backward tilt), the length of the hamstrings will vary when the body is in certain positions. For example, by tilting the pelvis while standing erect, one can change the angle of the hip, and therefore the length of the hamstrings, without having to change the position of the upper body as well. The length of the hamstrings will thus be affected by how the positions of the knee and hip joints work together, whereas the position of the hip joint (because the pelvis can move in different directions) is not directly related to the angle formed by the thigh and trunk.

Because of this 'three-cornered relationship' between the angle of the knee, the angle of the hip, and the length of the hamstrings, being able to improve the action of the hamstrings during functional movement is much more complicated in actual practice than would be the case for a monoarticular muscle. Learning to use the hamstrings well when moving (including during running) requires a great deal of effort. Hamstrings can therefore be called 'intelligent' in contrast, for example, to the 'dumb' gluteal muscles. Learning how to control the hamstrings well during functional movement is more important during training than trying to develop greater force. Being able to use the hamstrings accurately for running, especially at speed, will require sophisticated instruction about how the body moves (see also Sections 1.6.2–1.6.4).

The hamstrings have a pennate structure. However, their structure is less pennate than that of the rectus femoris. As suggested by the names of its medial segments (semimembranosus and semitendinosus), the hamstrings have large and important connective-tissue structures. Tendons run from both points of attachment, partially overlapping each other to become tendon plates. The fibers located between these tendon plates form an angle with the line along which the muscle works. The physiological cross-section is large, the length–force range is smaller than for parallel-fibered muscles, and the hamstrings are not suited for rapid shortening involving a low level of force. Due to the presence of passive structures, the muscle group is suited to working from prestretch.

As already stated, the hamstrings are biarticular, spanning the hip and knee joints. During the support phase of running, knee extension occurs simultaneously

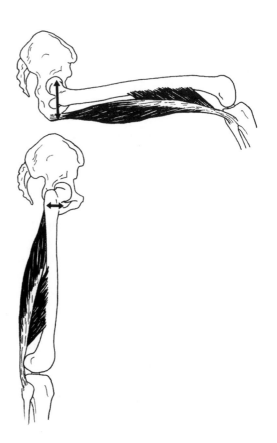

Figure 1.35 Function of the hamstrings (1)
In functional movement, the way in which the hamstrings work is determined by, for example, their lever arm with regard to the hip. This lever arm works best for forward flexion, being small for backward flexion. During running, this muscle group therefore works best at the beginning of push-off.

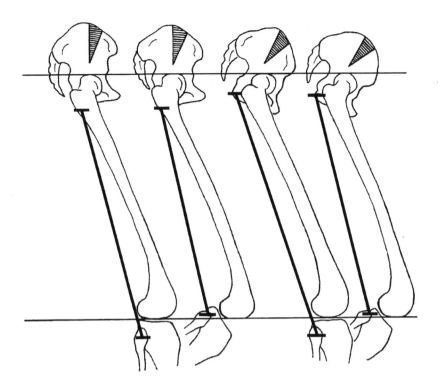

Figure 1.36 Function of the hamstrings (2)
The position of the thigh is identical
in each of the four drawings. Because
the pelvis can undulate forward and
backward, and the knee can bend and
straighten, the length of the hamstrings
will vary greatly for this one position of
the thigh. Therefore, the hamstrings are
coordinated by way of indirect factors, and
this coordination is thus a complicated
process.

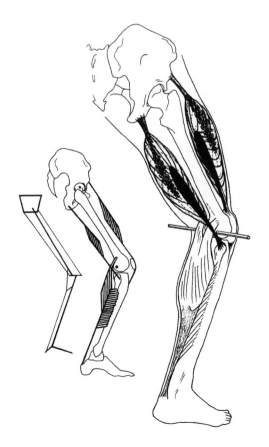

*Figure 1.37 Function of the triceps surae,
rectus femoris, and hamstrings*
During running, the triceps surae, rectus
femoris, and hamstrings have important
roles to play. What these muscles have
in common is their pennate structure,
elasticity in their important tissues (SEC),
and their biarticular character. Thus they
are able to store external energy and
release it during movement. These muscle
groups work as though they are superior
rubber bands.

with backward flexion in the hip. Elongating the muscles by extending the knee is compensated for when the muscles shorten during backward flexion in the hip. During stance, when the knee and hip are extended almost at the same time, the hamstrings can accordingly work reactively without having to change much in length. Therefore their structure is functionally appropriate.

As already discussed, the lever arm of the hamstrings with regard to the knee and hip is dependent on the positions of these joints. The lever arm is large when the hip is bent, and small when the hip is extended (backward flexion). This fact has important consequences for how the hamstrings function during the transfer of force when running. Hamstrings work chiefly at the beginning of the support phase.

The structure of the muscle, its biarticular character and its ability to move functionally are all closely interrelated. This combination of being biarticular and also having a pennate–elastic structure requires that the hamstrings be trained in a special manner. In this case, it is extremely important that the actions of passive and active tissues be well coordinated. Training the hamstrings in a manner that is incompatible with their structure and function will prove ineffective and may even cause injury. One is advised not to exercise with leg-curl equipment, with which the passive structures are strained non-functionally and the contractions are carried out close to the range of passive insufficiency.

Quadriceps femoris

The quadriceps femoris is composed of four parts. The rectus femoris is biarticular (spanning the knee and hip). Compared to that of the hamstrings, the lever arm of the rectus femoris is smaller with regard to the hip and larger with regard to the knee. This muscle is responsible for forward flexion in the hip joint and for extension in the knee. The patella serves as a turning point for quadriceps femoris, making the lever arm for this muscle group with regard to the knee larger than would ever be possible if the patella were not present.

The rectus femoris has a strongly pennate structure comparable to that of the hamstrings. The remaining three heads of the muscle are monoarticular and pennate with very large physiological cross-sections. For the quadriceps, force is more important than speed. Because the monoarticular segments of the quadriceps do not have important SEC segments, they do not work reactively, but rather specially with a great deal of force by which the angular velocity in the knee remains relatively low.

The quadriceps femoris is especially good at providing high force when the knee is bent. Therefore, for running, its action is especially important at the start, because significant stretch occurs during thrust when the knee is well bent. After speed is attained, the three monoarticular segments have only a stabilizing function. During running, the body's center of gravity not only moves horizontally during each step, but also undulates up and down vertically. During foot placement, the quadriceps femoris (together with other muscles) cushions the body's center of mass as it drops. However, the quadriceps femoris has little or nothing to contribute to the knee extension at the end of push-off. It is actually the gluteus maximus and gastrocnemius that play important roles during knee extension.

Adductors

The adductors in the thigh are the only group of muscles that remain active during the entire running cycle. Furthermore, their function is in particular to maintain balance because, in addition to adduction in the leg, they can also bring about forward flexion, backward flexion, lateral rotation, and medial rotation in the leg.

During propulsion, the role played by the adductors is neither explicit nor important (Mann et al 1986).

Soleus and gastrocnemius

Both the soleus and the gastrocnemius are attached to the Achilles (calcaneal) tendon. The soleus attaches to the bones of the lower leg and has short muscle fibers as well as a large physiological cross-section. The gastrocnemius, the two heads of which span the knee joint, is biarticular, like the hamstrings and the rectus femoris. The length of the gastrocnemius is therefore not directly related to the position of either the knee joint or the ankle joint; however, here one can also speak of a three-cornered relationship between muscle length and the positions of the knee and ankle joints. The gastrocnemius works functionally and its action is closely related to that of the hamstrings. Both muscles are able to slow the speed at which the knee is bent or extended. The Achilles tendon, which is about 37 cm long, attaches to the heel bone. It first becomes narrower, before widening as it moves upward, passing cranially under the gastrocnemius. The Achilles tendon, which attaches in the most dorsal area of the calcaneal tubercule, thus has a large lever arm with regard to the upper tarsal joint. The Achilles tendon is relatively long with regard to the muscle bellies of the two muscles. Because of the possibilities for stretch provided by the tendon, the muscle demonstrates important elastic properties (see Section 1.5).

The soleus is clearly pennate in structure, with short muscle bundles and a large physiological cross-section. Consequently, the muscle is able to work forcefully close to isometry over a limited range. The structure of the gastrocnemius is also pennate, but the angle between its fibers and line of action is smaller. Moreover, its fibers are longer than those of the soleus. Because both muscles have their insertion on the Achilles tendon, they must be well coordinated if they are to function optimally together.

The reason why the structures of the two muscles differ can be found in the fact that, in contrast to the soleus, which attaches to the lower leg, the gastrocnemius spans the knee joint and attaches to the femur. When movement is functional, such as during the support phase for running and jumping, activity in the soleus–gastrocnemius complex is accompanied by knee extension. This works eccentrically on the gastrocnemius and thus disrupts cooperation between the two muscles (knee extension does not affect the soleus). Because of the narrower angle and the longer length of the fibers, such disruption can be accommodated, so that collaboration between the actions of the gastrocnemius and the soleus with regard to the Achilles tendon, and therefore the ankle, can be timed well (see Section 1.6).

For that matter, when the knee is extended, the axis of the knee joint shifts forward from the rear so that the force moment of the gastrocnemius will increase with regard to the rotational axis (and, vice versa, the opposing moment of knee extension increases with regard to the gastrocnemius, which braces itself) (Lohman 1977, Rozendal & Huijing 1996).

Lower-leg muscles

In addition to the soleus and gastrocnemius, the lower leg also has a number of smaller muscles arising on the fibula and tibia that have terminal tendons crossing the ankle and attaching to the foot. These muscles have an important stabilizing function with respect to the tarsal joints, the arches of the foot, and the tarsal bone (Lohman 1977, Wingerden 1999).

During low-speed running, foot flexion is first plantar, then dorsal, then again plantar at the end of the support phase. Moreover, the entire arch of the foot flattens so that pronation of the foot occurs. The muscles (the tibialis anterior, extensor hallucis longus, and extensor digitorum longus) that pass anterior to the upper tarsal joint slow down the motion of foot placement. The dorsiflexion that subsequently develops is slowed by the muscles (the tibialis posterior, flexor digitorum longus, flexor hallucis longus medial, peroneus longus, and peroneus brevis lateral) that pass posterior to the axis of the upper tarsal joint. This is accompanied by strong activity in the soleus–gastrocnemius group. Elastic energy is stored in the muscle as the speed decreases and, at the end of push-off, is converted to extend the ankle.

Pronation and supination occur alternately in the lower tarsal joint, depending on the surface, on how the foot is placed on the ground, and in which direction the foot is moving. The above-mentioned muscles also have force moments with regard to the lower tarsal joint and they stabilize movement around that joint.

Finally, muscles in the lower leg have an important function with respect to the structural arches of the foot. The small muscles in the foot are not strong enough to absorb the large forces that can work upon the foot (sometimes many times the weight of the body). The tendons of the lower-leg muscles, together with the ligaments, absorb the forces working on the foot in a manner comparable to the

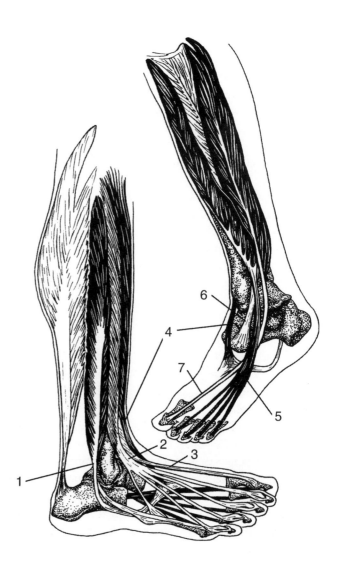

Figure 1.38 Muscles in the lower leg or shank

1 Peroneus longus and brevis.
2 Extensor digitorum longus.
3 Extensor hallucis longus.
4 Tibialis anterior.
5 Flexor digitorum longus.
6 Tibialis posterior.
7 Flexor hallucis longus.

mechanics of the lines of a cable bridge. Under high strain, the arches of the foot hang on the tightened tendons of the lower-leg muscles. The tibialis anterior, extensor digitorum longus, and extensor hallucis longus are attached from above on the arch of the foot. The tibialis posterior and peroneus longus have their insertions under the arch of the foot. The flexor digitorum longus and flexor hallucis longus run beneath the foot, extending to the toes. Together with, for example, the abductor hallucis and plantar aponeurosis, all these muscles not only ensure that the foot does not sag too far (about 1 cm) during foot strike, but they also can store energy that will be released when it is subsequently converted into the force of push-off.

All the lower-leg muscles have long terminal tendons that extend quite far cranially. Therefore, the fibers of the muscles are relatively short, and the muscles have a pennate structure. Consequently, these muscles are only suited to contract forcefully without much shortening. The range over which the lower-leg muscles can exert force is limited by their structure. Therefore, the foot can only tighten well when there is sufficient dorsiflexion (near the neutral position).

1.4.6   Summary

It can be concluded that it is of the utmost importance that muscles must be specialized if the body is to move well. In man, the muscle population of the locomotor apparatus can be compared to a zoo. There is a large diversity of types, each having its own uniqueness and specific characteristics. A zoo will only be successful if the different animals are nurtured in a manner fitting their individual behaviors. In the same way, functional movement will only be effective when the muscles are permitted to work according to their structure and ability. Both the zoo keeper and the trainer of athletes must take into consideration the diversity of populations. An animal must be fed food that fits the predisposition of its digestive system. A group of muscles must be physically exerted in a manner that fits its potential to adapt. The large differences between individual muscles are particularly important in strength training. Some muscle groups can be trained well by means of maximum concentric power training (e.g. the gluteal group). For other muscle groups (e.g. the hamstrings), using maximum concentric power training can be very detrimental, while using maximum isometric force and strength of impact will prove effective.

Considering the fact that many important muscles are pennate in structure, it is often a sign that the elastic properties of muscle are being put to good use when the extent of joint movement (particularly by spreading movement across several joints) as well as the angular velocity in joints can be limited.

1.5   ELASTICITY AND REACTIVE MUSCLE ACTION

During running, effort is exerted in order to overcome resistance. Of the total amount of energy generated, 5–10% is needed to absorb the shock of foot placement, 10–15% is required to overcome air resistance, and 80% is used to speed up and slow down the motion of the legs. The relationship between the amount of energy required for movement within the human motor (80%) and that for effective thrust (10–15%) makes the process of running extraordinarily energy inefficient. However, measurements have shown that during endurance running the body uses only about half the oxygen that would be needed to supply muscles with sufficient energy by way of aerobic metabolism (Cavagna et al 1964, Cavagna & Kaneko 1977, Williams & Cavanagh 1987). An important part of this energy requirement is not generated by the working muscle, but comes rather from elasticity. In other words, an important part of all the energy required can be produced by 'reusing' the kinetic and potential energy during the cycle of movement.

The elastic component also contributes greatly during high-speed running. In addition, the elastic components can partly absorb changes in muscle length (see Section 1.4.2). This characteristic is especially important during high-speed running. During a sprint, the angular velocity in the hip joint, as well as changes in the length of muscles around the hip, is very high per unit of time, and becomes a factor that can limit performance.

Of course, the elastic properties of muscle can be observed throughout the entire locomotor apparatus and exert a collective influence on the efficiency of movement. A number of structures deserve special attention when discussing running.

1.5.1   Elasticity in the foot

The configuration of the foot changes during the support phase of the running cycle. When keeping to a speed used by middle-distance runners, when the entire foot touches the ground, it appears that the arch of the foot flattens by about 1 cm halfway through the support phase. The energy that is loaded in the foot during foot placement is chiefly stored in the stretch of strong ligaments in the foot (e.g. in the plantar aponeurosis). These ligaments are mainly composed of collagen tissue with elastic properties similar to those of tendon. By the end of stance, the foot has regained its original form and has consequently returned about 80% of its stored energy. During stance, the foot works as a spring. To an important extent, the loading and release of energy from that spring is regulated by muscles in the lower leg. Being able to tense these muscles well before foot strike is closely related to the position of the foot (see Section 1.4.5).

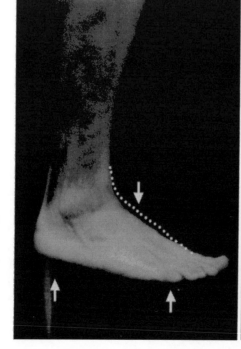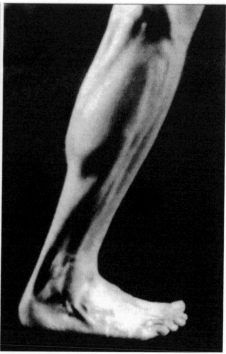

Figure 1.39   Elasticity in the foot
The arch of the foot drops by up to about 1 cm during foot strike. The cushion of the heel also becomes distorted under the calcaneal tubercle. Energy stored in ligaments, tendons (those of the peroneus longus and brevis are visible), etc., is released again as the body moves like a coiled spring. The entire foot has a spring-like function. On the right, the Achilles tendon appears taut and is loaded with potential energy. Approximately half of all the energy needed for push-off is supplied by the spring-like action of the foot and shank.

When the running speed is fast (say 5 m/s), the magnitude of the ground reaction force on the foot is of the order of 2.8 times the body weight. During the support phase, the total amount of kinetic and potential energy in the body first decreases before thereafter increasing. A runner can lose about 100 joule (J) in energy per stride due to eccentric muscle action (e.g. as the body slumps during the landing and as the pendular motion of the foot decelerates during the swing phase). A large portion of this energy is regained through elasticity. The arches of the foot have been estimated to contribute about 17 J to regaining this energy. In other words, about 17% of the total energy lost during each stride can be recovered through the spring-like action of the foot (Ker et al 1987, McNiell Alexander 1987). Moreover, more than 100 J are actually needed to execute the entire pattern of movement for running, because energy must also be generated for metabolic processes.

Whether the arches of the foot behave effectively as a spring depends not only on how precisely the lower-leg muscles maintain control, but also on the footwear worn by the athlete. Shoes are generally less suitable for supporting the spring in the foot. On one hand, this is because the foot sole can usually absorb energy well, but frequently demonstrates an inadequate or poorly timed spring. On the other hand, the spring-like action of the foot can be counteracted because the bed of the foot prevents the arches from sagging. In practice, however, it appears that running too frequently when wearing shoes that offer little absorptive potential can result in injury because the physical strain is one-sided. It is therefore necessary that an athlete seek a balance between trying to protect the foot against too much strain and training the spring-like movement of the foot. It is extremely important to alternate carefully the types of shoes worn when running (i.e. wearing spiked shoes while being taught reactivity and speed, but protective shoes when the foot must be spared strain). Running instruction through which the natural spring-like motion of the foot is optimized is therefore essential. Moreover, the foot itself has the ability to absorb shock during foot placement. Underneath the heel bone (calcaneum), lying in a double-spiral, 2-cm thick structures, are that can deform to absorb part of the landing energy (Snijders et al 1995).

1.5.2 Elasticity in the Achilles tendon

As the terminal tendon of the soleus–gastrocnemius complex, the Achilles tendon is particularly suited for returning elastic energy and for absorbing changes in muscle length.

During fast running (say 5 m/s), the Achilles tendon lengthens by about 5% during the support phase by which the pulling force upon the tendon can reach up to some seven times the weight of the body. The Achilles tendon is capable of returning a very high percentage of the stored energy. Measurements made on kangaroo tendon have shown that the return of energy can be as high as 93%. The human Achilles tendon is able to return about 35% of the total amount of energy that can be lost per stride and it also plays a central role for reactivity during running. Together with the 17% return attributed to the arches of the foot, this means that approximately half of the energy returned originates from the elastic components below the knee (McNiell Alexander 1987). The gastrocnemius has an important function in coordinating the energy flow discharged by the Achilles tendon. The gastrocnemius is most active when the knee is extended during the support phase, so its work must be well coordinated as the motion of the foot unwinds (see Sections 1.6 and 3.2).

1.5.3 Elasticity in the hamstrings

The structure of the hamstrings already demonstrates that this muscle group can work well reactively. In practice, the function of elasticity is difficult to chart during movement, notably during running. The reason for this is that the function of the hamstrings is extraordinarily complex during running (Chapman & Caldwell 1983). These muscles are biarticular, which means that a change in the length of the hamstrings is brought about by movement in two joints. If attention is paid to only one of these joints, no clues will be found to help explain how the hamstrings work reactively. In order to obtain an adequate model for explaining how the hamstrings work, one must consider the total complex of movements in the knee and hip (including pelvic tilt), as well as the accompanying changes in the lever arms. The hamstrings play an important role in the transfer of energy from the knee to the hip. During speed running, such a transfer of energy occurs very rapidly (in tenths of seconds). Reactivity is much more suitable for such rapid processes than is muscle action without absorbing a counteractive force moment. Being able to avoid the rise latency, and thus the need for pretension, when coping with a counteractive force moment is necessary if the hamstrings are to work rapidly. Another important point in the running cycle when one can adjust tension in the elastic and contractile segments of the hamstrings occurs during the outward pendular motion of the shank of the leading swing leg. Energy from the pendular motion is thereby stored as the elastic segments of the hamstrings are stretched.

1.5.4 Elasticity in the iliotibial tract

To a certain extent, the same can be said for the iliotibial tract as for the hamstrings. Their structures demonstrate that they are suited for elasticity which, in this case, is also quite complex. Because the pelvis can move in the frontal plane, the iliotibial tract can work to convert the drop of the body's center of gravity during foot strike into a rise at the end of push-off.

1.5.5 Reactivity during running

Based on the fact that, even at an early age, every healthy individual can run fast, one might easily assume that running is a simple coordinated pattern of movement. However, such a conclusion is far from true. The mechanics and coordination of running are made very complicated by the way in which elasticity functions to conserve energy. Muscle action during running is only partly directly related to the resistance that the runner must overcome. An important part of this work is indirect: i.e. creating prestretch in elastic tissues, transferring force across joints, and facilitating other muscles by stressing them eccentrically. Among other things, EMG data show that the most important muscles are active at the beginning of the support phase, thus at about the same time that ground reactive energy is being stored in elastic segments during landing. Running demands very precise timing because of this extreme use of elasticity. The total pattern of muscle actions is complex and certainly not more simple than for some other movements (e.g. backflip, swimming, and skating), which are much more difficult to learn. The fact that speed running is nevertheless a basic skill points to its having been given great priority by biological evolution.

The fact that everyone can learn a rough form of running more quickly than skating has caused some trainers in the field of athletics to attribute less value to the technique of running than to that of skating in the ice rink. This is certainly not correct. Even at the highest level of performance, reactivity still exerts a major influence on an athlete's ability to maintain and increase speed. This holds true not only for the sprinter, but also for the middle-distance runner. Much energy will be lost, frequently without compensation, for each stride and every several-thousandth of a second the athlete deviates from the optimum timing. Therefore, instructing a runner on the use of techniques will never be complete, and he will continuously profit by improving his skills.

1.6 HOW BIARTICULAR MUSCLES WORK

1.6.1 Biomechanical aspects

A large number of muscles in the body span not one but two or more joints. For some muscles, such as the soleus, which bridges the upper and lower tarsal joints, this has no practical consequence for movement. Because these joints lie very close together and their axes are approximately perpendicular to each other, the outcome of any motion in either joint will have either only a slight or no effect on the other joint. However, the situation is different when joints are located far apart and their axes are or can be parallel. In this case, the biarticular muscles demonstrate their special function in the mechanics of movement. Important biarticular muscles are the biceps brachii, the triceps brachii in the upper arm, the hamstrings, the rectus femoris in the thigh, and the gastrocnemius in the lower leg.

The process of charting the mechanics of biarticular systems is currently well underway, and that they are quite important is without question. The mechanics of biarticular muscles is slowly, but explicitly, being applied to opinions regarding technique for different sports. The most well-known example is the development of the 'clap skate'; these principles are also being incorporated in the construction of new-generation sprint spikes.

In addition to the hamstrings and rectus femoris, which are treated as the most significant muscles in the running model, the gracilis, sartorius, and, to a certain extent, gluteus maximus (via the iliotibial tract) also span the hip and knee. During

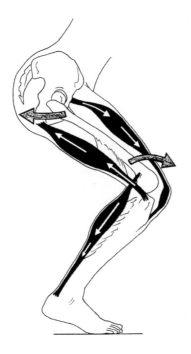

Figure 1.40 Mechanics of biarticular muscle groups 1
The biarticular muscle groups most important for running (i.e. the hamstrings, rectus femoris, and gastrocnemius) are colored black. Biarticular muscles can transfer energy generated by the monoarticular knee (quadriceps femoris) and hip (gluteus maximus) extensors from one joint to another. The white arrows indicate the direction of transfer in a closed-chain. The rectus femoris can slow down hip extension and convert it into knee extension. In turn, the hamstrings can slow down knee extension and convert it into hip extension, while the gastrocnemius can slow down knee extension and convert it into plantar flexion of the ankle.

running, in addition to the rectus femoris and the hamstrings, the biarticular character of the gastrocnemius, which spans the knee and ankle, is of major importance. Energy can be managed economically during running because of the way in which the biarticular muscles work, together with the potential for elasticity in the locomotor apparatus.

If all the muscles in the body were monoarticular, all movement not already being affected by the force of gravity would have to be slowed down by the forces generated by muscle. Energy generated by movement would be converted into thermal energy, because muscles would need to work eccentrically, resulting in a large loss of energy. In contrast, biarticular muscles are able to use energy that has been released by a counteractive force moment of one joint (when movement in that joint is decreased) in order to cause movement in the other joint (in the direction in which the muscle works). Biarticular muscles can therefore transfer energy from one joint to another.

During knee extension, the gastrocnemius works in a closed chain, through which the muscle is stressed by a counteractive joint moment. When the muscle tightens to resist eccentric movement, plantar flexion will occur in the ankle. In this manner, the gastrocnemius transfers energy from the knee to the ankle. The rectus femoris is responsible for the same type of transfer between the hip and knee joints. When the hip is extended, the rectus femoris wants to lengthen. However, when the muscle is tightened while its length remains unchanged, it exerts an extending force with regard to the knee joint. The hamstrings are knee flexors by which knee extension causes a counteractive joint moment. When the muscle is tightened but its length remains unchanged, an extending force moment is generated with regard to the hip.

By means of energy transfer, the rectus femoris and the hamstrings are able to coordinate extension and flexion in the hip with that in the knee. When a lot of energy is needed to extend the hip, the hamstrings assist by becoming taut in order to divert energy from quadriceps femoris for hip extension. Conversely, when a lot of energy is required by the knee extensors, the rectus femoris diverts energy from the hip extensors for knee extension. The mechanism by which biarticular muscles

Figure 1.41 Mechanics of biarticular muscle groups 2
In position A, a lot of energy is needed to extend the hip. By contracting the quadriceps, the hamstrings can be stressed by a counter-moment that can be converted into an extending moment with regard to the hip as the hamstrings tighten. In position B, a lot of energy is needed to straighten the knee. By contracting the gluteus maximus, the rectus femoris can be loaded eccentrically and then, by tightening, convert this energy into an extending moment with regard to the knee.

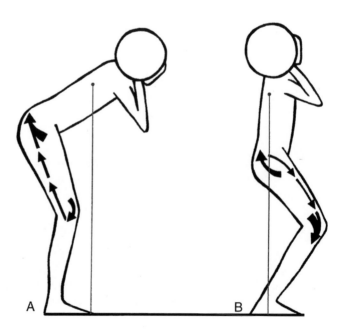

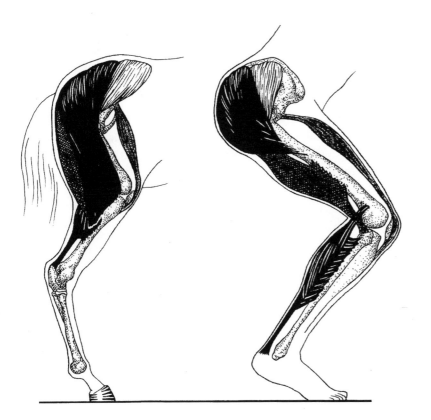

Figure 1.42 Comparison between the 'specialist' horse and the 'all-round' human In the horse, more muscle mass is grouped around the hip. Because almost no muscle mass is located in the distal parts of the legs, which oscillate during running, this movement uses little energy. Biarticular muscles make it possible for the body to have this type of structure.

transfer energy thus allows efficient and conservative management of energy for many types of movement. Running is such a pattern of motion that, through the way in which biarticular muscles function, can be executed efficiently and without loss of energy (Prilutskii & Zatsiorsky et al 1994, Doorenbosch et al 1997).

Furthermore, the function of biarticular muscles allows the body to be built in such a way that only a small amount of mass is needed in the distal leg (i.e. running becomes more efficient). In man, about 80% of all the energy required for running is used for the pendular motion of the legs, while 15% is used for propulsion. For the true specialist in running (i.e. high-speed beasts of prey), the relationship between these percentages is much more favorable. The back legs of a high-speed animal have been especially designed so that little energy is lost as the leg oscillates up and down during running. The muscle mass serving propulsion is grouped quite close to the pelvis. Because biarticular muscles have the potential to transfer force via long tendons, only relatively small or even no muscles will be needed around the distally located joints. Even the horse has biarticular muscles in which almost no muscle fibers can be found and for which, in fact, the term 'biarticular tendon' could well be applied. The leg of the horse can thus be long and thin with very little oscillating mass located distally. This structure therefore needs to use less energy. This holds true both for animals that must be able to run at high speeds (e.g. horse, ostrich and hare) and for animals that must cover large distances while using little energy (e.g. gnu and reindeer). The latter category of animal can even move forward without using the pelvis, thus conserving even more energy. Although the human body has not been built especially to run, even in man the nature of biarticular muscles offers possibilities for a number of adaptations that can greatly affect the total amount of energy needed to run. The lower leg is much thinner than the thigh and, even in man, the largest mass of tissue is located near the hips (the pelvis is that part of the body which has the most similar weight). The importance of limiting weight in distal parts of the body is also taken into consideration when designing running shoes. Because the foot accelerates and decelerates at extreme speeds when running, decreasing the weight of the foot even slightly can influence performance significantly.

That the body has been designed with as little mass as possible located in the limbs proves especially effective for endurance performance. When rapid acceleration, and thus much concentric force, is required, much muscle mass is needed around the limb joints (e.g. in the thigh of a sprinter) (Martin & Cavanagh 1990).

How biarticular muscles work during running is discussed below on the basis of a number of problems that occur during the support phase.

1.6.2 Magnitude versus direction of force at push-off

The amount of forward thrust during the support phase is dependent on both the magnitude and the direction of the force exerted by the foot on the ground surface. The greater the force and the better directed it is toward the rear, the more effective thrust will be. During speed running, directing the force of thrust to the runner's advantage is difficult when its magnitude is large. The reasons for this can be analyzed as follows.

It can be assumed that the body forms a closed chain (with the foot on the ground) and that its posture places its center of mass directly above the point of support, even when running at speed. One can assume that the trunk (including the pelvis) and the support foot are fixed points. The foot is fixed to the ground due to friction and the trunk is held stable due to mass inertia and movement of the arms (see Section 3.2). If only the muscles (e.g. the gluteus maximus) around the hip that provide backward flexion were active during the support phase, the force would pull the thigh backwards, resulting in joint moments in both the hip and knee. Both joints would experience a stretching force moment (knee extension, hip backward flexion) and the line of projection of the force upon the ground would be a continuation of the lower leg. When force is transferred from the leg to the ground, a reactive force develops in the opposite direction. In this case, the reactive force would pass through the ankle and knee. When the angle formed by the lower leg and the vertical plane is small, as during speed running, the direction of the reactive force is also vertical. If the force exerted by the hip extensors is large, the force unloaded to the ground is also large. When only the hip extensors are at work during running, the direction in which the body moves will never be favorable.

Force directed toward the rear is needed when running. When the force exerted on the ground is directed far enough to the rear, the ground reaction force will pass in front of the hip and knee. The ground reaction force moments tend to bend the hip and extend the knee. Moreover, the reactive force can be increased by simultaneously extending the hip while bending the knee more forcefully. If only monoarticular muscles were responsible for generating force for work around the hip and knee, the muscles would be working against each other simultaneously (i.e. the hip extensors would try to extend the hip and, indirectly, the knee, while the knee flexors would try to bend the knee and, indirectly, the hip). The muscles would work antagonistically, so that much energy would be lost as internal heat of friction (the heat generated when a muscle is stretched under resistance). Because the hip extensors work concentrically while the knee flexors work eccentrically, energy from the

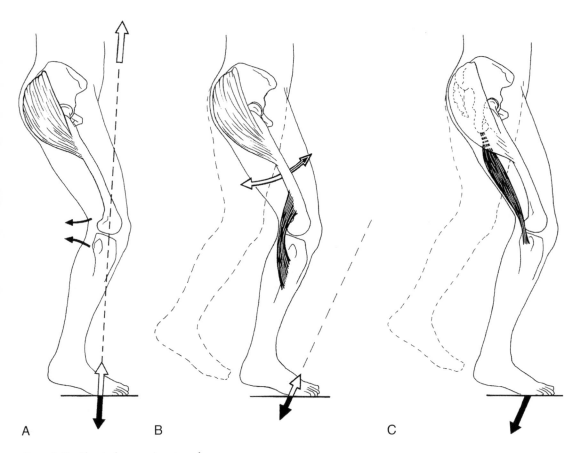

A   B   C

Figure 1.43   Thrust when running at speed
(A) If the gluteus maximus is the only muscle active when the body is held upright, then an extending
moment will develop in the knee and hip and the ground reaction force will pass through the knee.
(B) In order to direct the force of push-off toward the rear, force must be exerted to extend the hip
and bend the knee. Monoarticular knee flexors function just opposite the monoarticular hip extensors
(see the arrows at the thigh). If these flexors work simultaneously, little energy will remain. In a system
of monoarticular muscles, directing the force of push-off toward the rear will therefore always lead to a
decrease in the amount of energy available for thrust.
(C) The force that helps maintain the position of the gluteus maximus will have an extending effect
with regard to the knee. The hamstrings work to counteract knee extension and transfer energy from
the knee extension to the hip, thus helping to extend the hip. The hamstrings can direct force from the
hip extensors in a favorable direction without working against them. The hamstrings can create a
bending moment around the knee, without causing energy to be lost.

knee bend would be lost. This energy is generated by the hip extensors. Therefore,
when the monoarticular knee flexors are at work, the more the force is directed
toward the rear, the smaller this force will be. This is the reason why there are no
strong monoarticular knee flexors present in the locomotor apparatus.

The solution to this problem is provided by the structure of the hamstrings. Because
this muscle group spans both the knee and hip, it simultaneously works to bend the
knee and extend the hip. The indirect effect that the strong hip extensors (gluteus
maximus) have upon the knee (i.e. extending) is counteracted by the hamstrings.
The energy required to achieve this is not lost as internal heat of friction, but rather
can be diverted to the hip joint where it is used to strengthen hip extension. In this
way, the force on the ground can be directed toward the rear without there being a

loss of energy when speed decreases, as the knee must be extended. The hamstrings are able to divide the total force generated by the hip extensors between the knee and hip, as necessary.

In particular, during high-speed running, it is this mechanism that makes the hamstrings so important. At high speed, the time in which thrust can take place is necessarily very short, so that there is not sufficient time to compensate for forward or axial rotations. Forward rotation occurs when the trunk is allowed to lean toward the front. Therefore, the upper body should be held erect. Rotation around the longitudinal axis occurs when force is exerted at the end of the support phase. Therefore, propulsion must take place at the beginning of the support phase (see Section 3.2). Because the posture of the body is upright and because it is necessary to exert thrust at the beginning of ground contact, an imaginary line passing through the hip and foot at the moment of thrust will form a wide angle (about 90°) with the ground. When the force exerted on the ground is directed well to the rear, a large angle is formed by a line passing from the hip to foot and the intended direction of thrust. In this situation, much is being demanded of the force-directing potential of the hamstrings. These muscles are quite well suited to this task because, at the beginning of the support phase, they have a favorable lever arm with regard to the hip joint. By the end of this phase, however, this lever arm is no longer favorable. Thus speed running can also be called 'running on the hamstrings'.

When running at speed, the moment of thrust will occur at the beginning of the support phase. The reason for this is that the hamstrings can only function well as hip extensors if they have a large lever arm with regard to the hip. The lever arm is small when there is backward flexion and large for forward flexion. Although the angle formed by a line passing through the hip and foot in relation to the ground reaction force is somewhat more favorable by the end of stance, the lever arm of the hamstrings with regard to the hip is so small by that time that the hamstrings will barely be able to exert force upon the hip joint (Rozendal & Huijing 1996). EMG

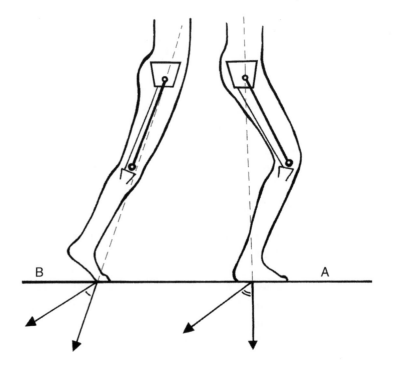

Figure 1.44 Running on the 'hamstrings'
During the first part of push-off (A), the hamstrings have a large lever arm on the hip joint, but likewise a great deal will be demanded of their strength and ability to direct the force of push-off toward the rear. At the end of push-off (B), less force is demanded because there is also less need to direct push-off. The lever arm of the hamstrings on the hip joint is now so small, however, that the hamstrings cannot work effectively. Therefore, the hamstrings only function during the first part of push-off.

research data also show that the hamstrings are especially active at the beginning of the support phase, which is in agreement with the demands being made by reactivity at the moment when elastic energy is being released.

1.6.3 Localization of body mass near the hip

As already stated, localization of mass in the distal part of the legs will not prove favorable for the economy of running. Furthermore, it is a fact that the chain of

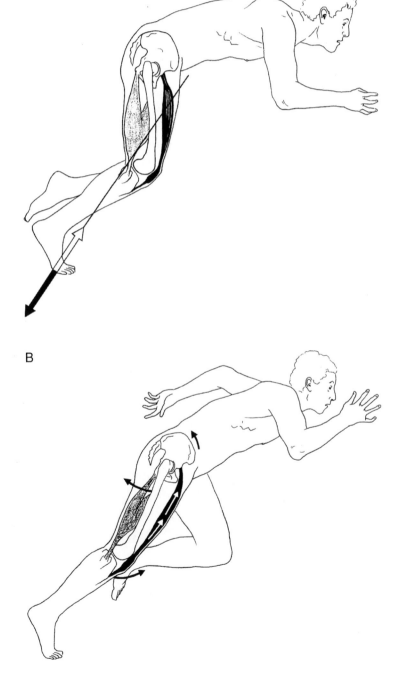

A

B

Figure 1.45 Forces surrounding the hip and knee

(A) At the start, when the body is hanging forward, the ground reaction force passes behind the knee and in front of the hip. Push-off can be strengthened further by extending the hip and knee simultaneously, without having to re-direct the force of push-off.

(B) Monoarticular knee extensors are able to exert less force than hip extensors. Hip extension creates a moment that counteracts the action of the rectus femoris, which will tighten and try not to lengthen. In this way, the rectus femoris has an extending moment with regard to the knee. Energy is transferred from the hip to knee. By regulating this transfer, one can coordinate hip and knee extension.

movement cannot tolerate the presence of a weak link. How much of the force generated around the hip joint can be exerted on the ground depends on the amount of force generated around the knee and ankle. If the plantar flexors of the ankle are very weak, the force generated around the hip is invalidated, 'draining away' as strong dorsiflexion (i.e. converted to frictional heat by way of eccentric muscle work). Through the transfer of energy from one joint to another by way of biarticular muscles, it is possible to generate a great deal of force around the ankle and knee without the need for the muscles themselves to be massive.

The rectus femoris has a relatively large lever arm with regard to the knee because of the presence of the patella (which functions as a pivot). The lever arm with regard to the hip is smaller that that of the hamstrings. Backward flexion in the hip is a joint moment opposite to the direction in which the rectus femoris works. When the rectus femoris is tightened, such a counteractive motion will result in an extending force on the knee. Therefore, the rectus femoris actively transfers energy, especially during movement that requires simultaneous backward flexion of the hip and knee extension. At the start, when a runner is leaning forward, the imaginary line passing through the hip and foot forms a relatively small angle with the direction of thrust. The reactive force therefore passes behind the knee and in front of the hip. Consequently, both hip and knee extension are mutually compatible, and the rectus femoris can actively transfer energy from the hip to the knee. The transfer of energy by the rectus femoris during the first strides of a sprint has been measured as contributing about 30% of the total force moment of the knee joint (Jacobs & Ingen Schenau et al 1992, Ingen Schenau et al 1995, Jacobs et al 1996). At speed, during the first part of the support phase, there is certainly no doubt that knee extension and backward flexion of the hip are mutually incompatible (in relation to

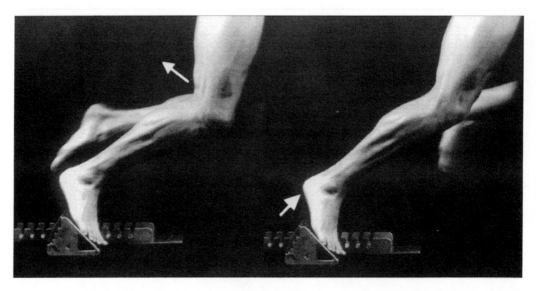

Figure 1.46   The function of the gastrocnemius during the start
When the knee extends rapidly, three problems arise: (a) the knee must eventually stop extending; (b) energy from the extension must not be lost; and (c) the direction of the knee at the end of extension is unfavorable with regard to the plane of progression. Knee extension imposes an eccentric moment on the gastrocnemius. By tightening, the muscle transfers energy from the knee extension to the ankle, which slows the knee extension and provides energy for plantar flexion in the ankle, which works to reinforce movement with regard to the plane of progression.

the directing of force by the hamstrings). The rectus femoris will therefore be less active, doing most of its work at the end of push-off.

The transfer of energy from around the knee to the ankle is provided by the gastrocnemius. Knee extension takes place at the end of push-off. The gastrocnemius becomes taut, with its tension being increased by knee extension. This results in plantar flexion in the ankle, which permits energy to be exerted on the ground. This force contributes 28% of the total force at the beginning of a sprint. The force with which plantar flexion is initiated in the ankle differs from one movement to the next. For a vertical jump on one leg, peak values for power with regard to the ankle joint have been measured to be about 1150 W; at the start of a sprint, peak values are 2050 W, and during running 2625 W. For a vertical jump, knee extension is relatively slow, so that tension in the triceps surae, as well as the pulling force on the Achilles tendon, is limited. Although it is true that there is a great deal of prestretch at the start of a sprint, the gastrocnemius is somewhat less active at this point than during running, possibly because if it worked too strongly at the beginning of the sprint it would counteract knee extension too much and have an unfavorable effect on how the force is directed to the ground. Energy transfer and elasticity contribute the most during running (Bobbert et al 1986, Jacobs et al 1993). The contribution from energy transferred during knee extension and from elasticity together can provide as much as 75% of the total power needed around the ankle joint during running. Because the lower-leg muscles need to shorten relatively little, they are able to have a strongly pennate structure and, moreover, need have little mass (Hof et al 1983, McNiell Alexander 1987).

1.6.4 Knee extension

In addition to being able to transfer energy, as discussed above, the gastrocnemius also provides the solutions for two other problems that arise at the end of the thrust phase.

First, the rapid knee extension just before the foot leaves the ground must be absorbed. If that were not possible by means of muscle strength, it would have to be managed by the passive structures, which are strong, rigid, and rather inflexible. The transfer of energy by the gastrocnemius (a knee flexor) has a knock-on effect that the speed of knee extension can be decreased without placing a heavy strain on the passive structures located in the hollow of the knee. Therefore, also in this case, energy is not lost as frictional heat, but can be 're-used'.

Second, the further knee extension progresses, the less it contributes to translating the body's center of mass. The force around the knee contributes increasingly little to acceleration in the targeted direction. When the transfer of force to the ankle has been timed well, thrust can continue to be directed correctly and is more effective.

The three functions (transferring energy, protecting the knee, and maintaining the direction of acceleration) of the gastrocnemius are closely interrelated.

1.6.5 Summary

In summary, it can be stated that the action of biarticular muscles and the elastic properties of the locomotor apparatus play a very important role during running. They help to make coordination more exact, making push-off more effective. Timing exactly when an action should be initiated is extraordinarily important. The lever arm with regard to the joint being moved must be favorable. The muscles must work in such a manner that the force of thrust is large and correctly directed.

When energy is being transferred, there must also be coherence between the force moments of the various joints. As already stated, together with the function of elasticity, an picture arises in which running can be seen as an extremely complex pattern of coordinated movements.

1.7 HOW RUNNING IS REGULATED

Locomotion or running is regulated by way of the central nervous system (CNS). The final pattern of movements is created by means of specially interwoven trajectories. The reason for this is that the locomotor system must not only adapt to the demands and possibilities dictated by its own structure, but it must also relate to the surroundings in which it must function. Adjusting the intended pattern to demands made by the surroundings will require great flexibility in dealing with the factors that affect the pattern of movement. Not only the body itself but also the environment will be influential. For example, during running, the motion of the swing leg must be adapted to that of the support leg (adaptation within the body) as well as to the demands made by the surroundings (e.g. adapting one's stride to conform with an uneven surface). The locomotor system can only be sufficiently flexible and expressive if the pattern of movement is not rigidly programmed. Therefore, many loops must be incorporated along the trajectory from program to implementation in order to give feedback and allow corrections to be inserted. Our understanding of the structure and function of the nervous system is still far from complete. In addition, after closer scrutiny, systems that were thought to be understood (e.g. how muscle spindles function and work) now appear to be more differentiated in their function than was formerly assumed. In the neurosciences, simplified models of reality are frequently used as a basis for study.

A very limited number of aspects of innervation are discussed below, with particular emphasis on their relevance to running.

1.7.1 Afferent and efferent innervation: locomotor and sensory systems

The nerve bundles that innervate the locomotor apparatus can be roughly divided into two groups.

- *Afferent bundles* carry information from the motor apparatus to the CNS (kinesthesia). By means of muscle spindles and sensors in the tendon and joint, information about changes in muscle length, tension in tendons, position of joints, etc., can be transmitted.
- *Efferent bundles* carry motor impulses from the CNS to muscles. All muscle fibers that are innervated by the same motor nerve form a single motor unit (MU), which can be either small or large. The force can be regulated in muscle by tightening few or many of these motor units. Small motor units are the first to be recruited when force must slowly be built up in a muscle; larger motor units are only switched on when much more force is needed. This so-called 'size principle' serves to adjust precisely the amount of force generated. The basis for controlling movement (Fox et al 1996, Cranenburgh 1997a,b) is to regulate the timing and the amount of force applied.

Information coming directly from the locomotor apparatus itself is supplemented by other sensory data. Visual, acoustic, tactile, and vestibular (equilibrium) information supplement kinesthetic information.

The locomotor and sensory systems are strongly interwoven. Motor impulses do not just descend from the brain without interference in order to effect movement. If this were true, then patterns of movement would be rigid and could not be adapted to the demands of one specific moment. A 'motor proposition' is made (an 'efference copy') that can be linked on many levels (sensory cortex, thalamus, reticular formation, dorsal columns, dorsal horn, and spinal cord) to available or expected feedback provided by the sensory organs. The motor impulse is altered on various levels and adapted to the situation in which the movement must be carried out.

Sensory information can be divided into two categories: one relevant to function and the other to locomotion.

- *Re-afference*: information originating within the locomotor system itself. Sensory information is created when the body moves (e.g. when a joint changes its position, from the inner ear's organ for balance, from the foot sole, or rhythmic sound of footsteps), and it is subsequently fed back to the interrelated motor–sensory systems and used for further adaptation in the locomotor system. Re-afferent information can also be acquired indirectly. An athlete need not observe directly what happens in his body, but can review feedback from his own achievements or from data stored elsewhere (e.g. on a video tape or through observations made by his trainer) to judge whether his technique is correct.
- *Exteroception*: information not resulting directly from motion (e.g. visual data about irregularities in the surface, an upcoming curve, an opponent's speed).
  - When running on an irregular surface (e.g. in woods, on hilly terrain), the exteroceptive sensory system plays a major role in the development of locomotion. Information (e.g. visual and acoustic) about irregularities in or the quality of the ground surface influences the amount of basic tension in the muscles and the changes in posture needed to maintain equilibrium.
  - When running under regular conditions (e.g. calm weather on an athletic tract), exteroceptive information is less influential. In this type of situation, an athlete would do better to concentrate on information from the re-afferent sensory system (e.g. Are my knees bent far enough. Is my foot strike sufficiently hard?).

When learning to run efficiently, an athlete can make use of both types of sensory systems. By means of exteroceptive information, a trainer can help an athlete alter his pattern of movement (e.g. by designating the length of stride, by using barriers – e.g. 15-cm high gates spaced 2.50 m apart – to accentuate flexion in the swing leg). However, when learning good running technique, the re-afferent sensory system is more important, because running is a cyclic motion. When a motion is cyclic, one movement will not be initiated from a new autonomous impulse (such as occurs when starting to throw something), but rather will develop out of the previous movement. The beginning of one cycle is actually the end of the previous cycle. Therefore, when a motion is cyclic, information obtained from the movement itself is more important than when the movement develops from an autonomous impulse. One can only develop an efficient running technique if the athlete is sensitive to re-afferent information. Even when external stimuli are introduced during training (e.g. the above-mentioned use of barriers), re-afferent stimuli will continue to be of greater importance when adapting a running pattern and must always be given adequate attention (i.e. running hurdles while maintaining good tension in the ankles, positioning the hips correctly, making short but hard ground contact). A good athlete will be sensitive to what happens within his body. Technique training

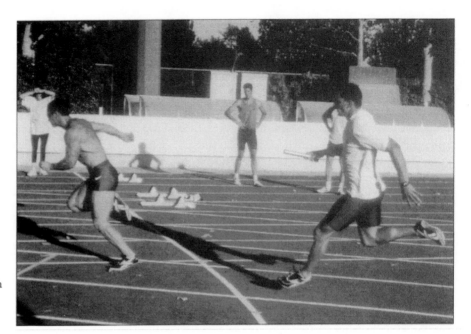

Figure 1.47 External and internal (re-afferent) information during a relay exchange
Re-afferent: coordinating movement in the right knee with extension of the left leg, and linking the ground contact time (long for the left-hand and short for the right-hand runner) with either a forward (left) or upright (right) posture of the upper body.
External: comparing one's own speed with that of the departing relay runner and anticipating when the baton should be handed over.

should focus on improving that sensitivity so that the athlete can continue to make good use of re-afferent information, even in situations where he may become distracted by external circumstances.

The following is an example of an athlete assigned to run at high speed while keeping the length of his stride very long (e.g. 2.50 m) and his ground contact time quite short (making only one ground contact between the 15-cm high gates placed 2.50 m apart). The athlete is able to complete this assignment (albeit with some difficulty). However, if his ground contact time is too long to achieve a single step, perhaps because his posture is incorrect, then he will find himself unable to make short ground contact during the following steps. The sensory feedback loop, which returns necessary information about the correct posture of and tension in the body, has been disrupted and will be unable to recover immediately. The athlete can learn to intuit exactly which step caused the targeted running pattern to fail and learn to maintain better posture and correct tension during speed running. The low practice gates can also be placed at longer distances from each other (beginning at 2.25 m and repeatedly increasing the space by 5 cm up to 2.75 m). The athlete's assignment remains the same: to run fast while keeping the ground contact time short. Using such an exercise during practice will help the athlete begin to realize how far he can increase the length of his step and still maintain short ground contact. By setting up practice hurdles (external stimuli) in this manner, an athlete can become sensitized to which combination of step length and ground contact time will prove to be optimal (re-afferent sensory system).

1.7.2 Myotatic and Golgi-tendon reflexes

The locomotor system is controlled according to patterns of excitation or stimulation, by which nerve impulses are transferred from one nerve cell to another and from one area in the nervous system to another. In addition, inhibition (i.e. inhibiting or blocking the transfer of a stimulus), plays an equally important role in the control of the motor system. At all levels of the nervous system, functionality is determined by the stimulus and how it is transferred, as well as by how the stimulus is extinguished or its transfer blocked (Burgerhout et al 1995, Fox et al 1996, Rozendal & Huijing 1996, Cranenburgh 1997a,b).

The nervous system can be subdivided into the central and peripheral nervous systems. The CNS (brain and spinal cord) will not be considered further here. However, several aspects of the peripheral nervous system (the division of the spinal cord into regions dealing with separate peripheral structures, such as muscle) that are relevant for the transfer of a stimulus are discussed.

Receptors arising from peripheral structures that are connected at the spinal-cord level can be subdivided as follows:

- interoceptors – sensors in organs (these are not discussed here)
- proprioceptors – muscle spindles, Golgi-tendon organ, joint sensors
- exteroceptors – sense of touch, pain, etc.

The muscle spindle is a receptor with a structure just a few millimeters long lying parallel to the fibers within the muscle. Because of its structure, the muscle spindle is sensitive both to the length and to changes in the length of the muscle. Afferent-1a fibers register and send information about how far and how rapidly a muscle increases in length. Afferent-2 fibers register and send information about any increase in muscle length. This information is supplied by stretch receptors located in the muscle spindle.

The length of a muscle spindle can change under the influence of efferent γ-motor neurons, which innervate muscle fibers located within the spindle. However, stretch receptors within the muscle spindle remain the same length, even though the length of the spindle itself changes. In this way, the receptors remain sensitive to stretch. Because it is possible to give the muscle spindle a certain length, one can adjust the stretch receptors to be sensitive to a certain length or change in length for the total muscle. For example, when the muscle spindle must be sensitized to changes in length of a greatly shortened muscle, then the muscle spindle itself must first be shortened by γ-motor neuron stimulation. Subsequently, the length of the muscle fibers within the spindle remains constant and any change in length of the total muscle is registered by the muscle stretch receptors. If thereafter the muscle must work from a more elongated position, the muscle spindles must themselves first lengthen before starting to measure the new position of the muscle through their stretch receptors.

Registration of muscle length, as well as any changes in length, by stretch receptors is sent to the spinal cord. In addition to sending information on to higher levels in the CNS, α-motor neurons become activated at spinal-cord level. Such activation results in the stimulation and contraction of the muscle. This is called the myotatic reflex. Moreover, the muscle spindle works to maintain length (i.e. a muscle that is rapidly stretched contracts involuntarily due to a signal from the muscle spindle).

Muscle can therefore be regulated by way of two different pathways: directly via α-motor neuron stimulation (driven from the brain) and indirectly via γ-motor neuron stimulation (resulting in a change in muscle-spindle sensitivity, which in turn leads to control of the γ-motor neurons). This latter mechanism is called α–γ co-activation.

In reality, how a muscle spindle functions and works is extremely complex. An active muscle spindle is linked to higher levels of the nervous system which, by adjusting the muscle spindle, have an important and influential effect on α–γ coupling and the myotatic reflex. When an isometric contraction has been carried out with awareness, muscle tonicity is supported by muscle-spindle activity. When a concentric contraction has been performed with awareness, muscle-spindle activity disappears (centrally driven). This phenomenon plays an important role for movements that are largely routine. The former idea that muscle spindles work either chiefly, or only, by way of reflexes at spinal-cord level must now be changed for a model that is much more complex, interactive, and flexible, and in which activity at the level of the spinal cord is only part of the whole story.

More important than the subject of reflexes, the muscle-spindle system (indirectly) offers a way to adjust the muscle to a certain predetermined length, independent of the external forces involved. When seen within the wider perspective of the locomotor system, this means that the muscle-spindle system can serve to exclude the influence of external factors (forces outside the body) from the behavior of the locomotor system. In this way, the system of movements is able to mold the locomotor system according to a predetermined plan, including those adaptations to external factors that are necessary for the successful implementation of a certain task.

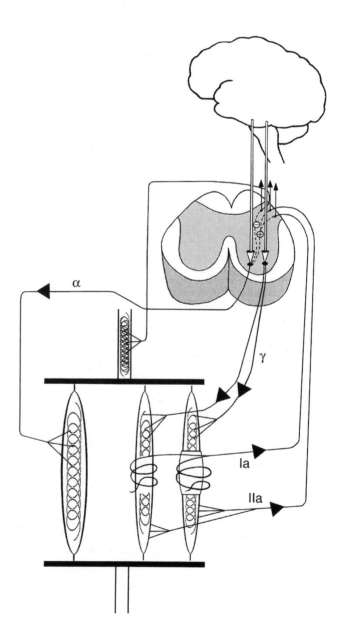

Figure 1.48 Scheme for the muscle-spindle system and α–γ coupling
There are two pathways along which signals from the brain can regulate muscles. One pathway (α) passes directly from the brain to the muscle via α-motor neurons. The second pathway (γ) is indirect; from the brain via γ-motor neurons to muscle spindles to sensitize them to changes in length within a certain range. Thereafter, during stretching, Ia and IIa fibers send signals that reinforce the activity of α-motor neurons. This indirect pathway makes the locomotor system nearly independent of external influences (the muscle reaches the intended length regardless of the external forces) and is therefore an important instrument for implementing movement in the manner intended.

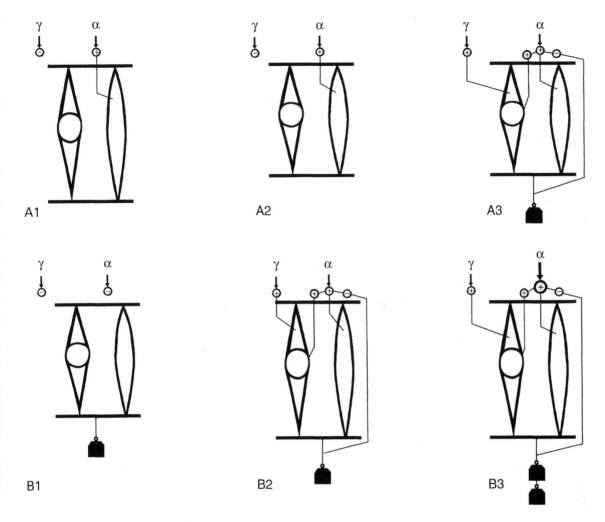

Figure 1.49   Two examples of α–γ coupling
(A1) A muscle is shortened to the length intended without much external resistance. (A2) Shortening ceases at the targeted length and (A3) this length is maintained, even when more external force is applied to lengthen the muscle further. α–γ Coupling maintains isometry. (B1) The muscle lengthens due to the external force without resisting. After having reached its targeted length, the muscle suddenly becomes fixed (B2) and no longer lengthens. This is caused by α–γ coupling. When external forces are stronger (B3), α–γ coupling maintains isometry.

Moreover, in addition to involuntary activation of its 'own' muscle, the muscle spindle has an inhibitory effect on antagonists. At spinal-cord level, inhibition is just as important as excitation. For example, activation of the muscle fibers in the gluteus maximus during backward flexion of the leg is accompanied by an inhibitory effect with regard to the fibers in the iliopsoas.

The Golgi-tendon organ works to limit tension. When a muscle is tightened, the tendon is stretched so that the Golgi-tendon organ becomes active. The Golgi-tendon organ works, among other ways, by feedback at spinal-cord level to inhibit the muscle. This system is much more sensitive than was previously assumed; i.e. the Golgi-tendon organ can register an increase in tension developing from the activity of a single motor unit.

The muscle-spindle and Golgi-tendon systems are in fact conservative by nature. They attempt to resist rapid and extreme changes in the length and tension of muscle. As already stated, the brain's motor system is capable of overruling these two conservative systems. This occurs best in situations in which the brain can anticipate which signals will be sent by the muscle-spindle and Golgi-tendon systems. In other words, when a movement is familiar, muscles can tighten and relax more rapidly, and with a greater difference between the tension and its release, than when a movement has not yet become routine. It is also true that, especially when a movement is cyclic, even when it is routine, unexpected influences coming from outside the body can disturb the ability of the brain to retain control. For example, during a 100-m sprint, an average tail wind of about 1.50 m/s will give a mechanical advantage (less resistance to overcome). Nevertheless, it makes quite a difference whether the wind is blowing regularly or in irregular gusts. When a tail wind of 1.50 m/s, but which is gusty and irregular, is actually measured during competitions, it often appears that all the athletes (especially those who are technically superior runners) clock greatly disappointing running times, despite the advantage of the tail wind. This is because the motor system is unable to anticipate alternating signals coming from the two conservative systems and therefore cannot utilize them optimally. Tension and the release of tension cannot be alternated optimally. The positive effect of having to work less because of the tail wind is partly negated when the motor pattern is disrupted. Measuring the wind during an athletic event is a method that will yield only very approximately correct data about the way in which an athlete's performance will ultimately be influenced by circumstances.

During the practice of athletic training, one perspective often emphasized is the influence of the muscle-spindle system, by way of the myotatic reflex arc. Springy stretching exercises are frequently discouraged because they are thought to increase tone. Some equipment even vibrates and is thought to help improve the athlete's level of strength by increasing tone. It would be useful to test any training methodology that strongly favors the implied dominant working of the myotatic reflex against changing insight into how muscle and tendon sensors work during functional movement.

1.7.3   Sensors in the joint

Joint sensors supply important information about the position of joints (e.g. sensitivity to the angle of the knee at foot placement during running). Such information is essential when comparing what one wants to achieve and what actually happens during running. Loss of information about the position of joints will lead the muscle to function less adequately. Therefore, rupture of the frontal cruciate ligament in the knee, where important sensors are located, can cause the knee to become unstable. Supporting the knee by means of braces or tape will only affect the soft outer tissue and, from a mechanical perspective, not the knee's stability. Such support is effective, however, through improving (facilitating) propioception of the knee-capsule and skin sensors. These sensors work to strengthen the effect of muscle tension and thus influence indirectly the joint's stability.

How exterosensors, especially those sensors in the sole of the foot, affect running technique is also significant. Wearing spiked shoes when running not only serves to increase a runner's grip on the ground surface, but also serves to transmit clear signals from the foot sole to the locomotor system. Running shoes designed with strong shock dampers have the great disadvantage that some sensory information from the foot is lost, which can lead to deterioration in muscle activity and technical skill.

Nowadays, sprinters make more of a differentiation between the spiked shoes worn for training and those worn for competition. Competition spikes are designed in such a way that the runner feels pressure earlier at the front of the foot. By means of such a (deceptive) stimulus, the cyclic movement of running is 'urged on'. Running proceeds as a matter of course. It is not advisable to wear such spiked shoes at all times because one must assume that the positive effect is only temporary and will disappear if applied too regularly.

1.7.4 Comparison of motor patterns

Excitation, as well as inhibition, plays important roles in motor patterns. Adjustment between the two factors will be more important for one pattern of movement than for another. For speed running, being able to control the conservative systems (muscle-spindle and Golgi-tendon organ) is very important, for a number of reasons:

- When running at speed, muscles are stretched quite forcefully before they contract powerfully thereafter. Adjusting the extent to which a muscle is stretched is especially important with an eye to retaining the elastic energy that accompanies the stretch. A muscle will strive to limit stretch to the elastic components connected in series, and a certain degree of conservatism in the length will therefore be necessary. However, too much conservatism will lead the body to cramp during running. An athlete must therefore know how to find a perfect balance between tension in the body in order to retain elastic energy and release of tension in order to permit rapid contraction.
- Running is a cyclic motion. This means that a previous movement will have a great influence on the following movement. The motor system needs information obtained from the previous step before taking the next step. The body is geared to copy patterns of motion continuously. This process is ongoing, as long as the information anticipated from the muscle receptors equals the information actually supplied. Therefore, it is easier to keep to a certain cadence while running than suddenly to change rhythm. The continuous copying of well-executed and effective strides leaves very little room for differentiation between anticipated and actual information (see also the effect of irregular wind on performance, Section 1.7.2). This fact is also used when jumping from one leg after making a running start. During the final steps before push-off, the stride frequency and degree of movement in both the hip and the knee are gradually increased so that the scissor movement of the legs during push-off can be executed more forcefully. The push-off is thus 'supercharged' (i.e. the wind-up technique) (Cranenburgh 1997a).

1.7.5 Stumble reflex

At spinal-cord level, there is a coupling between a muscle and its antagonist (an inhibiting action of each on the other). This system of excitation and inhibition also functions in the larger system of the stumble reflex. Imagine that someone walking along the street does not see a piece of pavement protruding. To avoid falling, the swing leg (which was in the process of moving forward) is caught hanging by the point of its shoe behind the protruding edge. In order to avoid falling, the stance leg, which was in the process of carrying out backward flexion (the foot moves backwards), shoots forward to support the body as it falls forward. Moving the support leg to the front was done without thinking or wishing it to happen (i.e. involuntary action). Apparently, unexpected backward flexion in one leg results in an equally unplanned forward flexion in the other leg. One can speak of an involuntary response not only in the case of antagonist muscles, but also in the case of one leg in relation to the other. This reflex (the stumble reflex) can be incorporated well in regular patterns of motion. In other words, when someone wants to carry out rapid backward flexion in the support leg (powerful push-off) then this can best be accompanied by a powerful forward flexion in the swing leg. Both motions are closely and involuntarily interrelated (Burgerhout et al 1995, Cranenburgh 1997a,b).

A similar involuntary reflex response is seen in the relationship between flexion in one leg and extension in the other leg (i.e. the inverse-extension reflex). When someone steps unexpectedly on a sharp object, the leg which receives the pain stimulus bends involuntarily, while the other leg stretches as a reflex response. Powerful extending of the support leg at the end of support can be strengthened by simultaneously bending the swing leg at the hip and knee more powerfully. It is particularly at the start of this sequence that the inverse-extension reflex proves to be quite important.

The sprint is a more precise implementation of both the stumble and inverse-extension reflexes. The level that can be reached using the support of a reflex is impossible to achieve any other way. Because excitation and inhibition (i.e. tension and the release of tension) occur so rapidly in succession and vary so greatly in peak during running, having developed a good reflex response becomes a condition sine qua non. When training techniques for speed running, push-off must be well coordinated with the action of the swing leg so that the reflex response can work optimally. Moreover, it is more than worth the effort during strength training to look for types of exercise in which involuntary movements can play a role. In particular, a training in which speed and force can be combined will thereby be facilitated with certainty. In practice, running instruction demonstrates that the two above-

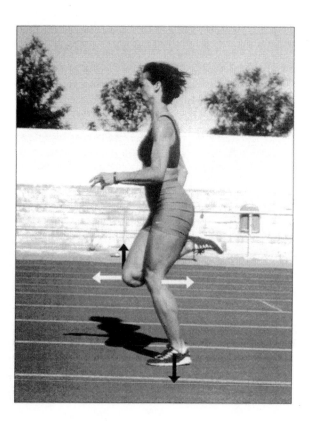

Figure 1.50 Stumble reflex
Stumble (white arrows) and inverse-extension (black arrows) reflexes during running when momentum is at its peak.

mentioned reflexes are closely interrelated (when the knee of the swing leg is bent forcefully at the beginning of swing, then forward flexion in the hip is also initiated with force). The best approach to teaching a running technique is therefore to begin with the total pattern.

1.8 ANATOMY AND TRAINING

In the previous sections, a series of anatomical data by which the performance of a runner can be determined has been reviewed. The data vary from the characteristic force–velocity relationship, as measured in isolated muscle fibers, to the effect of changes in the force moment of a muscle with regard to a joint, and to the effect that an involuntary movement can have on a muscle's output. One might assume that trainers and individuals knowledgeable in the theory of training would integrate as far as possible all these factors into a total training program. However, it has become almost a tradition, particularly when training for sprinting, to choose the force–velocity relationship for isolated muscle fibers as the most important starting point, particularly with regard to strength training. Therefore, the following theoretical arguments about and practical approach to strength training are proposed.

Running, especially the sprint, is characterized by the fact that an athlete must accelerate to the highest possible speed within the brief amount of time available. This means that acceleration must be maximal. The line of approach when training a runner is that it is actually the potential for acceleration that must be taught through strength training. In the field of physics, it has been known for centuries that a force (F) is needed to accelerate a mass (m): $F = ma$, where a is the acceleration. This implies that the higher the force, the greater the potential for acceleration. For example, applying maximum force at the start will help a runner achieve a higher speed. At that moment, because he is running faster, a runner will no longer have access to his absolute maximum power (Loo 1996). Another example is that of pumping a bar-bell along the body. The motion of the bar-bell is accelerated, whereby it is moved even faster just above the knees by the absolute maximum force of

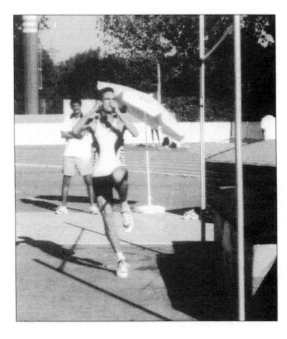

Figure 1.51 High-spring push-off
A technique that is almost never used today in which the extended leg swings upward. The mechanical advantage of keeping the swing leg extended (larger vertical impulse) appears inferior in practice to using the optimally enhanced inverse-extension reflex.

the stretch sequence. However, at the same time, the bar-bell has gained a speed at which it is no longer possible to apply the maximum force generated from that stretch sequence. Therefore, one can conclude that the ability to accelerate a mass (body) that has already reached speed will greatly determine performance in, for example, the sprint. Because time factors so strongly during a sprint, being able to generate the highest possible power is more important than being able to generate strength close to its absolute maximum level. In the field of physics, power is defined as the product of force and velocity ($P = Fv$). In strength training geared to runners, more attention is now being given to the component velocity as part of the power that a runner must deliver.

In practice, during strength training, the velocity at which an external load is displaced can be recorded using different instruments (Biorobot, Muscle Lab). Using a variable external load (e.g. a bar-bell disc), power can be calculated according to $P = Fv$. Instrumentation for measurement can be used to test or supply feedback during training. When an athlete is being tested, the amount of power generated can be recorded using, for example, five loads varying from very light to quite heavy. These data can be used to construct a force–velocity diagram and thus a power curve (Kraaijenhof 1994), and subsequent strength training can be organized on the basis of power. For example, a weight can be selected with which maximum power can be trained. Using computer software and a power range of 95–110% of the target power, one can determine whether an athlete's attempt was successful. Equipment will generally be used that supplies feedback in the form of sound or light signals that inform the athlete about the power he is providing. Thus if, for example, the level of power is too low, an athlete can choose to move more rapidly in order to reach the target level. Alternatively, the feedback may be used to end a series of trials prematurely when a runner is no longer able to achieve the level for which he was aiming. When power is assessed a second time using the same five weights and the same test, the effect of training can be determined according to changes in the force–velocity diagram and/or power curve. If the data plotted on the force–velocity

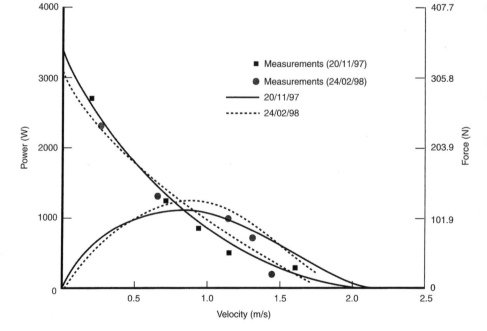

Figure 1.52   Force–velocity diagram and power curve
Force–velocity diagrams with power curves measured at two different times during a training season. Each force–velocity diagram and power curve has been constructed on the basis of five measurements using an ergometer. The measurements record the velocities of an external load varying from a light to a very heavy weight.

diagram are shifted upward and to the right, the training has been effective, although the maximum speed of contraction (without a load) remains the same.

One must now question whether the force–velocity relationship and the power curve for an isolated muscle fiber correctly represents how muscle is used during strength training aimed at runners. The representation is correct when considering the maximum contraction for monoarticular muscles (Poel 1993). Furthermore, one must stipulate that the load imposed on monoarticular muscles must remain constant along the entire trajectory of movement. When effort is submaximal, there appears to be no clear relationship between the force generated and the velocity. It was previously realized that the requirement that a muscle load be constant is impossible because both the lever arm (the shortest distance from the rotational axis in the joint to where the muscle inserts) and the relationship between force and muscle length are continuously changing. For still more complex movements such as running, biarticular muscles play a dominant role. It is impossible to predict the in vivo behavior of these muscles based on the force–velocity relationship using dissected muscle fibers (Poel 1993).

Apart from the fact that such information is not taken into consideration during power training, another factor that is also often ignored when using this training concept is the elasticity in SEC and PEC segments, and its implications for how CE segments function (see Section 1.4.2), and the way in which reflexes affect a muscle's ability to work.

Few muscles (only monoarticular) are built for power training, and one can question whether there is a factor lying within these muscles that limits their ultimate performance. Further attention is given in Chapter 6 to the implications of anatomical data with regard to planning strength training.

Placing too much emphasis on the force–velocity diagram with regard to organizing a strength training program can serve to illustrate the lack of interest in the world of athletics for other relevant anatomical data. As soon as such information has been integrated into how one now thinks about training, then new and useful insights and methodologies may result.

2
Generation of energy

2.1 INTRODUCTION

Traditionally, the basic motor properties of importance in condition training have served as the point of departure when investigating which factors might determine how successfully an athlete will perform across a certain running distance (Goolberg & Swinkels 1994). The way in which a training program is set up depends on the relative share designated to each basic motor property: force, speed, suppleness, and endurance. Using this approach, one can intuitively see that force and speed will be crucial factors when training sprinters, and endurance will be crucial when training middle- and long-distance runners. Generally, the four above-mentioned motor properties can be made more exact by making various combinations between them (Goolberg & Swinkels 1994), which will lead to the creation of complex sport-related motor properties, such as the ability to maintain force, the ability to generate force rapidly, and speed endurance.

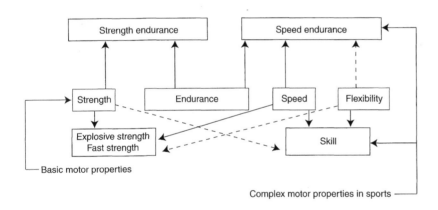

Figure 2.1 Scheme for motor properties relevant to the world of sports
The four basic motor properties can be fine-tuned by making combinations. In this manner, complex and difficult to define basic motor properties can be developed for sports.

Defining the latter characteristics is extremely problematic. Furthermore, even though it might be possible to define the basic motor properties in a simple way, it is just as difficult to determine them quantitatively as it is to define complex sport-related motor properties for running performance. In the literature on training, therefore, a further division is frequently made using various criteria that show how basic motor properties are manifested (Vrijens 1984, Kloosterboer 1996) in order to get some grip on which factors might possibly limit performance. For example, the basic motor property 'speed' can be subdivided into several of its manifestations: reaction speed, locomotor speed of force, maximum speed, and capacity to maintain speed (Swinkels 1980). Nevertheless, for most manifestations, it is almost impossible to delineate these concepts. Moreover, there is no consensus regarding how one can determine which manifestations are practicable, and thus one finds oneself confronting an impenetrable forest of phenomena. The first example that springs to mind is the locomotor property 'endurance' or 'stamina'.

Manifestations can be differentiated according to the amount of muscle mass applied, the type of muscle contraction, the anticipated effect of training, the duration of the competition, or dominant processes generating energy. Therefore it follows that endurance can be subdivided even further into: local versus general, static versus dynamic, general versus specific, short versus middle versus long, and anaerobic versus aerobic (Zintl 1995).

Because the relative contribution of each basic locomotor property and its manifestation during performance are still being used as the perspective from which to start when specifying performance-determining factors, this can lead to an incorrect choice of training challenges. In particular, it is the inadequate definition of basic locomotor properties and their manifestation that is the problem. For example, if one defines the basic locomotor property 'stamina' or 'endurance' as the capacity to resist feelings of fatigue (Zintl 1995), then it is this capacity that will determine the choice of challenges to be used during training directed at improving the stamina of, for example, a marathon runner. The ability to resist fatigue is focused on to such an extent that it becomes the goal, and thus during training a marathon runner must frequently be subjected to challenges leading to massive fatigue. It is self-evident that few more detailed demands will be made on the content of the training, because only its visible effect (i.e. that the runner is exhausted) will be considered important. Although the above-mentioned example is somewhat of an exaggeration, it does illustrate the fact that the use of basic locomotor properties and their manifestations to quantify performance-determining factors has many limitations and can lead to an incorrect interpretation of the training program.

Many of the problems described above can be avoided by taking a different approach when deciding which factors will determine performance. As there are a wealth of factors of varying importance that can be identified, it is difficult to obtain a clear perspective about where to start when deciding which training methodology should be followed. Reducing the factors to obtain one major influencing agent will give more clarity. The issue for an athlete striving to improve his running through training will always center around how to increase speed when running a certain distance. This is true not only for the sprinter, but also for the long-distance runner. The speed that can be realized during running becomes the central issue. This speed should not be equated with the absolute maximum speed that a runner can achieve, but rather represents an average running speed across a certain distance. Therefore, when planning a training program, the question that should always be asked first is that of how speed can be increased during running. In order to give a comprehensive answer to this question, one must first distinguish three phases for speed:

(1) at the beginning
(2) in the middle
(3) at the end.

Regardless of the phase, the focus will always be on how to deliver as much power as possible. Here power is defined as the work per unit of time that a runner can achieve. In Figure 2.2, one can clearly spot the differences between a trained and an untrained athlete. First, the trained runner is able to deliver more power, which results in a higher maximum speed. Second, the trained runner appears to cope more efficiently with energy generated at submaximum speeds. At most submaximum speeds, an untrained runner will use more energy. When the power generated is exactly sufficient to overcome opposing forces, the runner can maintain speed.

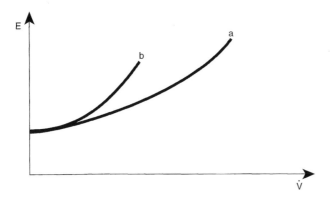

Figure 2.2   Graph showing the relationship between energy and velocity
The energy (E) generated (i.e. power) is plotted against velocity ($\dot{V}$) for untrained (b) and trained (a) runners.

If the runner is able to exert more power than the amount consumed by antagonistic forces, the runner will accelerate. Therefore the aim of a training program will always be to increase the power that can be provided. For the terminology to be correct, it is necessary to specify further the concept of power. One needs to differentiate between power that is generated metabolically and that which is generated mechanically. Power that is generated metabolically is the energy released from the breakdown of foodstuffs such as glycogen and fat. Only part of the energy released in this way can be used to move the body forward during running (i.e. provide mechanical power). The percentage of energy contained in foodstuffs that eventually

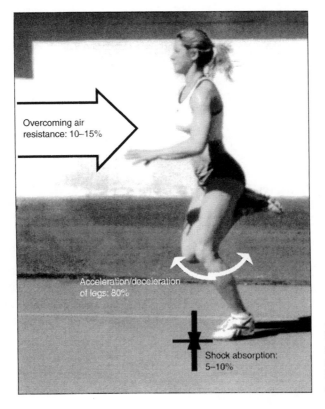

Figure 2.3   Power needed for running
Most of the power generated will be consumed as the legs accelerate and slow down. Any remaining power will be used to absorb shock and overcome air resistance.

provides mechanical energy is called the mechanical efficiency (Ingen Schenau & Toussaint 1994). At muscle level, mechanical efficiency is estimated to be about 25–30%; a large portion of the energy released from foodstuffs is lost as heat.

The speed of movement is chiefly determined by how the central nervous (CNS), locomotor system, and vegetative system function. Of the vegetative systems (i.e. those directed at keeping the body alive), only the cardiorespiratory system (heart, blood circulation, and lungs) is discussed in this book. The cardiorespiratory system decreases in importance as the running distance becomes shorter, and is no longer a performance-determining factor for an athlete running 100 m. Energy is needed if the CNS, locomotor system, and cardiorespiratory system are to function. In this chapter we discuss the role played by energy-generating processes and by the cardiorespiratory system in trying to deliver as much power possible. The ways in which the CNS and locomotor apparatus function have been discussed in Chapter 1.

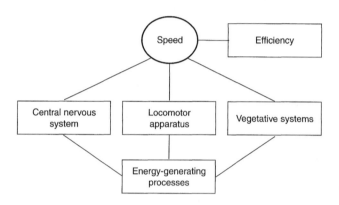

Figure 2.4 Factors determining running speed
Different factors, and their interrelationships, which determine speed.

2.2 ENERGY

Energy is an abstract concept that can be defined as the capacity to perform work. Energy exists in six primary forms:

- thermal
- chemical
- mechanical
- electrical
- radiation
- atomic.

In the human body, it is chemical and electrical energy in particular that are used to move the body (muscle contraction), provide active transport, and carry out biosynthesis (the creation of certain molecules) (Stryer 1995). During the process of converting one form of energy into another, energy is neither created nor destroyed. In general, conversion of energy (the transformation of one form of energy into another) is a rather inefficient process. For example, when chemical energy is converted to mechanical energy in the human body, much of the chemical energy becomes thermal energy or heat. Unfortunately, the human body is not equipped to convert heat into other forms of energy. From this perspective, it can be said that thermal energy has no value for the human body. Nevertheless, thermal energy is essential for biological systems. Many processes, such as muscle contraction and enzymatic reactions, are greatly dependent on temperature. These processes can only function optimally in a narrow temperature range around 37°C. Although, theoretically, muscle should be able to contract more rapidly near 50°C than at 35°C, in reality this is impossible due to denaturation (the distortion of structure) of proteins in muscle at such high temperatures (Brooks et al 1996). Furthermore, heat is used to maintain body temperature at about 37°C. In summary, energy exchange in the human body results in conversion of energy to a form useable for performing work and to thermal energy, expressed as heat, which cannot be used for work. In a biological system, the useable form is called 'free energy'.

2.2.1 Enzymes

In a biological system, chemical reactions are essential in order to transfer energy to various sites within the system (Silverthorn 1998). To gain more insight into the various energy systems, one must examine more deeply the chemical reactions that take place within the human body during energy exchange. The chemical processes by which energy is generated and stored in the chemical bonds of biomolecules are called metabolism. In a chemical reaction, molecules react to form other molecules. New products are formed via the breaking of the molecular bonds in the substrates. One example of such a chemical reaction is shown below, where products C and D are formed from substrates A and B:

$$A + B \rightarrow C + D$$

The products can have a higher energy level than that of the substrates, which means that energy must be added during the reaction. Such a reaction in which small molecules are synthesized into larger molecules is called endergonic. For example, the formation of glycogen from molecules of glucose is an endergonic reaction.

When the products have a lower energy level than the substrates, then energy has been released and the reaction is called exergonic. When glycogen is converted into glucose, the energy that has temporarily been stored in the bonds of the glycogen molecule is released. Thus the glucose–glycogen reaction can run in two directions. The glucose $\rightarrow$ glycogen reaction is endergonic, while the glycogen $\rightarrow$ glucose reaction is exergonic. A chemical reaction that can take place in either direction is called reversible, and this is the type of reaction that occurs most frequently in a biological system. A double arrow pointing in opposite directions is used to show that the reaction is reversible.

$$A + B \leftrightarrows C + D$$

An irreversible reaction is characterized by a large exchange of energy. The reaction will run in one direction because a lot of energy is either being released or must be added. There is very little chance, therefore, that a reaction in which a great deal of energy is released will spontaneously begin to react in the opposite direction, because this reversal would require the addition of a large amount of energy. Irreversible reactions seldom occur in a biological system (see following paragraphs). One feature of metabolism is that it links endo- and exergonic reactions. Therefore, metabolism can be compared to a network of coupled reactions.

The speed of a chemical reaction is measured by the speed in which substrates A and B disappear and products C and D appear (see above formula). Because the temperature (37°C) of the human body is relatively low, one might expect most chemical reactions to run quite slowly. At low temperatures few collisions take place between molecules, thus decreasing the chance that one substrate will 'meet' the right partner needed for a particular reaction. In order to start many chemical reaction, one must first add a certain amount of (activation) energy.

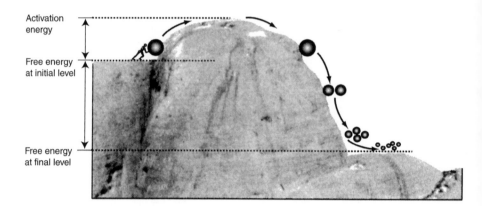

Figure 2.5 Activation energy
In the human body, a certain amount of energy (i.e. activation energy) must be added before most chemical reactions can take place. The substrates involved must first be brought to a higher energy level, illustrated here as a stone being rolled uphill. The stone shatters into a number of smaller pieces as it rolls back downhill. This comparison can be made for products formed during a chemical reaction.

In order to convert certain substrates in such a way that the products intended are formed in one reaction, so much activation energy would be required that the temperature of the human body would become too high. The body's ingenious solution to this problem is to convert molecules by using many small steps in which only a small amount of activation energy is used each time. Enzymes play an important role in speeding up chemical reactions by lowering the energy of activation. A chemical reaction that requires a lot of activation energy will either fail to occur or run slowly without enzymes. Without the catalytic (accelerating) action of enzymes, the human cell would be unable to survive. An example using numbers will show how enzymes are essential to life. The presence of one molecule of an enzyme can accelerate a reaction in such a way that, within 1 s, 1 million molecules of product can be formed, while in the absence of the enzyme only one molecule of product could be formed in 100 s. Enzymes act to bind substrates in such a way that they come to be ideally positioned to take part in a chemical reaction. Without enzymes, it would be left to chance for substrates to bump into one other while correctly positioned. An enzyme is only able to catalyze a certain chemical reaction or a group of closely similar reactions. Furthermore, when an enzyme takes part in a chemical reaction its own structure does not change. Chemical reactions within an energy system are usually a chain of enzymatic reactions. The products, or intermediate products, formed at each step can regulate the activity of certain enzymes in the chain reaction.

Two types of regulatory, or modulatory, processes also have an influence on chemical reactions. First, a chemical product or its intermediates can function as competitive inhibitors by using a site on the enzyme intended as a binding site for a substrate. The number of enzyme–substrate complexes decreases as the number of possible binding sites for the substrate declines. Second, enzyme activity can be stimulated or inhibited by a product, or its intermediate products, which acts as an allosteric modulator. Such a modulator binds to the enzyme at a site not intended for the substrate, the allosteric modulator bond can affect a possible binding site in such a way that it will either become active or inactive for binding with the substrate. In addition, there are many other factors that can influence the activity of an

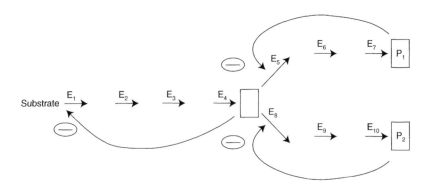

Figure 2.6 An example of an enzymatic chain reaction
The products P_1 and P_2 exert an inhibiting effect on enzymes E_5 and E_8, respectively, so that fewer byproducts F and H can be formed. Furthermore, byproduct D has a negative effect on enzyme E_1.

enzyme. For example, the presence of hydrogen ions and an increase in temperature (>37°C) alter the spatial structure of enzymes, thus inhibiting enzyme activity (Newsholm et al 1994).

The concentration of enzymes and substrates in a cell directly affects the speed of a chemical reaction. A higher concentration of enzymes makes more binding sites available for the catalysis of substrates. The number of enzyme molecules available is regulated by the speed of their production, on one hand, and the speed of their breakdown, on the other. When the concentration of enzymes remains constant, the speeds of production and breakdown are equal (i.e. there is equilibrium). In such a situation, when the substrate concentrations are low, the speed of reaction will increase linearly with an increase in substrate concentration. When the concentration of a substrate reaches a certain level, all available enzymes will be saturated with substrate, and the speed of reaction will reach its maximum value ($\dot{V}_{max}$). The properties of enzymes in this respect are shown in Figure 2.10, where the speed of reaction is been plotted against substrate concentration.

Each enzyme has specific characteristics, which can be expressed by $\dot{V}_{max}$ and the substrate concentration that leads to one-half the maximum speed of reaction (K_m).

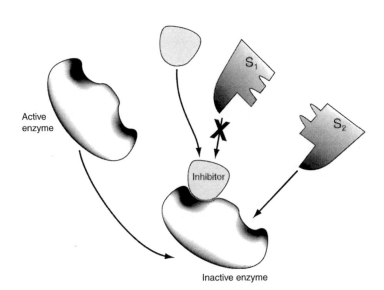

Figure 2.7 Bonding of a substrate to an enzyme 1
A competitive inhibitor binds to an enzyme at a site intended for the substrate.

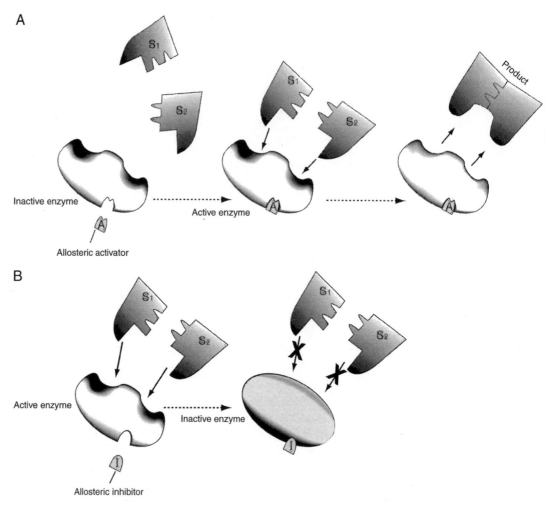

Figure 2.8   *Bonding of a substrate to an enzyme 2*
An allosteric modulator binds to the enzyme at sites not intended for the substrate. However, the modulator alters suitable binding sites for the substrate in a way that makes them either active (A) or inactive (B) for further reaction with the substrate.

Figure 2.9   Bonding of a substrate to an enzyme 3
Due to an increase in hydrogen ions (when the pH is lowered), some negatively charged groups on the enzyme are exchanged for positively charged groups, so that it will be difficult for a positively charged substrate to form a bond.

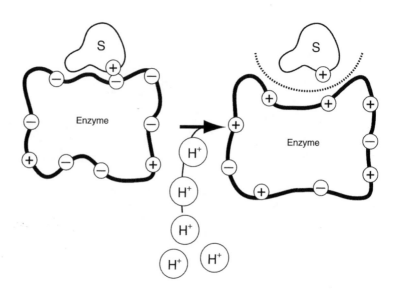

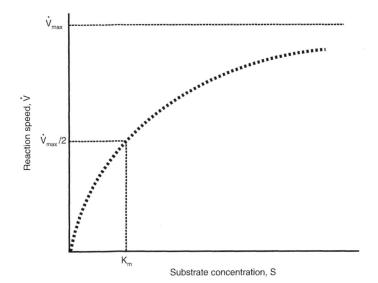

Figure 2.10 Bonding of a substrate to an enzyme 4
Most enzyme properties can be quantified using the terms K_m and V_{max}. K_m is the substrate concentration which leads to one-half the maximum speed of a chemical reaction. $\dot{V}_{max}$ is the maximum speed of reaction. This is attained when the substrate is so concentrated that all available enzymes have become saturated.

Around K_m only a slight change in substrate concentration is needed to bring about a substantial change in the speed of the reaction. An increase in the substrate concentration around $\dot{V}_{max}$ will have almost no effect on the speed of the reaction.

2.2.2 Adenosine triphosphate (ATP)

Because energy exchange occurs in nearly every cell in the human body, a substance is needed to help store the useable energy that has been produced as well as to release it for processes requiring energy. Adenosine triphosphate (ATP) almost always fills this intermediate position in the human cell, thus forming the link between catabolic and anabolic reactions. Catabolism is the breakdown of energy-rich bonds, which leads to lower energy products and a release of energy. In an anabolic process higher energy products are formed, and thus a supply of energy is required.

The energy required by anabolic reactions is supplied indirectly by the useable energy released from catabolic processes. The fact that energy is supplied indirectly here relates to the role played by ATP. In these processes, energy-rich bonds function simultaneously as both the energy receiver and the energy donor. Energy is released during the breakdown of lipids (or fat) and carbohydrates, but the energy released cannot be used directly for muscle contraction, because too little energy is released to allow muscle contraction to take place. The useable energy released during these catabolic reactions is temporarily stored in the form of ATP.

Subsequently, ATP functions as the universal provider of energy for muscle contraction. Muscles can be compared to chemical machines: the mechanical work that they do relies on the supply of chemical energy. The energy needed for a muscle to work originates from the breakdown of ATP. Compare the function of ATP with that of money in our society. When labor is provided, money is paid, which can later be spent according to one's wishes. ATP is the means used to exchange intracellular chemical energy. Energy-producing systems synthesize ATP from adenosine diphosphate (ADP) and inorganic phosphate (P_i), after which energy-consuming systems break down the ATP, creating ADP and P_i:

$$ATP + H_2O \rightarrow ADP + P_i + H^+ + energy$$

Because ATP is only present in muscle in low concentrations, it must be continuously resynthesized by catabolic reactions at the same speed in which it is being consumed. No more than 100 g of ATP is stored in muscle cells, while it has been calculated that, after completing a marathon, an athlete will have consumed 75 kg of ATP (Newsholme et al 1994). Because the cellular reserve of ATP is low, using even a very small amount of ATP results in a relatively large decrease in its concentration. The result of this is an immediate stimulation of catabolism, eventually in combination with a decline in anabolic processes.

In addition to functioning as an 'energy bridge' between energy-demanding and energy-providing processes, among other things ATP also works to control the coordination of anabolic and catabolic processes. To complete the picture, it must be stated that the intercellular concentrations of ADP and P_i also play important roles. Metabolism is regulated by the phosphate potential, which is the relationship between ATP, on the one hand, and ADP and P_i, on the other. In other words, the phosphate potential coordinates both the production and the use of energy.

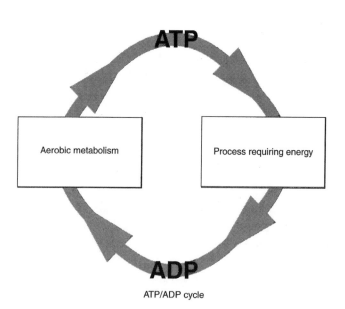

Figure 2.11 ATP/ADP cycle
The ATP/ADP cycle is a continuous process by which ATP is consumed and then resynthesized. This example shows the aerobic metabolism of foodstuffs.

2.2.3 Resynthesis of ATP

Four processes are constantly at work in the body in order to resynthesize ATP. The general process used to store energy through the formation of energy-rich bonds is called phosphorylation. The four processes that allow phosphorylation to take place in the human muscle cell are:

- creatine–phosphokinase reaction
- adenylate kinase reaction
- glycolysis
- aerobic pathway.

Although the four processes that regenerate ATP occur simultaneously, their relative contribution depends on the duration and intensity of physical exercise (Thoden 1991, Spurway 1992). The muscle cell has the ability to always be able to regenerate a sufficient amount of ATP, regardless of the situation – whether exercise is brief and explosive or long and of low-intensity. This phenomenon is referred to as the energy-continuum concept. The resynthesis of ATP by the four energy systems can be compared to a small bath (the supply of ATP in muscle) from which water is poured via a faucet (the use of energy) that can be regulated. The water level in the small bath must be kept constant by using four inflowing water faucets (four energy systems), each having an opening with a different diameter and water reservoirs of varying capacity. The diameter of the faucet's opening is equal to the power, and the size of the water reservoir is equal to the capacity of an energy system. Both concepts are discussed later in this chapter.

Creatine–phosphokinase reaction

It is almost without exception the breakdown of creatine phosphate (CrP) that is mainly responsible for the resynthesis of ATP during short-term maximum exercise. During the first seconds of exercise in particular there is very rapid breakdown of CrP (Greenhaff et al 1993). The initial supply of ATP in muscle cell is very low, and measurements have shown that the supply is almost constant in spite of maximum stress. Consequently, should the demand for energy increase within several milliseconds by a factor of 500, then ATP must be resynthesized rapidly.

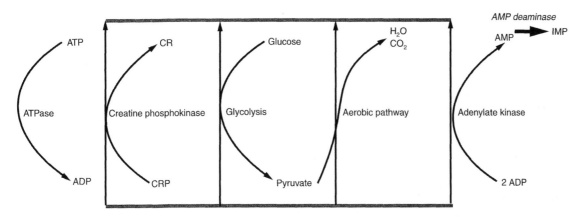

Figure 2.12 Resynthesis of ATP (1)
The four processes responsible for resynthesis of ATP are the creatine–phosphokinase, glycolytic, adenylate kinase, and aerobic pathways.

The primary function of the creatine–phosphokinase reaction is thus as providing an ATP buffer. In this manner, metabolism can cope with the delay of several seconds that occurs before energy is provided by glycolysis (Meyer et al 1984, Marsh et al 1993, Balsom et al 1994, Greenhaff 1995). Rapid resynthesis of ATP can be realized because not many enzymatic reactions are required and because CrP is situated in the cytoplasm of the muscle cell (see comparison of reactions). However, the supply of CrP is limited.

A second function of the creatine–phosphokinase reaction is to buffer protons (hydrogen ions) in the muscle cell, which result from the breakdown of glycogen to lactate (Harris et al 1992, Maughan 1995, Vandenberghe et al 1996):

$$CrP + ADP + H^+ \rightarrow Cr + ATP$$

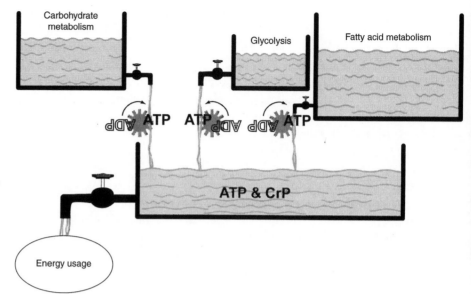

Figure 2.13 Resynthesis of ATP (2)
Depending on the amount of energy used, the four energy systems are responsible for a corresponding resynthesis of ATP (the water level in the lower bath must remain constant). The different faucet diameters and volumes of the water reservoirs represent the power and capacity, respectively, of each energy system.

In this way, the intramuscular buffer capacity can be raised so that the degree of acidity will rise (i.e. the pH will decline) less rapidly in the direction of the critical value. When the intramuscular pH declines, Ca^{2+} will bond less easily to troponin-C and the enzymatic processes in the muscle cell will be inhibited. The creatine–phosphokinase reaction negates somewhat the decline in intramuscular pH.

The third function of the creatine–phosphokinase reaction is to facilitate the transfer of energy from mitochondria to sites where ATP will be used (Harris et al 1992, Maughan 1995, Vandenberghe et al 1996). ATP must be able to travel to the myofilaments, for example, from the mitochondria, where much ATP is resynthesized by the aerobic pathway (see Section 2.2.3). In comparison to ATP, CrP is a much smaller molecule and therefore can move (via diffusion) much more easily through the muscle cell. An additional advantage is that only those structures that possess enzymes used to transport the phosphate group of CrP to ADP can profit from this energy shuttle (Billeter & Hoppeler 1991). Myofilaments are equipped with such an enzyme in order to make use of the CrP shuttle.

The availability of CrP in muscle is considered to be one of the performance-limiting factors for short-term high-intensity muscle activity, because depletion of CrP should result in a situation in which ATP can no longer be resynthesized rapidly enough (Greenhaff 1995). However, the results of research on the concentration and degree of depletion of CrP in muscle are not consistent (see Section 2.3).

Adenylate kinase reaction

There is another, directly available, source of energy present in muscle cell. The enzyme adenylate-kinase, called 'myokinase' in muscle, is able to form one molecule of ATP from two molecules of ADP:

$$ADP + ADP \xrightarrow{\text{myokinase}} ATP + AMP \text{ (adenosine monophosphate)}$$

In this way, a high phosphate potential can be maintained. The adenylate kinase reaction takes place during heavy physical exercise. One disadvantage is that the total number of phosphate-rich bonds with adenosine (ATP, ADP, and AMP) tem-

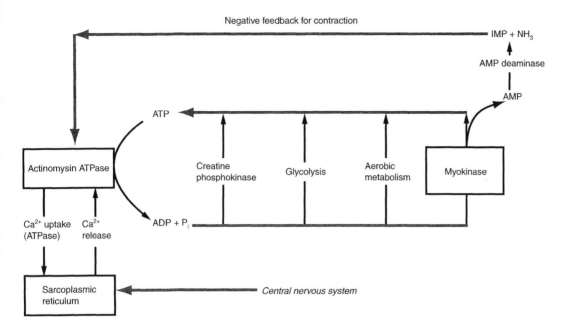

Figure 2.14   Adenylate kinase reaction
Inosine monophosphate (IMP), which is formed during the adenylate kinase reaction, appears to be involved in giving negative feedback for the cross-bridge cycle.

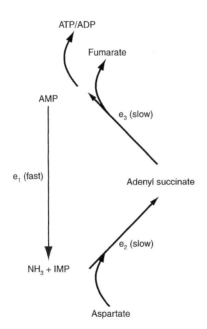

Figure 2.15   Resynthesis of ATP and ADP from AMP
When ATP and ADP are resynthesized from AMP, the first step in the chain reaction in which IMP is synthesized occurs rapidly, while the following steps are slower.

porarily decreases. The AMP formed during this reaction is, in turn, converted into inosine monophosphate (IMP) and ammonia (NH_3). IMP appears to give direct negative feedback for the interaction between actin and myosin during muscle contraction (Westra 1993).

In this way, an expensive energy carrier is discarded. The enzymes involved in the resynthesis of ADP and ATP from IMP are slower than the one which converts

AMP into IMP. Restoration of ATP and ADP does not actually get going until a period of rest. The practical consequence of this fact is that the best running performance for middle and long distances will be achieved by running as evenly as possible. When the start is too rapid, IMP is formed immediately, thus impeding muscle contraction throughout the remainder of the race. At that time, less power can be generated because converting the concentration of IMP in the muscle cell into ADP and ATP is a particularly slow process.

Glycolysis

The creatine–phosphokinase reaction can only guarantee that ATP will be resynthesized for a brief period (5–15 s). The adenylate-kinase reaction functions as an emergency system that can only resynthesize ATP briefly and in small quantities. Other non-oxidative sources of energy must also be rapidly called upon to resynthesize ATP. Glucose and glycogen in the muscle cell are broken down into pyruvate, by which energy is released in order to resynthesize ATP.

Glucose/glycogen → pyruvate

Depending on the substrate used, these processes are called glycolysis (substrate: glucose) or glycogenolysis (substrate: glycogen). In muscle cells, the concentration of free glucose is low, so that the non-oxidative source of energy consists essentially of glucose in its stored form (i.e. glycogen). In addition, however, glucose can be supplied via blood flowing from the liver or gastrointestinal tract.

Figure 2.16   Glycolysis (greatly simplified)
In the muscle cell, glucose and glycogen are broken down into pyruvate, thus releasing energy for the resynthesis of ATP from ADP.

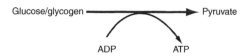

From the moment that pyruvate has been formed, the reaction can proceed in two directions. Pyruvate can: (1) be transported into the mitochondrion, a bean-like organelle in the muscle cell, where the aerobic pathway takes place, or (2) be converted directly into lactate and hydrogen ions with the help of the enzyme lactate dehydrogenase (LDH). For a long time it was thought that the only criterion affecting the fate of pyruvate was the presence of oxygen. Without oxygen (anaerobic), pyruvate is converted into lactate and hydrogen ions. In the presence of sufficient oxygen (aerobic), pyruvate is introduced into the aerobic pathway. Later in this chapter, it will become clear why for such a long time the presence of oxygen here was held to be the only criterion.

Like the energy systems discussed below, glycolysis also takes place in the cytosol of the muscle cell. The distance to the myofilaments, where ATP is converted into ADP, is also small for this energy system. In comparison to the creatine–phosphoskinase reaction, the rate at which energy is released through glycolysis is somewhat lower, because the breakdown of glucose and/or glycogen is a more complex process. The creatine–phosphokinase reaction takes place rapidly because it runs without the assistance of many special structures in the muscle cell. Compare this

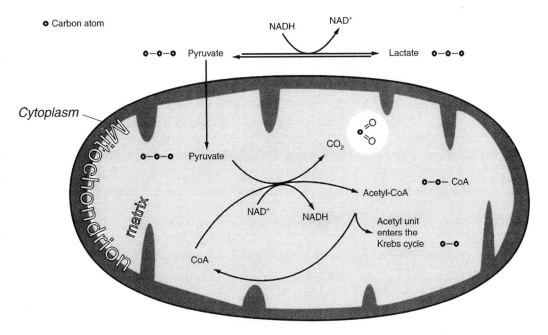

Figure 2.17   Pyruvate synthesis from glycolysis
Pyruvate formed during glycolysis can follow one of two pathways: it can either be converted into lactate with the help of the enzyme lactate dehydrogenase; or it can enter the mitochondrion, where it will continue to be processed in the aerobic pathway.

reaction to that of glycolysis, which only takes place after a series of 12 enzymatic reactions in the cytosol.

From an historical perspective, glycolysis is always divided into two forms:

(1) anaerobic
(2) aerobic.

Famous scientists such as Pasteur, who studied the metabolism of single-cell organisms, introduced the terms 'aerobic' (with oxygen) and 'anaerobic' (without oxygen). Both terms have led to much confusion within the areas of the physiology of exercise and the practice of athletic training. Pasteur discovered that lactate was formed under experimental conditions when no oxygen was present. This observation was then applied to muscle-cell metabolism – if lactate was formed, then it must be the result of a shortage of oxygen in the muscle cell. Even today, views about training for endurance are still limited by this incorrectly extrapolated observation.

The presence of insufficient oxygen in the muscle cell is only one of the causes of lactate formation. Lactate (1.0–2.9 mmol/l) is also produced in a resting state, under completely aerobic conditions (Connett et al 1990). The production of lactate during rest is related to the indirect manner in which glucose is stored by the liver as glycogen. The liver and muscles are the storage sites for glycogen. During exercise, glycogen stored in the liver is converted back into glucose so that it can be absorbed by muscles via the bloodstream to be converted further into a useful source of energy. After eating a carbohydrate-rich meal, the liver can absorb glucose directly from the bloodstream and store it as glycogen. However, the liver has another metabolic pathway at its disposal, in which lactate is converted into glycogen, for storing glycogen. Because muscles, due to their high glycolytic enzyme activity, are able to convert a large amount of glucose into lactate, this becomes an indirect way for the liver to replenish its supply of glycogen. This phenomenon is called the glucose paradox.

Other ways in which lactate functions are discussed later in Section 2.3.2. For the moment, it is essential that we no longer regard lactate as an end-metabolite (i.e. a waste product). The importance of lactate for energy is indeed too great for it to be considered merely as a useless leftover of anaerobic glycolysis.

The terms 'anaerobic' and 'aerobic' glycolysis are incorrect, because they suggest that there are two dissimilar types of glycolysis and that one of these processes would take place in the presence of oxygen, while the other could occur when there is no oxygen. However, regardless of whether sufficient oxygen is present in the muscle

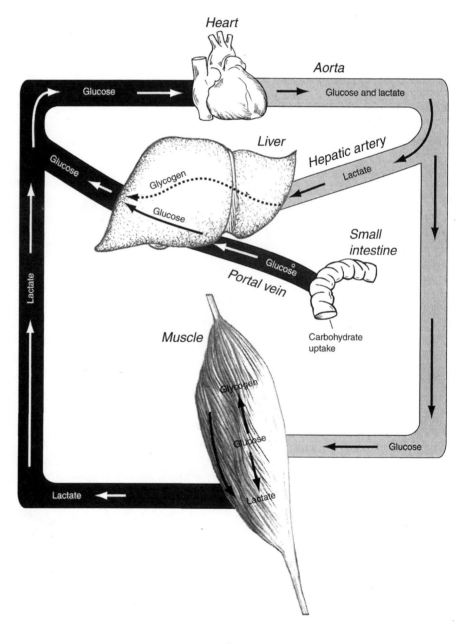

Figure 2.18   The glucose paradox
In addition to being a direct reservoir for storing blood glucose as glycogen, another indirect metabolic pathway is available to the liver. Namely, glucose can be converted into lactate in muscle, due to its high glycolytic enzyme activity. Subsequently, lactate is removed from the bloodstream and stored as glycogen in the liver.

cell, glycolysis is a chain reaction by which glucose is converted into pyruvate. Oxygen is not involved in this metabolic pathway. In order to emphasize this fact, glycolysis is described by the term 'non-robic' in some literature (Brooks et al 1996).

'Fast and 'slow' glycolysis

Here we discuss the conversion of glucose, via pyruvate, to lactate and hydrogen ions. The metabolic pathway through which pyruvate is transported to the mitochondrion is discussed below (see pp. 95–99).

It has already been stated that the energy released during catabolism is transferred to ATP. The transfer of energy generally proceeds indirectly via carriers of energy-rich electrons. One of these electron carriers, NADH (nicotinamide adenine dinucleotide) plays an important role in glycolysis. In the middle of the enzymatic chain reaction (step 6) of glycolysis, energy-rich electrons are transferred via NAD^+ to NADH.

During rest, or when exercise is not too heavy, the electrons and H^+ bonded to NADH are transported into the mitochondrion. However, when the activity of the mitochondria is still low at the beginning of exercise, or when it is insufficient during a heavy load, there will either be no or too little resynthesis of NAD^+ via the mitochondria. The concentration of NAD^+ in the cell is limited, and whether or not NAD^+ is formed is completely dependent on the surrender of electrons and H^+ from NADH. An alternative way to regenerate NAD^+ so that glycolysis does not come to a halt is the conversion of pyruvate to lactate, by which lactate acts as the acceptor for the electrons and H^+ of NADH.

$$\text{pyruvate} + \text{NADH} + \text{H}^+ \xrightarrow{\text{enzyme LDH}} \text{lactate} + \text{NAD}^+$$

Therefore, whether or not lactate is formed is related to the relative activity of the mitochondria, and not to the presence or absence of oxygen. In this case, it is better to speak of 'fast', rather than anaerobic, glycolysis during the conversion of pyruvate to lactate. Once glycolysis has reached its maximum, but mitochondrial activity is too low to utilize the NADH being supplied, then much of the pyruvate present is converted to lactate by LDH, which is the glycolytic enzyme with the highest $\dot{V}_{max}$. After pyruvate has entered into the mitochondrion, it will turn up in the aerobic pathway. The processes through which it must pass proceed 2.5 times more slowly

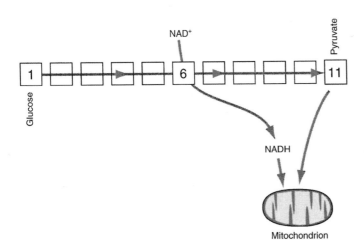

Figure 2.19 Slow glycolysis
Halfway through the glycolytic pathway, energy-rich electrons are transferred from NAD^+ to NADH. When the running intensity is not too high, mitochondria can act as acceptors for NADH and pyruvate. In this manner, NAD^+ can be resynthesized, so that glycolysis does not come to a halt after the sixth step in the pathway.

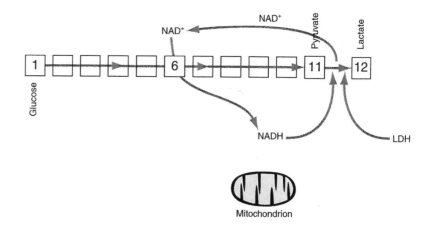

Figure 2.20   Fast glycolysis
When the mitochondria cannot work
adequately due, for example, to low
enzymatic activity, NAD^+ is resynthesized
because lactate accepts electrons and H^+
from NADH.

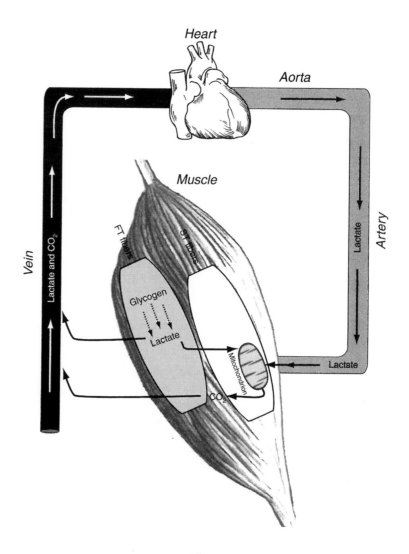

Figure 2.21   The lactate shuttle
Lactate produced in FT muscle fibers
can be transported to adjacent ST muscle
fibers, where it is used as a source of
oxidative energy.

than in 'fast' glycolysis, and therefore the name 'slow' glycolysis for the aerobic breakdown of glucose or glycogen.

The amount of ATP obtained from 'fast' glycolysis is greater than the amount produced by the creatine–phosphokinase reaction, but much less than what the aerobic pathway yields. The breakdown of 1 mol glucose nets a yield of 2 mol ATP for 'fast' glycolysis, while a net yield of 36–38 mol ATP is produced by the aerobic pathway. Glycolysis is the dominant energy system at the beginning of (maximum) exercise and remains dominant from the first several seconds to about 1 min.

As a product of 'fast' glycolysis, lactate dissociates rapidly at the prevailing pH. The hydrogen ions released have the adverse effect of lowering the pH, which, in the muscle cell, has a negative effect on enzymatic activity and lowers the affinity of troponin-C for calcium. The lactate that has built up in the muscle cell diffuses, with some delay, into the bloodstream and surrounding muscle fibers. The hydrogen ions in the blood are buffered so that any lowering of the pH there remains marginal.

The ability of the blood to buffer is discussed later in this chapter. What happens to the lactate produced is becoming increasingly clear. Formerly, lactate was thought to be an end metabolite or waste product of 'fast' glycolysis. However, if the body were to produce a high-energy substrate, such as lactate, as a useless end product, this would indicate poor energy economy. Lactate can diffuse into the bloodstream, where it is taken up by the liver and converted to glycogen. Moreover, lactate is used as fuel by the heart and, especially, by slow-twitch (ST) muscle fibers. It even appears that lactate produced in type-IIb muscle fibers diffuses into the surrounding type-I fibers, where it can be used directly as an oxidative source of energy. Lactate produced in this way will not come into contact with venous blood. This phenomenon is called the 'lactate shuttle' (Brooks 1985). Because of this, the concentration of lactate in the blood shows major limitations as an indicator of the contribution of 'fast' glycolysis.

Lactate measurements

The concentration of lactate in (capillary) blood can be measured using simple equipment. During the practice of sports training, whether during a field test or under laboratory conditions, the blood lactate concentration can be determined at

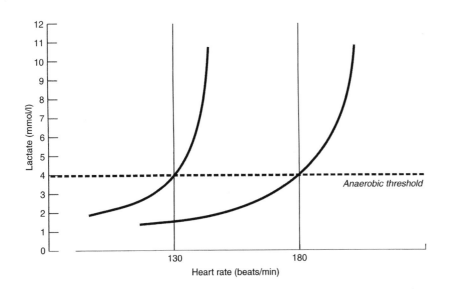

Figure 2.22 Anaerobic threshold
The characteristic change in the concentration of blood lactate as running intensifies. In the literature, the start of the exponential increase in concentration (here at 4 mmol/l) is often called the 'anaerobic threshold'.

various running speeds using different test protocols. The test results are used to determine the optimum running intensity, particularly for endurance exercise, and, when re-testing is done, to follow how performance is progressing. Interpretation of the results is guided by the characteristic pattern formed when the lactate concentration is plotted against running speed. When running intensity increases, the concentration of lactate first remains relatively low and constant before increasing exponentially at a certain running intensity. In the literature (Brooks 1985, Anderson & Rhodes 1989, Tanaka 1990, Ohira & Tabat 1992, Spurway 1992, Loat & Rhodes 1993, Myers & Ashley 1997, Basset & Howley 2000), various names have been given to this sudden increase in lactate concentration, such as 'onset of blood lactate accumulation', 'lactate threshold', 'anaerobic threshold', and 'aerobic–anaerobic transition'. The explanation for this is that, at a certain running intensity, the aerobic energy system becomes inadequate and must be assisted by 'fast' glycolysis, thus causing lactate to accumulate in muscle cells and diffuse into the bloodstream. In other words, the concentration of lactate in blood can be used to quantify the contribution of 'fast' glycolysis to the total delivery of energy.

A number of facts are overlooked when metabolic processes are simplified in this way. First, the blood lactate concentration is the result of the production minus the elimination of lactate. Statements about lactate production are dubious because one cannot ascertain exactly how much lactate has been taken up and removed for use by the heart, liver, and ST muscle fibers. Second, no account is taken of the delay that occurs when the lactate produced diffuses into the bloodstream. Third, it is impossible to gain insight into the contribution of 'fast' glycolysis over time. For the graph shown in Figure 2.23, the only interpretation possible from points 1 and 2 is that 'fast' glycolysis has not contributed. Fourth, it appears that the way in which a test protocol is set up will greatly affect the concentration of blood lactate measured. For example, dividing a workload into discrete steps and then varying the duration of its increments will cause a substantial difference in the concentration of blood lactate when the running speed remains unchanged. Plotting concentrations of

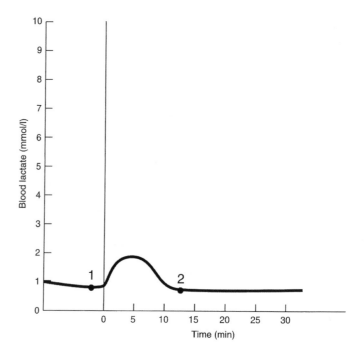

Figure 2.23   Lactate concentration
The change over time in the concentration of blood lactate, from a resting state followed by a low-intensity running workload. Based on the equal values measured at coordinates 1 (resting state) and 2 (after running 10 min), it would appear that 'fast' glycolysis has made no contribution.

blood lactate against the running speeds of many different test protocols gives a scatter of points, demonstrating a weak correlation between these two parameters.

Choosing the optimum intensity (e.g. for duration of effort) on the basis of lactate measurements appears to be a precarious undertaking (Hoogeveen et al 1997). Lactate concentrations measured repeatedly under standardized conditions (e.g. identical test protocols) can be only be compared insofar as they are recorded in the same way (i.e. they can be compared as higher or lower). Thus any interpretation that goes further and any attempts to make a statement about the contribution of 'fast' glycolysis or the shortcomings of the aerobic pathway are not justified.

So far, with the exception of the test protocol applied, other external variables that can cause interference with lactate measurement have not been taken into account. Among such variables, here we consider temperature, fatigue, and nutrition. The latter two variables are concerned with maintaining the level of the glycogen supply in muscle. Because glycogen is the most important substrate for 'fast' glycolysis, when less of it is available there will be a low blood lactate concentration when the submaximum running speed remains constant. The maximum running speed recorded in an earlier test will not be achieved while the maximum blood lactate concentration is lower than in that test. This phenomenon is called the 'lactate paradox' (Jeukendrup et al 1992). Advocates of lactate measurement will consider the effect of training to be positive when the lactate curve moves toward the lower right, yet the curve will shift in the same way when the store of glycogen in the muscle has not been completely filled.

Aerobic pathway

In contrast to the aerobic pathway, the energy systems described above are not dependent on the presence of oxygen in order to provide energy for ATP resynthesis. It is in the mitochondria located in muscle cells that several processes are

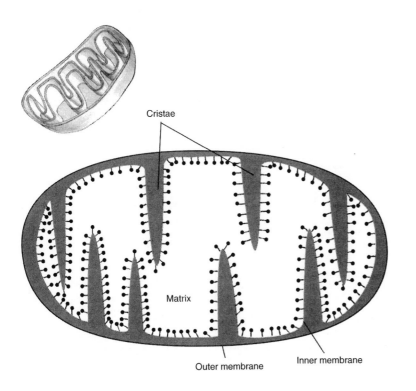

Cristae

Matrix

Outer membrane

Inner membrane

Figure 2.24 Structure of a mitochondrion
A mitochondrion has a smooth outer membrane and a strongly folded inner membrane. The folds, or projections, are called cristae. The interior of a mitochondrion is called the matrix; a number of energy-generating aerobic processes take place here.

brought together: nutrients are decomposed, oxygen is taken up, and the levels of ATP and CrP are maintained. The aerobic processes in mitochondria for providing energy, also called 'cellular respiration', depend on whether the heart and lungs function optimally. The cardiovascular system, which from the perspective of anatomy, is located relatively distant from the locus of aerobic cellular metabolism, is responsible for the transport of oxygen to the mitochondria. This is a delaying factor as the aerobic pathway starts up, because it takes a while for hormones and the nervous system to prime the heart and lungs. Mitochondria also need time to become active. It is thought that the aerobic pathway is only fully active after 2 min.

When the mitochondria have become sufficiently active, the pyruvate formed during the final step of glycolysis is transported into the mitochondria via a carrier. Pyruvate must pass through the smooth outer and strongly folded inner mitochondrial membranes for further use within the matrix. In the muscle cell, mitochondria are located close to the myofilaments, which require energy, and also alongside the muscle membrane, where the energy-consuming active transport of ions and metabolites takes place. In this book, particular attention is given to the intermyofibrillar mitochondria located next to the myofibrils.

The degree of activity shown by mitochondria depends on the ATP/ADP ratio. Thus a number of conditions must first be met before mitochondrial activity can

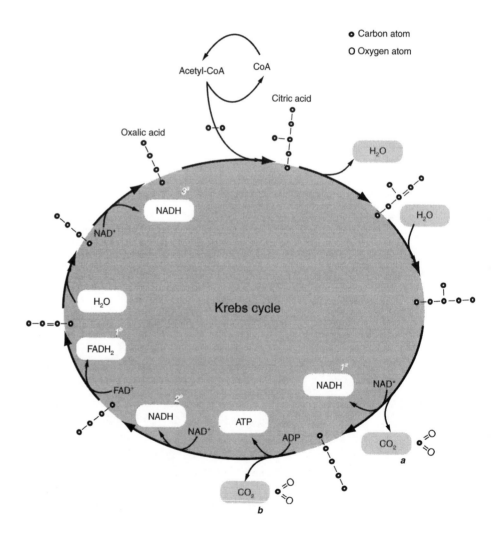

Figure 2.25   Krebs cycle
The Krebs cycle is a continuous round of enzymatic reactions, which in each cycle generate one molecule of ATP, two molecules of CO_2, and energy-rich electrons bonded to three molecules of NADH and one molecule of FAD-H_2, which is a similar electron acceptor.

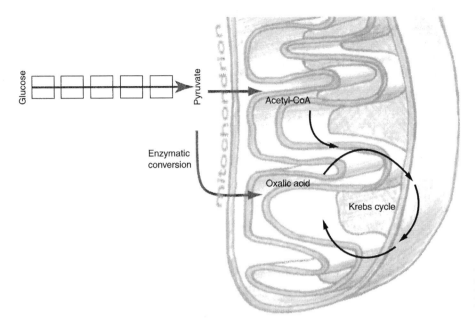

Figure 2.26 Metabolic pathway by which oxalacetate enters the Krebs cycle
Here pyruvate is converted into oxalacetate, which can be fed into the Krebs cycle.

actually increase. These requirements are the presence of oxygen, substrate, and ADP. Among the processes providing energy, mitochondrial activity always lags behind those energy delivering processes that are directly available in the sarcoplasm. Using energy that is directly available will decrease the concentration of ATP, which by lowering the ATP/ADP ratio will activate the mitochondria. When interval training is aimed at improving 'slow' glycolysis in particular, it is important not to pause too long between repetitions. A 5-min pause of low intensity allows resynthesis of ATP to be completed, through which, during the next repetition, the contribution of 'fast' glycolysis will be increased at the start. If the pauses are shorter, then the phosphate potential will not recover completely and the mitochondria will remain active, so that in total the delivery of energy by the aerobic pathway will dominate.

In the mitochondrial matrix, pyruvate is converted into acetyl coenzyme-A (CoA). During this exergonic reaction, carbon dioxide is released and NADH is formed. The acetyl unit (two carbon atoms) enters the Krebs cycle, where it bonds with oxaloacetate, thus forming citric acid. The Krebs cycle is an unending circle of enzymatic reactions in which, during each cycle, are generated one molecule of ATP, two molecules of carbon dioxide, and energy-rich electrons bound to three molecules of NADH and to one molecule of FAD-H_2 (a related electron acceptor). The speed of the Krebs cycle depends on the concentration of oxaloacetate, which must be increased during physical exercise. The increase in oxaloacetate originates primarily from glycolysis, in which pyruvate is converted to oxaloacetate by enzymes via a metabolic pathway. By way of a number of conversions (see Section 2.2.4) fats also pass into the Krebs cycle as acetyl units. However, it is not possible to use only energy from fatty acid oxidation, even when there is a shortage of muscle glycogen, while running a marathon. Without the contribution from glycolysis, the concentration of oxaloacetate would decrease and the Krebs cycle would come to a halt, causing acetyl-CoA to accumulate in the muscle cell. Combustion of fat without the metabolism of glycogen is thus impossible, and would lead to an energy crisis within the cell. If the concentration of oxaloacetate decreases, then too much acetyl-CoA is converted into ketones. If the rate of fat metabolism is high, ketones will

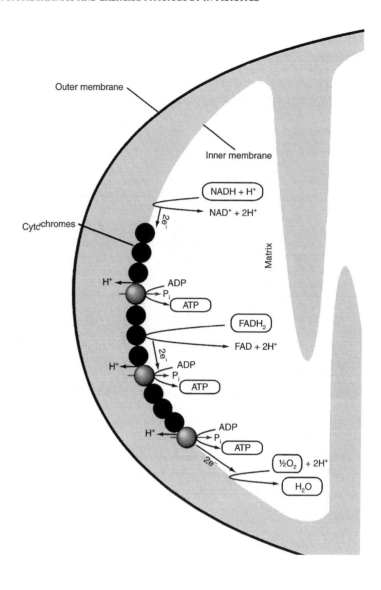

Figure 2.27   Respiratory or electron-transport chain

always be formed due to incomplete oxidation. This phenomenon can be recognized by the odor of acetone (a type of ketone), which some long-distance runners emanate after lengthy physical exercise. The practical consequence is that glucose must definitely be consumed during the second half of the marathon.

During a single Krebs cycle, one molecule of ATP is formed. More important is the yield of energy-rich electrons bonded to NADH and FAD-H_2, which can be re-used in the following step (oxidative phosphorylation) of the aerobic pathway. It is not until this step has been reached in the aerobic pathway that large quantities of ATP are generated. The principle of oxidative phosphorylation is the transfer to ATP of the energy that has been obtained from the binding of hydrogen to oxygen, when water is formed (Vander et al 1994). During this part of the resynthesis of ATP, hydrogen ions are obtained from the NADH and FAD-H_2 formed during the Krebs cycle. In order to keep the Krebs cycle going, NAD^+ and FAD^+ are needed to act as electron acceptors. If oxygen is not present, NAD^+ and FAD^+ cannot be formed by oxidative phosphorylation. Both the Krebs cycle and oxidative phosphorylation would come to a halt, because mitochondria are unable to produce NAD^+ and FAD^+ from NADH and FAD-H_2 by any alternate route.

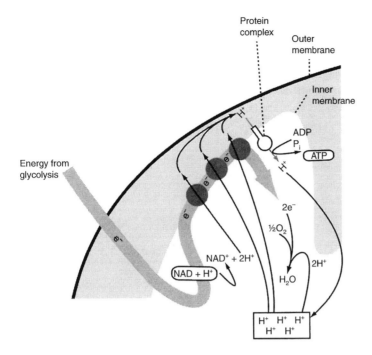

Figure 2.28 Resynthesis of ATP via the respiratory chain
H$^+$ ions are pumped out of the inner mitochondrial membrane and then flow back into the matrix by way of a protein complex. Energy released from this influx is used to resynthesize ATP.

The protein structures that are involved in the last stage of oxidative phosphorylation can be found in the inner mitochondrial membrane. Because the majority of these proteins (cytochromes) contain iron and copper, they are able to function like a conveyor belt for electrons. The electrons are transported in a chain to or from an iron or copper ion before finally being taken up by an oxygen molecule (Vander et al 1994), thus the name 'respiratory' or 'electron-transport chain'. At the beginning of the respiratory chain the electrons are stripped of their hydrogen ions, which were obtained from the NADH and FAD-H$_2$ formed in the Krebs cycle. FAD-H$_2$ follows NADH by one step in the electron-transport chain. Because energy is released during each step in which electrons are passed onto the next cytochrome, FAD-H$_2$ provides somewhat less energy in total than NADH, because it misses the first step in the chain. In the respiratory chain energy is always passed on in small increments. With the help of this energy, hydrogen ions are actively pumped from the matrix into the space formed by the outer and inner mitochondrial membranes. The resynthesis of ATP occurs at three locations in the respiratory chain and proceeds according to an ingenious mechanism. Because of the concentration gradient that develops, hydrogen ions that have been pumped out can now stream back into the matrix by way of canals made up of protein complexes. Energy created by the motion of hydrogen ions is subsequently used to form ATP from ADP and P$_i$. By way of the respiratory chain, one pair of electrons transferred from one molecule of NADH can be used to form three molecules of ATP, while one pair of electrons from FAD-H$_2$ can be used to form two molecules of ATP.

2.2.4   Metabolism of fat

In the human body, 80% of the total energy supply is stored as fat in the form of triglycerides, which in turn are stored in subdermal and other fatty tissue, skeletal muscle, and the liver. The capacity of this energy source, which is estimated at 70,000–75,000 kcal, can be regarded as inexhaustible. Nevertheless, the mobilization of fatty acids up for oxidation in the mitochondria progresses slowly. The efficient storage of fat in the form of triglycerides in, for example, subcutaneous fatty tissue requires a large number of conversions in order for energy to be transfered to and utilized by the muscle fibers. Only a small supply of triglycerides is stored in and around the muscle fibers. Together with the triglycerides stored subcutaneously and in deeper adipose (fatty) tissue, these triglycerides form the most important sources of energy for the metabolism of fat. Triglycerides cannot be used directly in the aerobic pathway. A series of reactions is needed to transform them into molecules of acetyl-CoA, which can enter the Krebs cycle directly (Fox et al 1997). From this point in the cycle, fat is metabolized along the same metabolic pathway as for 'slow' glycolysis. Before they can be transported to muscle, subcutaneous triglycerides must first be converted into glycerol and free fatty acids. Because fats are either poorly soluble or insoluble in water, free fatty acids must be coupled to the protein albumin for transport in the blood. Rapid uptake into muscle fibers is facilitated by specific fatty acid receptors located on the sarcolemma. Once inside the muscle cell, the fatty acid is first brought to a higher energy level by linking with CoA. The reaction, which costs one molecule of ATP, creates an activated fatty acid called acetyl-CoA, which is passed through the mitochondrion by a carrier. Two carbon atoms are repeatedly split off the end of the long carbon chains of the activated fatty acids. With the help of CoA, acetyl-CoA is made to fit into the Krebs cycle. This

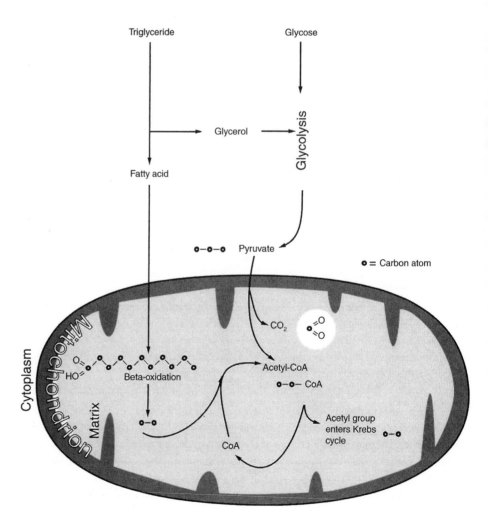

Figure 2.29 Beta-oxidation
Converted fatty acids can also participate in the Krebs cycle.

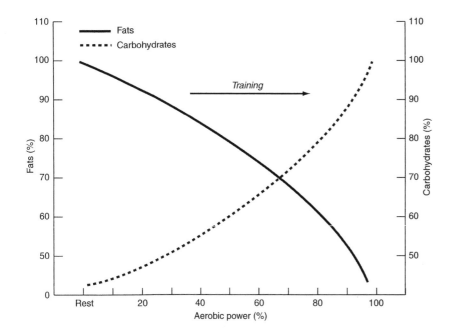

Figure 2.30 Influence of training on the use of substrates
The contribution of fats and carbohydrates to the total delivery of energy at different running intensities. Training directed at raising the aerobic potential increases the contribution of fatty-acid oxidation in the generation of energy when the running load is submaximal.

cycle repeats itself until the carbon chain has been exhausted. The cycle of reactions by which activated fatty acids are converted into acetyl-CoA in the mitochondrion is called beta-oxidation.

Palmitic acid, a fatty acid with 16 carbon atoms that frequently occurs in the body, can pass through such a cycle seven times. During each cycle, one molecule of NADH and one of FAD-H_2 are formed. As already shown, by way of oxidative phosphorylation, this will provide a total of five molecules of ATP. After passing through the Krebs cycle and respiratory chain, each molecule of acetyl-CoA will have provided 12 molecules of ATP. In total, the breakdown of one palmitic acid molecule results in 129 molecules of ATP $[(7 \times 5 = 35) + (7 \times 12 = 84) = 129]$. During the metabolism of fat a great deal of ATP is resynthesized, because a large amount of acetyl-CoA is formed during the breakdown of a fatty acid. However, because the speed of resynthesis is slow, glycogen becomes the preferred substrate when the effort to run is intense. Fat metabolism is the dominant process during lengthy low-intensity exercise and during rest. Fat metabolism provides 50–60% of the total energy in a resting state. Up to an intensity that is 50% of the maximum oxygen uptake ($\dot{V}O_{2\ max}$), the amount of energy provided by lipids increases. At higher running intensities, this portion remains constant or decreases. The preference for either glycogen/glucose or fatty acids as the substrate for the resynthesis of ATP is regulated by the blood lactate concentration and the amount of citric acid formed by beta-oxidation. The conversion of glycerol into free fatty acids is inhibited when the blood lactate concentration increases, and this results in a decrease in the amount of free fatty acids in the blood. In this way the metabolism of fat is inhibited. Similarly, glycolysis can be inhibited when the activity of phosphofructo-kinase, the key enzyme for glycolysis, is held in check by the concentration of citric acid formed by beta-oxidation.

As a result of training directed at increasing the aerobic capacity, fatty acid oxidation will contribute an increasingly larger share of energy when the running effort is submaximal. This will have a glycogen-saving effect for long-distance runners, which will benefit their performance over long distances. Depletion of the glycogen supply in muscles is one of the causes for the appearance of fatigue and the accompanying decrease in performance. The effect of the training previously described can be explained by an increase in mitochondrial activity for the oxidation of fatty acids. A doubling of such mitochondrial activity, compared to untrained individuals, has been found after training. In addition to the importance of being well trained, the percentage of ST muscle fibers in the total muscle mass is also of importance. The capacity of ST muscle fibers to use fatty acids as the substrate is 8–10 times greater than that of fast-twitch (FT) fibers. Considering the fact that, to a great degree, heredity defines how muscle fibers are distributed between different types, the contribution of energy from fat metabolism will depend on heredity, on one hand, and on the degree of training, on the other. In comparison to glycogen, the breakdown of fat requires more oxygen, because processing a large number of carbon atoms from fatty acids demands more oxygen. For each molecule of oxygen, one molecule of fatty acid will provide 5.6 molecules of ATP, while one molecule of glycogen will provide 6.3 molecules of ATP. In contrast to the breakdown of glycogen, fat metabolism is a purely aerobic process. Should the amount of available oxygen become insufficient, the electron-transport chain would stop, neither NAD^+ nor FAD^+ would be produced, and the Krebs cycle would come to a halt. At that time, there would be no other possibility to continue the oxidation of fatty acids.

2.3 CAPACITY AND POWER

In practice, it is standard to employ the concepts of 'capacity' and 'power' when training energy systems. Capacity can be defined as the supply of energy-rich substrates, and power as the energy that can be released from energy-rich substrates per unit of time. Another frequently used definition of capacity is the duration for which power can be maintained (Bon 1998). The metaphor of a silo fitted with a conveyor belt can give insight into the concepts of capacity and power. Capacity is the content of the silo, and power is the width of the conveyor belt. Now, by linking the above three energy systems to the concepts of capacity and power, one can create six parameters that can be influenced by training:

- *Alactic anaerobic power*: this can be seen as the energy obtained from the creatine–phosphokinase reaction per unit of time.
- *Alactic anaerobic capacity*: this is the supply of CrP in the muscle cell.
- *Lactic anaerobic power*: here the requirement is to produce as much lactate, as quickly as possible. In other words, what is important is the speed with which 'fast' glycolysis generates energy.
- *Lactic anaerobic capacity*: strictly speaking, this should be the supply of glycogen in muscle and liver. Usually this parameter is equated with the time in which 'fast' glycolysis can claim the greatest portion of the total delivery of energy.
- *Aerobic power*: the energy provided by the aerobic pathway per unit of time.
- *Aerobic capacity*: the supply of glycogen and fat.

The goal is now to increase both the capacity and power of the most relevant energy system needed for a certain running distance. Training to increase the capacity of an energy system generally precedes similar training for power. The intention is first to increase the supply of energy-rich substrates before increasing the power of an energy system through training. However, working in reverse (i.e. first increasing the power of an energy system and thereafter its capacity) is also possible. The argument here is that, when there is more power, the capacity of an energy system can become further exhausted during training. With a larger overload, the effects of training are translated into enlarging the capacity of the energy system under stress. This way of working is only applied sporadically, because the intensity of training directed at increasing power is greater than the intensity of training directed at increasing capacity. Thus increasing the power before increasing the capacity of an energy system is an illogical sequence for training.

The question is whether, from the perspective of physiology, it is correct to link the three energy systems with the concepts capacity and power, which will have far-reaching consequences for the interpretation of means and methods for training. The most important point for criticism is that each energy system appears to have an 'exclusive' character, by which it should be possible to train each system independently. According to the concept that energy is a continuum, all three energy systems supposedly begin simultaneously during maximum exercise, having a certain duration, but differ in their contribution over time. The aerobic pathway is the slowest energy system to get started, while the creatine–kinase reaction proceeds at high speed.

Figure 2.31 shows the relationship between power and capacity for each of the three energy systems. The creatine–kinase and aerobic pathways, in which fat is the substrate, are the extremes. The most energy, but with the smallest capacity per unit of time, is generated by the creatine–kinase reaction. Although it is true that the breakdown of fats in the aerobic pathway yields little power, the supply of stored triglycerides is nearly inexhaustible.

It is difficult to determine whether a training procedure is directed at the power or capacity of an energy system. For example, identical training methods (e.g. 30-min tempo endurance) can be used to increase both aerobic power and aerobic capacity. This training can be aimed at increasing the glycogen supply (capacity) as well as at increasing aerobic power.

Moreover, making a division between the capacity and power of an energy system becomes artificial when considering 'fast' glycolysis as an energy system. The supply of substrate used is not the limiting factor. Furthermore, the enzyme LDH, which is

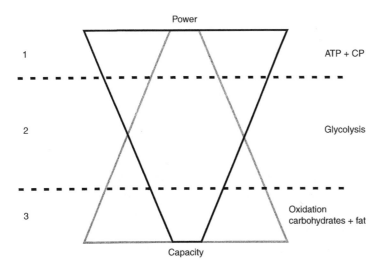

Figure 2.31 The power and capacity of energy-generating systems
Schematic illustration of the power and capacity of three energy-generating systems.

involved in converting pyruvate to lactate, has a very high $\dot{V}_{max}$, and thus an increase in the concentration of substrate will have little effect on the speed of conversion.

Previously in this chapter it was made clear that the speed of a chemical reaction is directly influenced by the concentration of the enzyme and the substrate. The power of an energy system is thus dependent on both these concentrations. Therefore, it is impossible to differentiate between power and capacity if the capacity is equated with substrate concentration. It is thus impossible to apply training methods for the purpose of influencing either the capacity or power of an energy system. In the following three sections we examine the possible effects of training on the concentrations of substrate for the three energy systems. Based on what has just been discussed, the terms 'power' and 'capacity' are synonymous.

2.3.1 Training the creatine–phosphokinase reaction

It is impossible to train the creatine–phosphokinase system in isolation. After a 2–2.5 s effort, 'fast' glycolysis is already providing 50% of the total energy. In much of the literature about training, the impression is given that the creatine–phosphokinase reaction can only claim to provide energy for the first 10–15 s of maximum effort. After this period, the supply of CrP in the muscle cell has been exhausted and will only be almost completely replenished after a 2-min pause. The capacity of the creatine–phosphokinase reaction is considered to be a performance-determining factor when the effort of running lasts for 10–15 s. From this perspective, an important goal for training 200-m runners is to increase the supply of CrP in muscle cells. For example, the training procedure for increasing alactic anaerobic capacity is composed of three series of four repetitions over 60 m, with a 2-min pause between repeats and 6-min pause between series, at a speed of about 95% of the maximum for 60 m. The adaptation resulting from this form of training should lead to a greater supply of CrP in the muscle cell. An 'overshoot', such as occurs in the supplies of liver and muscle glycogen after a 'glycogen-exhausting' training, is also expected to occur for the supply of CrP in muscle.

Data obtained from much scientific research (Cheethan et al 1986, Tesch et al 1989, Söderlund et al 1992) shows that the supply of CrP in muscle during an all-out (sprint) effort is certainly not totally exhausted. A range of concentrations has been reported in the literature for CrP measured in muscle tissue in a resting state as well as after maximum short-term exercise. It appears that this range can be partly ascribed to interindividual variability (Maughan 1995). In addition, the methods used to determine the concentrations have some limitations. In order to discover what is taking place within the muscle fiber, a biopsy of muscle tissue must first be taken. After applying a local anesthetic, a hollow needle is used to remove a small piece of tissue (biopsy) for investigation. The tissue sample is analyzed using histochemical and biochemical techniques. There is always a lapse of time between the end of exercise and taking the biopsy, and at the moment when the muscle biopsy is being taken resynthesis of CrP is already in full swing. Therefore, the values found for the depletion of CrP are most probably an underestimate. Although there appears to be a strong relationship between all-out exercise, the concentration of CrP, and power generated, no causal link has been found. It cannot be demonstrated biochemically that a depletion of CrP is alone responsible for a decline in the power generated. In spite of low concentrations of CrP in the muscle, the concentration of ATP remains at a high level (Hitchcock 1989). Furthermore, one must differentiate between the concentration of CrP in ST (type-I) and that in FT (type-II) muscle fibers in a resting state and after maximum short-term exercise. The resting-state concentration of CrP is generally higher in FT fibers. In sprinters who have a high percentage of FT fibers, higher concentrations of CrP have been measured in the quadriceps (Bernús et al 1993). However, in long-distance runners, it has been found that the resting-state concentration of CrP is higher in ST fibers (Rehunen et al 1982). The explanation given for this observation was that, because of the low intensity of their duration training, long-distance runners in particular should be able to influence their ST fibers through training. This should lead to improved use, resynthesis, and storage of CrP in ST fibers. The speed with which CrP is used during all-out exercise is higher for FT than for ST fibers.

No agreement has been reached regarding the speed of resynthesis of CrP. The period of time required before the supply of CrP has almost recovered its level varies from 2 to 7 min. The recovery curve followed has both a rapid and slow component (Balsom et al 1994). During the first part of recovery, which is rapid, the supply of CrP is restored to 50% of the resting-state value within 1 min. Complete resynthesis during the second part of recovery proceeds exponentially; 60 min after ending a maximum 30-s exercise, the resting-state value has yet to be reached (Tesch et al 1989). Even in this case, the division of muscle fibers can influence recovery. In runners whose muscle has a high proportion of ST fibers, the supply of CrP is restored more rapidly. This is because the recovery of the CrP level is dependent on oxygen. ST fibers are better supplied with blood, and thus with oxygen, than FT fibers.

2.3.2 Training the lactic anaerobic reaction

Strictly speaking, training the lactic anaerobic capacity should aim at increasing the supply of glycogen in muscle. Theoretically, 'fast' glycolysis provides 2–3 molecules of ATP per molecule of glycogen. 'Slow' glycolysis is capable of providing about 12 times as much ATP per molecule of glycogen. There is sufficient glycogen present in the liver and muscle to resynthesize ATP in about 75 min via 'slow' glycolysis. Using these data, it can be calculated that 'fast' glycolysis can release energy from glycogen present in muscle for about 6 min (1/12 of 75 min) (Newsholme et al 1994). However, 'fast' glycolysis can only run at full speed for about 45–90 s. Unfavorable changes in the internal environment due to the release of energy from 'fast' glycolysis leads to a lowering of the pH, which results in negative feedback for phosphofructokinase (i.e. the enzyme that determines the speed of glycolysis) (Zintl 1995).

2.3.3 Capacity of the aerobic pathway

Energy-rich substrates are supplied by fats and glycogen. It has already been stated that oxidation of fatty acids is impossible without glycolysis. However, a severe depletion of glycogen during long-distance running must be seen as a performance-limiting factor. A trained runner can generate energy for 60–90 min with the help of 'slow' glycolysis. For a reasonably accomplished runner, this will mean that he can complete half a marathon without depleting his supply of glycogen. The situation is quite different if he has not performed warming-up exercises or if he has made a very rapid start. In that case, 'fast' glycolysis makes a much greater contribution during the first half of the marathon. In order to generate the same amount of ATP, 'fast' glycolysis needs 18–19 times more glycogen. The great share of activity undertaken by 'fast' glycolysis during the first kilometers knocks a sizeable hole in the supply of glycogen in the muscles. Glycogen in muscle supplies at least 80%

of substrate for glycolysis, and here lies one of the most important causes of the fatigue that can develop during long-duration exercise.

The effect of training on the capacity of the glycogen supply is not minor. In untrained individuals, there is about 80 g of glycogen stored in the liver and 350 g stored in muscle. In trained runners, these values can be as high as 120 and 650 g glycogen, respectively (Zintl 1995).

2.4 CARDIORESPIRATORY SYSTEM

The most important function of the cardiorespiratory system is to supply the body with oxygen (Zintl 1995). Because the aerobic processes that provide energy are dependent on oxygen, the cardiorespiratory system has a great influence on endurance performance. In particular, the quality of the heart and lungs has a great effect on the level of $\dot{V}O_{2\,max}$, which can be defined as the maximum capacity to absorb oxygen through the lungs and to transport it in the blood for use in the muscles. The heart and lungs are not only responsible for the exchange of oxygen but also for the exchange of carbon dioxide between the body and atmospheric air.

The transport of oxygen and carbon dioxide by the cardiovascular and respiratory systems takes place via four independent processes (Costill & Wilmore 1994, Martini 1998):

- respiration
- diffusion, by which gases are exchanged between the lungs and the blood
- transport of oxygen and carbon dioxide in the blood
- capillary exchange of gases (between capillaries and, e.g., active muscle tissue).

2.4.1 Respiration

One of the aims of ventilation, or respiration, is to exchange oxygen and carbon dioxide between the blood (pulmonary capillaries) and atmospheric air (Brooks et al 1996). To do this, air must constantly be refreshed in the lungs by means of air movement. Air in the lungs is regularly refreshed by the movement of respiration (i.e. inhalation and exhalation).

Inhalation is an active process, during rest as well as exercise, directed at increasing the volume of the lungs. Pressure in the lungs decreases as the pulmonary volume increases, so that a difference in pressure develops with the atmospheric air.

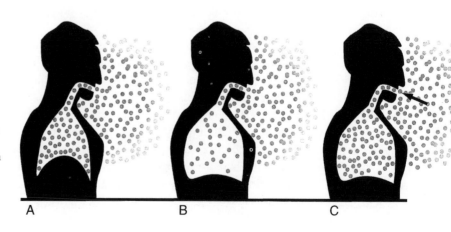

Figure 2.32   The process of inhalation
(A) In a resting state, the pressure in the lungs is equal to that of atmospheric air.
(B) By increasing the volume of the lungs (e.g. by contracting the diaphragm), the pressure in the lungs becomes lower than that of atmospheric air.
(C) Atmospheric air streams into the lungs until the difference in pressure is equalized.

A   B   C

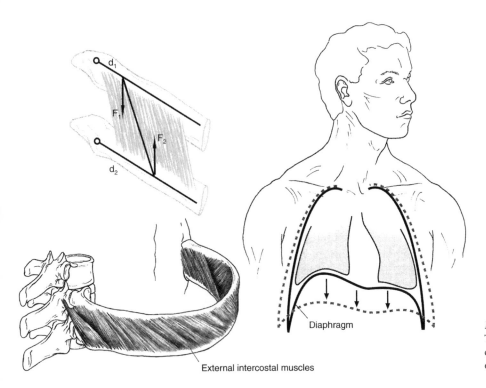

Figure 2.33   Enlarging the thoracic cavity
The thoracic cavity is enlarged as the diaphragm and respiratory muscles (the external intercostal muscles) contract.

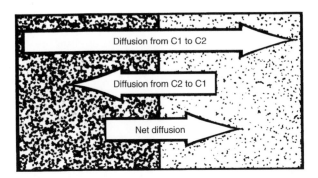

Figure 2.34   Diffusion of gases
The nature of a gas is to disperse from a high to low concentration until reaching a state of equilibrium.

The result is that external air streams into the lungs until the pressure difference levels out. The increase in the volume of the lungs is chiefly due to the activity of the diaphragm and the respiratory muscles, located between the ribs (external intercostal muscles), which enlarge the thorax cavity with which the lungs are indirectly joined by their membranes (pleura). When the stress of running is high, enlargement of the thorax cavity is still supported by auxiliary respiratory muscles such as the serratus anterior and the sternocleidomastoid.

Exhalation while the body is at rest is a passive process. However, during physical exercise, the process becomes active, with the help of the abdominal muscles and the muscles that lie between the ribs (the internal intercostal muscles). Exhalation during rest takes place when the thorax springs back elastically under the impact of gravity.

Top runners are able to ventilate at a rate of 150–200 l/min, giving rise to a pressure gradient (between the air in the atmosphere and the air in the lungs) of −30 and +100 mmHg during inhalation and exhalation, respectively. When the body is at rest, the pressure gradient is –1 mmHg during inhalation and +1 mmHg during exhalation. More attention is given ventilation as a performance-limiting factor for middle- and long-distance runners later in this book (see Ch. 4).

2.4.2 Diffusion of gases

One characteristic of gases is that they diffuse from an area of high concentration to an area of low concentration until equilibrium is reached (i.e. until the concentrations of the gas in two interconnected compartments are identical). In the field of physiology, one usually speaks of the partial pressure rather than the concentration of a gas. Air that is inhaled consists of a mixture of gases, each of which exerts a certain pressure depending on its concentration. The total pressure of a gas mixture is the sum of the partial pressures of the gases present in the mixture. Outdoor air, for which the barometric pressure is 760 mmHg, is composed of 79.04% nitrogen, 20.93% oxygen, and 0.03% carbon dioxide. The partial pressures of nitrogen, oxygen, and carbon dioxide are 600.7 (0.7904×760), 159.0 (0.2093×760), and 0.3 (0.003×760) mmHg, respectively. From this perspective, gases flow from a high to a low partial pressure. The difference in pressure between two interconnected compartments is also called the pressure gradient. The greater the pressure gradient, the more rapidly gases diffuse from one compartment into the other. At a different barometric pressure, for example at 2000 m above sea level, although the proportion of oxygen may be the same as that at sea level (20.93%), the partial pressure of oxygen will clearly be lower in comparison. The barometric pressure at 2000 m is 596 mmHg, which gives a partial pressure for oxygen of 124.9 mmHg. Because the partial pressure of oxygen in atmospheric air is lower at higher altitudes, the speed at which oxygen diffuses from the alveoli (sacs in the lung) into capillary blood is decreased. It will no longer be possible to completely saturate with oxygen the cap-

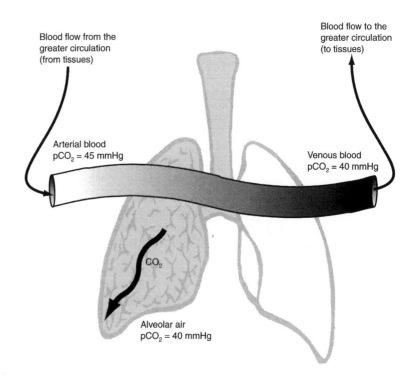

Figure 2.35   Oxygen diffusion
The change in the partial pressure of oxygen in the blood of a pulmonary capillary.

illary blood flowing along the alveoli, despite the fact that the proportion of oxygen is identical to that at sea level. When explaining physiological processes in which gas diffusion plays an important role, using the partial pressure, rather than the proportion, of gases yields more useful data.

At sea level, the partial pressure of oxygen in the alveoli is about 105 mmHg. The partial pressure of oxygen decreases from 159 to 105 mmHg, because atmospheric air is being mixed with air already present in the lungs. Even when the body is experiencing maximum exertion during running, the partial pressure of oxygen can be held at 105 mmHg through ventilation. The oxygen-impoverished capillaries supplying blood to the alveoli have a partial oxygen pressure of 40–45 mmHg. The resulting pressure gradient of 55–65 mmHg is sufficient to almost completely saturate the blood with oxygen. Blood flowing out of the lungs and returning to the heart therefore has a partial pressure of about 100 mmHg.

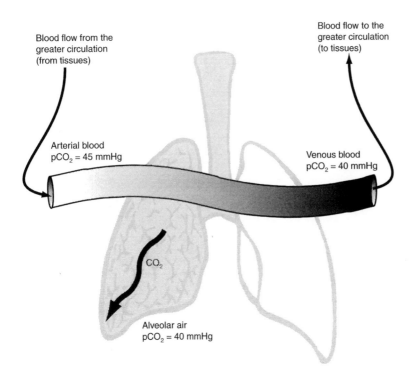

Blood flow from the greater circulation (from tissues)

Blood flow to the greater circulation (to tissues)

Arterial blood pCO$_2$ = 45 mmHg

Venous blood pCO$_2$ = 40 mmHg

CO$_2$

Alveolar air pCO$_2$ = 40 mmHg

Figure 2.36 Carbon dioxide diffusion
The change in the partial pressure of carbon dioxide in the blood of a pulmonary capillary.

At 5 mmHg, the pressure gradient of carbon dioxide in the alveoli is much lower than that in capillary blood, which is low in oxygen. However, the diffusion of carbon dioxide across the respiratory membrane (the barrier between the capillary and the lung sac) is much more rapid than that of oxygen, because carbon dioxide is 20 times more readily dissolved in blood.

2.4.3   Transport of oxygen and carbon dioxide in blood
All the processes that have been described so far involve the transport of gases from atmospheric air to the lungs and blood, and vice versa. In this section, attention is paid to the way in which oxygen and carbon dioxide are transported in the blood

(e.g. how oxygen is supplied to and carbon dioxide is removed from the active muscle tissue where it was produced). The cardiovascular system plays a major role in the transport of carbon dioxide and oxygen. Consequently, the mechanisms responsible for adaptation in the cardiovascular system, so that the exchange of gases remains optimal during exercise, are discussed at length.

Oxygen transport

Blood leaving the lungs is 96–98% saturated at sea level. Most of the oxygen taken up in the blood is bound to hemoglobin in red blood corpuscles (erythrocytes). Only 3% of the oxygen can be dissolved directly in blood, due to its poor solubility in blood plasma. The extent to which oxygen will bind to hemoglobin depends on the partial pressure of oxygen in the blood and the affinity between hemoglobin and oxygen (Costill & Wilmore 1994). The relationship between the partial pressure of blood oxygen and the degree to which hemoglobin is saturated with oxygen can be plotted on an oxygen-dissociation curve.

A number of factors influence the affinity of hemoglobin for oxygen, and therefore the shape of the oxygen dissociation curve. An increase in blood temperature and a decrease in blood pH, conditions frequently encountered in active muscle tissue, lower the affinity of hemoglobin for oxygen. In other words, under such conditions the oxygen dissociation curve shifts toward the right; oxygen is surrendered more easily to active tissues by hemoglobin and the percentage saturation of hemoglobin with oxygen decreases in these regions.

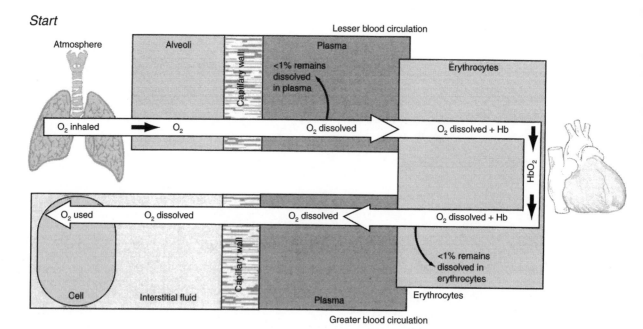

Figure 2.37 The transport of oxygen from atmospheric air
Oxygen is transported by way of the lungs (lesser blood circulation) to tissues (greater blood circulation).

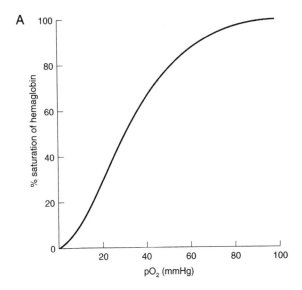

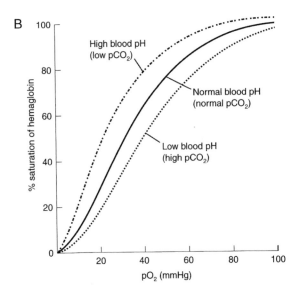

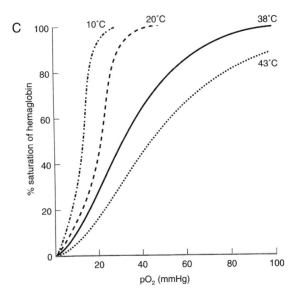

Figure 2.38   *Dissociation curve for oxygen*
(A) The relationship between the partial pressure of blood oxygen and the degree to which hemoglobin is saturated with oxygen.
(B) The effect of changes in blood pH on the oxygen dissociation curve.
(C) The effect of changes in blood temperature on the oxygen dissociation curve.

Carbon dioxide transport

Traditionally, hemoglobin has been strongly associated with the transport of oxygen in blood and much less with the transport of carbon dioxide. The reason for this is probably due to the fact that only 25% of the carbon dioxide produced can bind in that form to hemoglobin to create the complex called carbaminohemoglobin. Of the carbon dioxide produced, 70% is removed as a bicarbonate ions (HCO_3^-) and only 5% is dissolved in blood plasma. This means that most of the carbon dioxide produced will diffuse into erythrocytes, where it binds directly to hemoglobin to form, together with water (H_2O), carboxylic acid (H_2CO_3) which is unstable and rapidly breaks down into HCO_3^- and hydrogen ions (H^+):

$$CO_2 + H_2O \rightarrow H_2CO_3 \leftrightharpoons HCO_3^- + H^+$$

Subsequently, hemoglobin functions as a buffer by binding with H^+. When blood has reached the lungs, where the partial pressure of carbon dioxide is low, the reaction reverses direction so that carbon dioxide can be passed into the alveoli.

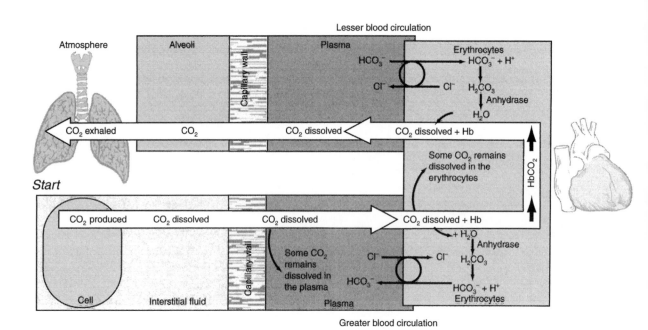

Figure 2.39   Carbon dioxide transport
Carbon dioxide is transported from atmospheric air by way of the lungs (lesser blood circulation) to tissues (greater blood circulation).

Cardiovascular system

The transport of oxygen and carbon dioxide in blood is strongly dependent on the capacity of the cardiovascular system to transport these gases. Assuming, when 96–98% hemoglobin is saturated with oxygen, that 100 ml of blood will contain 20 ml of oxygen, then the transport of oxygen will depend directly on the volume of circulation (V_{circ}) (i.e. on the number of liters of blood pumped through the body by the heart measured per minute (l/min)). During exercise, if V_{circ} is 40 l/min, then 6 l of oxygen can be transported per minute (20 ml of oxygen/100 ml of blood $\times$ 30 l

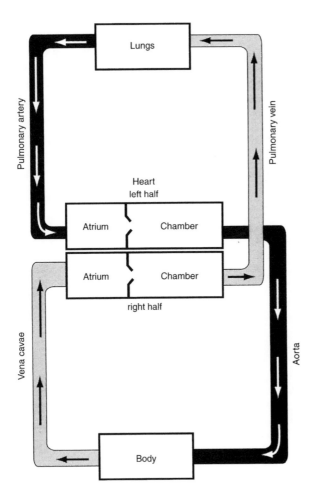

Figure 2.40   Schematic illustration of the blood circulation
The heart can be compared to two pumps connected in series.

of blood/min = 6 l of oxygen/min). The actual oxygen uptake is clearly less, because venous blood flowing back into the heart still contains a substantial amount of oxygen (Brooks et al 1996).

The value of V_{circ} is determined by both the heart rate and by the stroke volume (V_{stroke}) (i.e. the amount of blood ejected from a ventricle with each beat of the heart). V_{stroke} is the difference between the end-diastolic (V_{ED}) and the end-systolic (V_{ES}) volumes. V_{ED} refers to the amount of blood with which the heart ventricles are filled just before the start of each heart beat. The heart can be seen as two interconnected serial pumps, by which the venous and pulmonary blood flowing back to the heart enters the right or left atrium, respectively. After being transported from the atria to the ventricles of the heart, the blood in the left ventricle is propelled into the aorta, while blood from the right ventricle flows into the pulmonary artery. The volume of blood remaining in, for example, the left ventricle, after the heart has contracted is the end-systolic volume. V_{stroke} is therefore the difference between V_{ED} and V_{ES}:

$$V_{stroke} = V_{ED} - V_{ES}$$

When an athlete is running at low-intensity, it is mainly V_{stroke} that increases in order to increase V_{circ}. The heart rate does not increase linearly with the intensity of effort exerted. Up until the heart rate reaches about 120 beats/min, V_{stroke} continues to increase as V_{ED} increases and V_{ES} slightly decreases. When the heart rate exceeds

120 beats/min, the relationship between heart rate and intensity of effort is linear. The increase in V_{stroke} during physical exercise is partly an automatic process. When V_{ED} is increased, the wall of, for example, the left ventricle of the heart becomes more stretched, causing it to react by contracting more strongly. This is called the Frank–Starling mechanism. The linear relationship between heart rate and running intensity, when the heart rate exceeds 120 beats/min, can be used to help determine the correct intensity of training, using the heart-rate parameter (pulse rate). Thus the running intensity can be determined based on a percentage of the maximum heart rate (HR_{max}) or on the heart rate reserve (HRR), which is the number of heart beats by which the resting heart rate (HR_{rest}) can increase until HR_{max} is reached. In other words, HRR is the difference between HR_{rest} and HR_{max}.

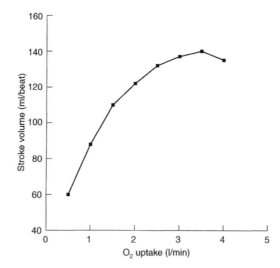

Figure 2.41 The relationship between stroke volume and running intensity
The relationship between stroke volume and running intensity expressed as oxygen uptake. When the intensity of the running load is low, the volume of blood pumped by the heart per minute is generally increased by increasing the stroke volume.

Example *The HR_{max} of runner A is 200 beats/min and his HR_{rest} is 50 beats/min. His HRR is determined by subtracting his HR_{rest} (50) from his HR_{max} (200), yielding a value of 150 (200 − 50 = 150). This shows that his heart rate can increase by 150 beats from a condition of rest before his HR_{max} is reached. Training for endurance running with an intensity of 60–70% of his HRR shows that his heart beat may increase by 60–70% of 150 beats, i.e. an increase of 0.60 × 150 = 90 up to 0.70 × 150 = 105. Obviously, these values must still be added to the HR_{rest}: 90 + 50 = 140 and 105 + 50 = 155. The optimum intensity for this endurance training for runner A is a heart rate somewhere between 140 and 155 beats/min. Determining intensity in this way is appropriate when the workout requires most of the energy be derived from aerobic processes. A workout that makes great demands on the energy contributed by anaerobic pathways cannot be regulated by using the heart rate as a guide. Later in this book (see Ch. 4) more attention is paid to the application of heart rate as a measure of intensity, using various ways and means of training.*

2.4.4   Capillary exchange of gases

The exchange of oxygen between capillary blood and active muscle tissue depends on the partial pressure of the oxygen in the blood, the pH and temperature of the blood, and the supply of blood to muscle tissue. The increased demand for oxygen by active muscles during the start of exercise is met when more oxygen is supplied as the pH is lowered and the blood temperature rises.

The measure of the extraction of oxygen from the bloodstream by muscle tissue is the difference between the arterial and venous oxygen contents ($_{a-v}VO_2$). In a resting state, arterial blood contains about 20 ml of oxygen per 100 ml of blood. By the time blood has reached the veins, this value has decreased to 15–16 ml of oxygen per 100 ml of blood. In a resting state, $_{a-v}VO_2$ is about 4–5 ml, indicating that the tissues supplied with blood have taken up 4–5 ml of oxygen per 100 ml of blood. During maximum physical effort, $_{a-v}VO_2$ can be as high as 15–16 ml. In particular, the low partial pressure of oxygen in active muscles facilitates the delivery of oxygen by hemoglobin in this situation.

Carbon dioxide formed in the aerobic pathway is taken up in the blood by means of diffusion. The carbon dioxide pressure gradient between muscle tissue and blood determines the diffusion of carbon dioxide into the blood.

2.5 MAXIMUM OXYGEN UPTAKE

It is intriguing why some athletes can run faster than others. This question could be answered quite simply by assuming that faster runners are merely more talented. However, talent is only part of the total picture. Training also influences an athlete's running performance, and one runner may be able to run faster because of his training.

In order to research the influence of training on endurance performance, physiologists studying physical exercise sought a single criterion for evaluation (Costill & Wilmore 1994). This criterion might then also serve as a predictor of talent for endurance sports. Most physiologists studying physical exercise have considered $VO_{2\,max}$ to be the most suitable criterion for evaluation. The question is now to what extent the value of $VO_{2\,max}$ is able to supply information in order to determine the quality of a runner and to what extent this criterion is applicable on a practical level as a guide to training.

2.5.1 $VO_{2\,max}$ as a predictor of running talent

Determining $VO_{2\,max}$ is one of the tests most frequently carried out in the physiology laboratory. It is generally accepted that this is the best measure for determining the functional capacity of the heart and lungs (Howley et al 1995). Being able to cover large distances rapidly is largely determined by the level of $VO_{2\,max}$ (Arts & Kuipers 1994). Studies have demonstrated that when the $VO_{2\,max}$ is taken in proportion to body weight, the highest values are found in runners who are the most accomplished (Noakes 1988). Therefore, in practice, the value of $VO_{2\,max}$ can be applied during training as a way of measuring talent in runners. When $VO_{2\,max}$ is scaled to body weight, the value is the relative $VO_{2\,max}$ and is expressed in milliliters per kilogram body weight per minute (ml/kg/min). Absolute $VO_{2\,max}$ is not dependent on body weight and is expressed in milliliters per minute (ml/min). Because during running the body's weight must constantly be 'carried', the relative uptake of oxygen is the most relevant parameter. Later in this section, when we speak of $VO_{2\,max}$, it will always be the relative $VO_{2\,max}$ to which we refer.

However, using $VO_{2\,max}$ to predict talent for endurance running has its limitations. One limitation is that, while $VO_{2\,max}$ is a good predictor for runners heterogeneously grouped together according to their performance level for endurance, the parameter remains a relatively poor predictor for more homogenous groups (Costill

& Winrow 1970). It is possible that individuals who can run a marathon in the same time will still demonstrate clear differences in their levels of $\dot{V}O_{2\,max}$. It is assumed that such differences can be explained by variations in the expenditure of energy during running and by the different percentages of $\dot{V}O_{2\,max}$ at which the entire race can be run. A marathon is generally run at an average of 82% (range 76–87%) of $\dot{V}O_{2\,max}$ (Noakes 1991).

There are many factors that have an influence on the economy of running, for example: the athlete's running technique; biomechanical factors, such as leg length; the distribution of body weight; and the ability to make good use of landing energy. The term 'landing energy' refers to the energy that is stored in the body's elastic structures, such as the tendons, each time the leg makes contact with the ground surface. This energy is re-used for the subsequent push-off. The difference between runners in terms of their ability to use landing energy appears to be important, and might possibly provide an explanation for individual variations in the expenditure of energy during running.

On average, the $\dot{V}O_{2\,max}$ measured in untrained healthy young men is 45–55 ml/kg/min (i.e. their muscles are able to absorb 45–55 ml of oxygen per kilogram of body weight per minute). Values of about 80 ml/kg/min have been found in top runners. The level of $\dot{V}O_{2\,max}$ detected must be seen in context of the progression detected in $\dot{V}O_{2\,max}$ through training. Values ranging from 5% to 20% have been documented in the literature. This implies that, even after receiving the most optimum training, young untrained men whose $\dot{V}O_{2\,max}$ is 45–55 ml/kg/min will never be able to achieve a value anywhere near the values measured in top runners. In other words, an individual's talent for becoming a good long-distance runner is to a large degree genetically determined. However, while the $\dot{V}O_{2\,max}$ value can be used to differentiate between athletes with or without a talent for running, it is of no use for detecting small variations in the level of performance.

2.5.2 $\dot{O}_{2\,max}$ as a guide for training

In practice, a trainer is constantly searching for information that can be used to optimizing the process of training. In addition to evaluating the effects of training for which an athlete has been striving, an important aspect is to determine which training intensity will help that runner improve more rapidly his capacity to perform. The central question, therefore, is whether values of $\dot{V}O_{2\,max}$ can be used in optimizing the intensity of a (chiefly) aerobic workout during training.

2.5.3 $\dot{O}_{2\,max}$ to determine optimum training intensity

To date it appears that using $\dot{V}O_{2\,max}$ has little to offer for the total training process. However, the research done by Billat et al (1994) has presented a positive perspective for the use of $\dot{V}O_{2\,max}$ in regards to determining the optimum intensity to use during intensive training sessions. In their study, these authors did not look at the $\dot{V}O_{2\,max}$ itself but rather at the speed or velocity of trained runners when their first $\dot{V}O_{2\,max}$ was being determined ($_v\dot{V}O_{2\,max}$). Subsequently, a second test was run in which, after a warm-up, the running belt was brought directly up to speed in order to study how long a runner could maintain this speed ($_{t\,lim\,v}\dot{V}O_{2\,max}$). Based on these two variables ($_v\dot{V}O_{2\,max}$ and $_{t\,lim\,v}\dot{V}O_{2\,max}$) for performance, the most intensive and therefore often the most important training session of the week could be drawn up. For clarity, these two variables can be defined as follows: $_v\dot{V}O_{2\,max}$ represents the minimum running speed at which $\dot{V}O_{2\,max}$ can be achieved, and $_{t\,lim\,v}\dot{V}O_{2\,max}$ represents the time during which $_v\dot{V}O_{2\,max}$ can be maintained.

An efficiency factor is already embedded in the concept $_v\dot{V}O_{2\,max}$, to which $_{t\,lim\,v}\dot{V}O_{2\,max}$ adds another important component representing endurance. In this manner, one can sidestep the problem of the variations in energy expenditure seen between runners with identical $\dot{V}O_{2\,max}$, who therefore demonstrate large differences in their levels of performance. Determining only $\dot{V}O_{2\,max}$ or only energy expenditure during running is of little use, and both are embedded in the term $_v\dot{V}O_{2\,max}$. In this manner, $_v\dot{V}O_{2\,max}$ and $_{t\,lim\,v}\dot{V}O_{2\,max}$ become good instruments for explaining differences in the levels of performance between runners and for predicting talent for endurance. An additional advantage is that $_v\dot{V}O_{2\,max}$ and $_{t\,lim\,v}\dot{V}O_{2\,max}$ can be used to determine the optimum intensity and magnitude of the interval workload needed for training. From the research of Billat et al (1999) it appears that the effect of training will be very positive when an athlete completes a once-weekly session consisting of five repetitions at an intensity set at $_v\dot{V}O_{2\,max}$, with a magnitude one-half the endurance time of $_{t\,lim\,v}\dot{V}O_{2\,max}$, and with a workload/recovery ratio of 1:1. In Billat et al's study of eight trained athletes, $_v\dot{V}O_{2\,max}$ improved by 3% (from 20.5 to 21.1 km/h), energy expenditure during running improved by 6%, and the heart rate during submaximum exercise (70% $\dot{V}O_{2\,max}$) decreased by 4%. There was no change in $\dot{V}O_{2\,max}$.

3
Running techniques

3.1 INTRODUCTION

Running is an exceptionally flexible form of movement, the pattern of which can be adapted to numerous environmental factors, such as wind direction (running with or against the wind) or degree of incline (running up or down a slope), and the quality of the ground surface (hard, soft, uneven or smooth). Step length, cadence, and body posture can be changed in order to adapt as optimally as possible. In some situations it may be useful to bend the upper body forward, while in other cases it might be better to hold the body erect. Sometimes the surface will require that the ground contact time be kept brief, while in other situations a longer thrust with an accent on the end of the support phase will be needed. It is not feasible to include all the influencing factors in the analysis of a running technique (thus also when describing what is understood by 'optimum technique'). Therefore, a certain degree of standardization is necessary. When describing a running technique, one can assume that the athlete will be running straight ahead on a hard, flat, and even surface. The influence of wind and air resistance, or drag, are not taken into account.

After excluding environmental conditions, two groups of factors remain that will determine which technique to use: (1) the influence of, and eventual changes in, velocity; and (2) the influence of the morphology and function of the locomotor apparatus. The situations in which the velocity (change in speed) can be expected to affect how one runs can be categorized as follows:

- high-speed running
- start and acceleration
- constant low-speed running.

The structure and function of the locomotor apparatus demonstrate many similarities but only a few differences between individuals. In fact, the similarities are extraordinarily predominant. In nearly all humans the construction of the locomotor apparatus follows the same blueprint. This becomes evident when considering the anatomy of the skeletal musculature. We all have hamstrings with a pennate structure and femoral epicondyls shaped like a snail shell. In addition, control of the locomotor system, as well as locomotion itself, follows nearly the same pattern in every individual. Collaboration between muscles and reflexes, and the conversion of elasticity into kinetic energy during locomotion are also carried out in the same way in all individuals. These similarities form the basis for describing a correct running technique. That there are differences between individuals is clearly obvious: one person may be tall and heavy, while another is short and light; one individual may have long limbs that can act as levers; and so on. Such variations lead to individual differences in the implementation of a certain technique: to an individual style of running.

Style and technique are interrelated during running. An individual style is only considered acceptable and correct if it does not impede on correct technique. A runner who allows a great deal of landing energy to ebb away with each step may not uphold the excuse that it is a question of his personal style, but should rather admit that his running technique is not good. Therefore, a trainer must have the skill to be able to gain insight into the relationship between an athlete's technical ability and his personal style. In other words, it is important to make a distinction between those patterns of movement which may be seen as personal style (and therefore need not be corrected) and those which must be labeled faulty (i.e. are contrary to morphology and function) and corrected by training. In addition to correcting errors, it is important to understand to what extent optimizing an athlete's good qualities will actually contribute to an improvement in his performance. For example, would it prove helpful for a middle-distance runner to train the reactive properties of his muscles to the highest possible level, or is there no added value to be gained beyond a certain level?

In a sense, the locomotor system can be described as a kernel (the plan for movement) surrounded by a number of outer shells. When we observe from the outside how the body moves, we see partial body segments oscillating, translating, rotating, accelerating, and decelerating. The components that can be observed externally belong to the first, or outermost, shell of the locomotor system. There is a second shell beneath this outermost one. Movement is brought about through the cooperation (i.e. intermuscular coordination) of various muscles, which can frequently be quite complex, such as the teamwork seen between monoarticular and biarticular muscles. Such teamwork will seldom be observed from the outside. Using electromyography (EMG), focus can be shifted in part to the activity taking place within the body, thus making visible the second, or middle, shell. There is also a third, or innermost, shell in the locomotor system, i.e. that for intramuscular coordination. With regard to this shell, one can describe the interplay between the active and passive parts of a muscle for which phenomena such as pretension and elasticity play a large role.

What actually happens during running can only be derived in part from the data obtained from measurements. Much is still unknown about this subject. Most measurements and research directed at understanding running have only been conducted outside the body (i.e. on the outermost, or first, shell). For example, attempts

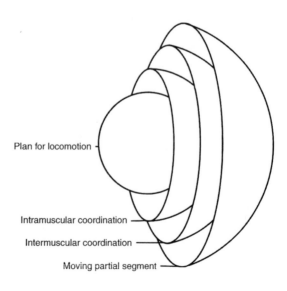

Figure 3.1 Build-up of coordination
The way in which coordination functions is illustrated schematically as a kernel surrounded by three outer shells. The center represents the plan for or design of the movement. In the first (outermost) shell are all of the oscillating body parts. This shell is placed on the outside because only the movement of partial segments can be observed on the body's exterior. In the second shell, coordination between muscles is determined. In the third (innermost) shell, both active and passive tissues within individual muscles are regulated.

Plan for locomotion

Intramuscular coordination

Intermuscular coordination

Moving partial segment

have been made to discover which segments can be seen as an unchanging unit and how those segments behave during the motion of running. Some information can be gained by studying the upward and downward oscillating motions of partial segments, but there are also very important biomechanical events taking place within the body (see Section 1.1). The most important joints are usually bridged by a large number of muscles. It is nearly, if not totally, impossible to determine exactly which muscle is contributing to which movement by observing the body's exterior (the so-called problem of underdetermination in the second shell). Even EMG will not provide complete insight into what is happening within the body. Opinions on the technical aspects of running are, therefore, never more than models for movement into which one attempts to fit as many pieces of data as possible.

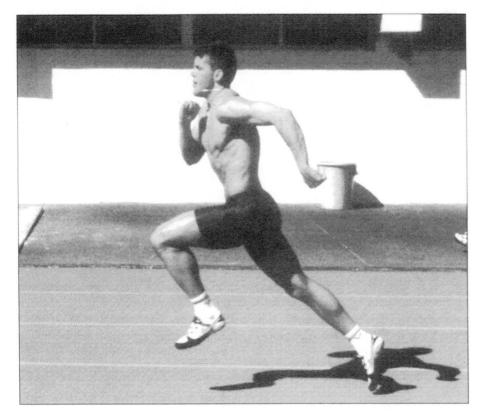

Figure 3.2 Moment of toe-off
Generally, the moment of toe-off is used to illustrate push-off during running. However, toe-off is not relevant to propulsion, and the position of the body at the moment of toe-off gives little indication of the quality of the running technique.

In the models currently used to study technique, for a long time absolutely no consideration was given to the elastic potential of muscles (i.e. the third shell: intramuscular coordination). With regard to the technique used for endurance running, a particular attempt was made to find the most efficient way to use energy by making the cyclic motion proceed in as 'circular' a fashion as possible (by imitating the motion of a wheel). The stride should roll, foot placement should be as soft as possible, and much emphasis was placed on how the motion of the foot was completed.

During a sprint, emphasis was always placed on the thrust at the end of push-off. To illustrate this, photographs taken at the moment of toe-off were used, although they had often actually been taken during the acceleration phase. Once at speed, running looks quite different and other factors have determining influence. For many reasons, during speed running (up to the pace for 800 or 1500 m), thrust takes place at the beginning of the support phase. A model was employed in which the motion of running was divided into three phases: landing, thrust, and swing. During the landing phase, the energy generated had to be able to flow away, while thereafter, during thrust, by working concentrically the muscles could bring about forward propulsion. Because it gradually became clear that the model designed for the push-off, swing, and landing phases was not in agreement with what was actually happening, another more detailed model, including forward and backward support and swing phases, was proposed. However, this model was very mechanical and poorly integrated. What makes running efficient lies precisely in the mutual cooperation between all the actions that take place during running (i.e. between the swing and support legs, arm movement and axial rotation in the trunk, pelvic tilt and push-off, etc.). Therefore, a more integrated model was needed.

The level of knowledge about the biomechanical aspects of running has lagged behind what is known about aspects of physical exercise. Of all sports, athletics has the reputation of being one of the most highly developed. However, in the area of biomechanics, athletics research still suffers from a substantial backlog. Future research will undoubtedly provide new data on the mutual cooperation between various movements.

In this chapter, the technique of running is analyzed from a total perspective. Among other things, we observe which roles are actively played by the trunk, pelvis, and swing leg during forward thrust, and how the reactive properties of the body's musculature can be optimized during the motion of running. This approach should provide a model that can have far-reaching consequences for the exercises used to practice running techniques and for forms of power training.

3.2 HIGH-SPEED RUNNING

Patterns of movement proceed from one decisive moment to the next. A moment is decisive when a motion is either initiated or greatly changed. Such decisive moments are not necessarily chosen fully consciously, but can also be regulated automatically during the movement. When a movement is non-cyclic, successive decisive moments can be recognized easily. For example, the motion of throwing proceeds sequentially: the pull-back is initiated, the front support leg is blocked, the motion of throwing begins, the ball is released, and the motion of the arm slows after its outward swing. Here one can speak of an obvious series of decisive moments that are integrated into an automatic progression of movements. Running is a cyclic motion, and thus the transitions between the sequence of phases occur less abruptly and the decisive moments are more difficult to identify. Therefore, it is somewhat problematic to begin an analysis of running randomly within the cycle. Nevertheless, a choice has been made to use the individual characteristic phases of running as the point of departure for describing why a technique is correct. Repeatedly, however, one will be reminded how a phase is affected by the previous phase and will itself have an influence on the following phase. Here, the starting point chosen is the moment when the foot of the stance leg leaves the ground at the end of push-off (i.e. at the moment of toe-off).

The following analysis of running uses the concepts 'swing phase' and 'floating phase'. 'Swing phase' is used to describe leg movement alone. Therefore, the swing phase is that period of time for which the foot of the relevant leg is off the ground (i.e. the period between toe-off until the foot of the same leg returns to the ground surface). The term 'floating phase' is used to describe the period for which the entire body is briefly suspended in mid-air. The floating phase lasts as long as both feet are off the ground.

3.2.1   Posture of the trunk

During high-speed running, the posture of the trunk can only be varied to a certain degree, from being bent very slightly forward to very slightly backward. Frequently, leaning backward is interpreted as being technically incorrect, but one can question to what extent this opinion is correct. Besides the fact that the arguments supporting this opinion lack rigor (supposedly push-off will not be as good), it appears that a number of the world's best sprinters, fully consciously or not, tend to lean their shoulders slightly backward (especially in the last part of the 400 m). In any case, it is clear that the trunk should be held more or less upright when running at speed, which is preferable for a number of reasons.

(a) If the trunk is bent toward the front, the line of projection of the body's center of mass reaches the ground in front of the body's point of support at the moment of foot placement. As gravity will have a lever arm in regard to the point of support, a forward rotation moment will develop. Threatening to topple forward, the runner will be forced to compensate for this in one of two ways:

    (1) The runner can exert extra force in the opposite direction (up and backwards). When there is sufficient time, such as during the first strides at the start of a race, a runner can find adequate compensation for such a forward rotational moment. In addition to directing force toward the rear, the runner will also be able to generate an extra vertical force. When running at speed, however, the ground contact time will be very short (0.07–0.11 s at high speed). Generating extra force to compensate for forward rotation, in addition to the force that is thrust toward the rear, will be impossible when ground contact is brief, and so the runner will have to use less force for thrust in order to direct more force vertically, thus decreasing his forward speed.

    (2) The runner can place his foot further ahead, so that the line of projection of his center of mass does not fall in front of his foot placement. In this way no forward rotational moment will develop. However, the runner has now assumed a posture (foot and shoulder forward, hip to the rear) in which the landing energy loaded during foot placement can no longer be 're-used' properly for thrust. Because the foot has been placed too far in front of the hip, a hard foot strike, which is necessary to prevent landing energy being lost, will slow the runner down. He must wait until his foot is located beneath his hip so that a great deal of energy will be lost (see also Section 3.3.4).

(b) As already stated, when running at speed, the ground contact time is very short. In addition to there being no time to compensate for forward rotation, there is no time to compensate for rotation around the longitudinal axis, which must thus be avoided as far as possible. Such axial rotation usually develops at the end of push-off, when a lot of force is being exerted. If this occurs when the right leg is considerably extended, axial rotation will develop, with the right shoulder moving to the front and the left shoulder to the back. Rotation around the long axis can only be compensated for by lengthening the next stride. The foot must be placed on the ground further in front of the body. During foot strike, the foot will be far in front of the hip. Foot placement must be soft, because a hard foot strike would break the runner's speed. By making the landing soft, the energy released cannot be stored in elastic tissues, but will 'ebb away' or be cancelled out. Such loss of energy is detrimental, as already stated. Because the body rotates around its long axis at the end of push-off, it is important to release the foot from the ground promptly at the end of the support phase. Releasing the foot from the ground can be regulated by keeping the upper part of the body well upright: in this way, prestretch develops early in the iliopsoas and especially in the abdominal muscles. In particular, the abdominal muscles work as sensors and begin the transition from a closed to an open chain when there is sufficient prestretch.

Rotation around the long axis must not be confused with torsion. When there is torsion, the right shoulder moves forward while the left shoulder moves backward as the runner pushes off with his right leg. For rotation, however, shoulder movement compensates for movement in the pelvis in the opposite direction (medial rotation in the hip of the push-off leg). In contrast to rotation around the longitudinal axis, the rotational moment of the body is equal to zero

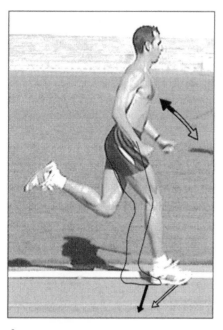
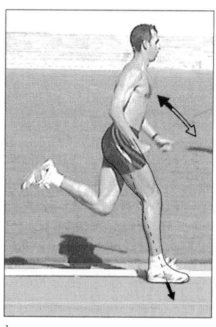
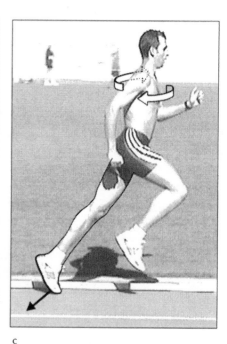

a b c

Figure 3.3 Position of the trunk during speed running

(a) The trunk leans forward when running at speed. As a result, a forward rotation moment will develop. When the foot is placed directly beneath the hip, push-off must be directed more vertically to compensate for rotation. For this reason, the direction of thrust will be less favorable.

(b) The forward rotation moment can also be compensated for by placing the foot on the ground in front of the hip. When the foot strike is hard, the body will decelerate. When the foot strike is soft, landing energy will be lost.

(c) By holding the upper body forward, push-off toward the rear can be lengthened. Exerting force at the end of thrust will cause rotation around the long axis. When the left foot pushes off, the left shoulder will rotate to the front. The disadvantage of such axial rotation is that it must be compensated for during the next step.

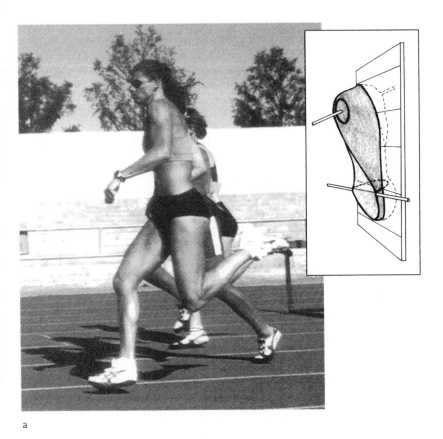

a

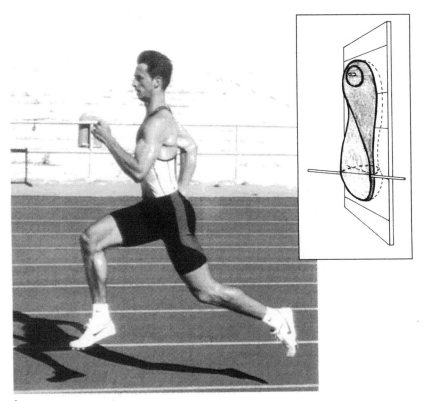

b

Figure 3.4a,b   The difference between long-axis rotation and torsion
When the body rotates around its long axis (a), forward rotation of the (left) shoulder will not be compensated for by a counter-active movement of the (right) hip. When torsion is perfectly balanced (b), the sum of the shoulder and hip rotations is zero. Therefore, during the next support phase, no compensation will be required.

for torsion. Medial rotation in the hip (and thus also torsion) takes place during the first part of the support phase. At the end of support, the hip is strongly retroflexed and the possibility for medial rotation is limited. Consequently, one can speak of torsion during the first part of the support phase and axial rotation at the end of support. Torsion in the trunk, but not axial rotation, is desirable during running.

(c) At the end of the swing phase, just before foot placement, there is powerful backward flexion in the hip. This movement can only be carried out forcefully if forward flexion takes place forcefully in the opposite leg. Such forward flexion is initiated directly after the transition has been made from a closed to an open chain. By holding the trunk upright, the muscles that will initiate this movement can receive the necessary tension through prestretch. If the trunk is allowed to lean far forward, forward flexion will not take place fast enough.

When running at speed, it is not only important that a great deal of force be exerted, but also that this force be built up rapidly. Loss of time in order to compensate for rotation around the longitudinal or lateral axes should therefore be avoided. Learning to avoid rotation will have a greater impact on whether a runner performs well than was previously thought possible. Keeping the trunk upright is therefore an important requirement for high-speed running. Moreover, no arguments can be found in the above reasoning to support the opinion that the trunk must not be allowed to lean slightly backward.

3.2.2 Electromyography

Muscle activity can be measured by means of EMG. EMG measurements of muscle motor-unit activity during running have been frequently recorded. Unfortunately, EMG for the iliopsoas muscle is almost always missing from any series of muscle groups recorded. Because this muscle lies deep within the body, its activity can only be measured with difficulty using skin electrodes.

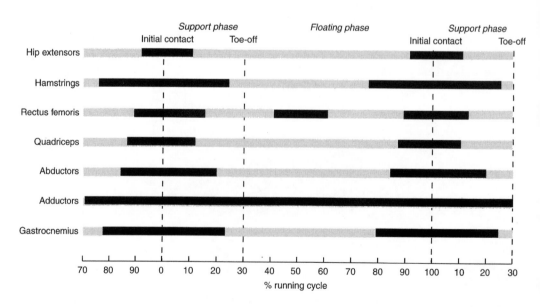

Figure 3.5 An EMG recorded during running
The most important muscles are especially active at the end of the floating phase and at the beginning of the support phase. (EMG data from Novacheck 1995.)

In addition, different EMG measurements show different patterns of generated activity or inactivity. Muscle fibers contract neither only once nor simultaneously throughout the entire muscle, but rather according to a certain pattern. Apparently it makes quite a difference exactly where along the muscle the recording electrodes are placed (Mann et al 1986, Hinrichs 1990, McClay et al 1990, Miller 1990, Jacobs et al 1993). Therefore, an EMG will fail to give complete insight into what is actually taking place in muscle during running.

Furthermore, an EMG is nearly always recorded when the running speed is not too fast. When the speed changes, however, the range in which a certain muscle group is active within the running cycle also shifts. Generally, when speed increases, muscle activity tends to shift to an earlier point in the running cycle (e.g. as speed increases the hamstrings become active earlier in the swing phase). In addition, as speed increases, the muscles are active for a greater portion of the cycle.

When studying an EMG that has been recorded during running, it is immediately apparent that the most important groups of muscles for the hip and leg no longer show any electrical activity by the end of push-off. This is not only true for the muscles responsible for important backward flexion in the hip joint; the knee extensors are also electrically inactive by the end of push-off. From this observation it is obvious that an athlete should not try to give extra push-off force at the end of the support phase. Furthermore, it is also noteworthy that the activity of the monoarticular heads of the quadriceps femoris is limited at the end of the support phase. During the support phase, these muscles only play this important function during the initial moment when the weight of the body must be carried.

At the end of the swing phase, activity can be observed in many muscles. The foot of the stance leg is consequently placed on the ground with much tension already present in the muscles. Because there is a great deal of activity just before and after the foot makes initial contact with the ground, it can be concluded that the use of landing energy for reactive muscle activity is apparently very important. This aspect is given a prominence in the following description of running techniques.

Data obtained from EMG provide evidence for and the importance of avoiding rotation around the long axis by not exerting force at the end of the support phase. The principle of loading and unloading the elastic capacity within a very brief time span also fits well with the idea that propulsion is best carried out at the beginning of the thrust phase. This fact forms the basis of the technical model for running described below.

3.2.3 Description of the running technique

Toe-off: last moment of the support phase

The posture of the body at the moment of toe-off is determined by two requirements: that rotation around the long axis be avoided and that the transition from a closed to an open chain be rapid. The position of the trunk is important in order to avoid axial rotation; i.e. the trunk should be held erect. Holding the trunk upright will also serve to provide good pretension and timely action in the muscles (iliopsoas and abdominal muscles) responsible for initiating forward flexion in the hip during the swing phase. In addition to the position of the trunk, tension around the ankle also plays a role in the rapid initiation of swing. In the ankle, dorsiflexion first develops during the support phase, before becoming plantar flexion at the end of push-off (the exact progression depends on the running speed). When there is sufficient activity in the calf muscles, plantar flexion at the end of push-off will either be slight or perhaps not occur at all. In that case, the mechanism for transferring energy from the knee extension to plantar flexion in the foot (via the gastrocnemius; see also Section 1.6.1) will not be working optimally. As a result, transition from a closed to an open chain is delayed. After the foot has left the ground, the swing leg experiences a moment of inertia or dead moment, just before forward flexion in the hip begins. When tension in the ankle is correct (and the trunk is held correctly upright), forward flexion in the hip can be forceful and initiated immediately after toe-off. During this process, patterns of reflexes probably play a determining role.

The angle of the knee at the moment of toe-off varies somewhat among technically skillful runners. The knee of one athlete may clearly appear to be bent, that of another may appear to be straight until viewed in delayed video images, and the knee of a third runner is actually completely extended. Even runners who extend the knee completely can avoid inconvenient rotation around the long axis by not exerting force at the end of push-off. Knee and hip extension will take place more or less passively, and the swing phase will thereby be initiated later. Because the swing phase lasts somewhat longer, such a variation in technique requires that the stride be long. This technique is somewhat 'dangerous', especially when fatigue has set in, because an athlete will want to exert extra force for push-off, therefore causing more rotation around the long axis. For a discipline such as the 400 m, in which loss of coordination due to fatigue can be a great problem, runners tend to keep the knee relatively more bent at the moment of toe-off. Trying emphatically

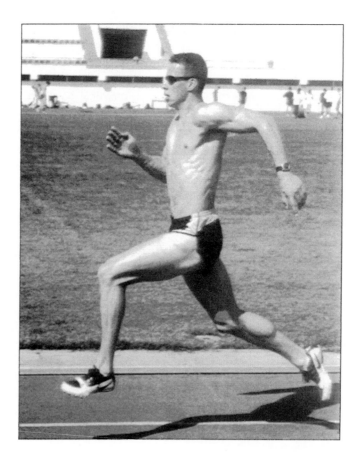

Figure 3.6 Correct body posture at toe-off
The trailing leg does not reach complete extension and the upper body is held in a good upright position. In this way, long-axis rotation can be avoided and the swing leg moves forward linearly. The arms are moved correctly toward the rear, to create torsion. The leading foot is positioned correctly so that foot strike will be hard and reactive.

to avoid rotation around the long axis is apparently an important aid in the struggle against decreasing speed along the last straight stretch of track. It is noteworthy that a runner who clearly holds his knee at an angle and whose foot leaves the ground early will always hold the upper part of his body erect, often even leaning somewhat backward.

The position of the trunk, the angle of the knee at toe-off, and the tension around the ankle are all closely interrelated. Therefore, when instructing an individual how to run these three aspects should always be tackled together. For example, changing the position of the trunk will have a limited effect on the moment of toe-off when there is insufficient tension around the ankle.

Errors during toe-off

- There is no tension around the ankle. The runner is sitting quite deeply. The ground contact time is long due to too much dorsiflexion in the ankle, the vertical component of push-off is small so that ground contact will be long, and the swing phase is brief, compelling the athlete to run at a high stride frequency. Because there is a lack of tension, the swing leg does not move rapidly enough following release from the ground.
- The trunk is held too far forward, so that the swing leg is not brought forward immediately after leaving the ground. As a result, the swing leg arrives too late for the next landing. In order to hold the upper part of the body quite erect when running fast, the runner must be able to maintain a great deal of tension in the trunk. Frequently the abdominal muscles are unable to perform this task well

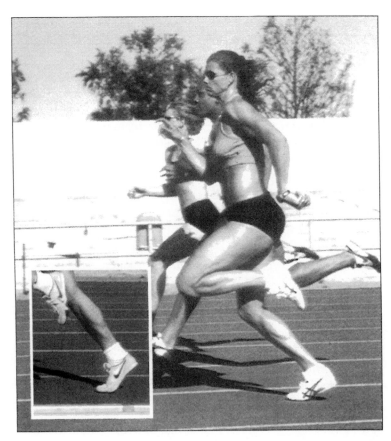

Figure 3.7 Dorsiflexion during the stance phase
Half way through push-off there is too much dorsiflexion in the foot of the stance leg (main photograph; compare with correct position in the inset). As a result, thrust will last too long and too much rotation will develop around the long axis (see also Figure 3.4a).

enough, and the runner will lean forward to take the strain off them. Morphology is also extremely important during running.

- The runner tries to exert thrust at the end of the support phase. He then actively reaches through with his knee. The shoulder on the side of the stance leg moves forward so that the motion must be compensated by medial rotation in the hip of the push-off leg. Torsion in the trunk should take place. Because the leg is strongly flexed backward, such compensation is nearly impossible, and the rotation that has developed around the long axis will have to be compensated for during the following stride.

Swing phase

In many respected opinions about the technique of running, it is thought that the swing leg should be observed moving in isolation. Then the most important function of the swing phase would be to get the leg back into position after toe-off before the following step. Generally it is recognized that, during the second part of the swing phase, the free leg also serves to assist the stance leg at push-off. Otherwise, little connection has been found between the movements of the two legs. The leg (swing) that is in an open chain remains relatively passive, while the leg (support) in a closed chain does the work.

The function of the swing leg, both during swing and during stance in the other leg, is quite complex. The action of the swing leg is of utmost importance if the force of thrust is to be unloaded rapidly and directed to the runner's advantage. For a good analysis of how the swing leg works during the swing and support phases, it is necessary to determine how the various movements are interrelated. Until such an interaction has been elucidated, the effect of swing cannot be determined.

Floating phase: suspended in mid-air

During the floating phase, the hip and knee of the trailing leg are flexed, while the hip and knee of the leading leg are extended. The scissor-like movements of the two legs are involuntarily related as a reflex. This scissor movement is nothing more than a combination of the stumble and inverse-extension reflexes. In other words, bending the hip and knee of one leg strengthens extension in the other hip and knee, and vice versa. This involuntary, reinforcing effect is important. The pendular action of the leading leg just before foot placement is carried out with more force because of such reinforcement. During the outward pendular motion, the hamstrings experience strain from a counteractive force moment. When the muscle fibers are able to maintain their same length as well as possible, the elastic muscle components will stretch. These components will be preloaded so that the contractile segments of the muscle can rapidly attain a high level of power (see Section 1.4).

When running at about 5 m/s, the hamstrings are already exerting force on the tibial plateau during the outward pendular motion of the lower leg which is equal to the weight of the body. When running at high speed, this force increases further. The pretension that thereby develops in the muscles (i.e. in the hamstrings) is needed in order to be able to push off reactively and in the appropriate direction after the landing. Because changes in the knee-joint moments occur very rapidly during landing (within 25 m/s), it is impossible for the runner to react to these changes and have an effect (Bobbert et al 1992, Pink et al 1994). Therefore, sufficient tension must already be present in the muscles by the end of the floating phase and the runner should anticipate any rapid changes expected to develop during the landing. In order to carry out the pendular motion and build up tension optimally, it is neces-

A

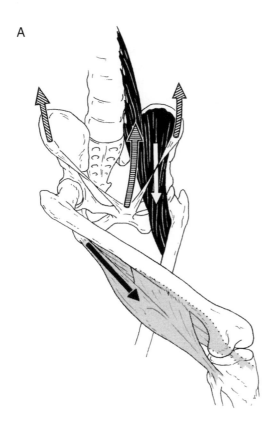

B

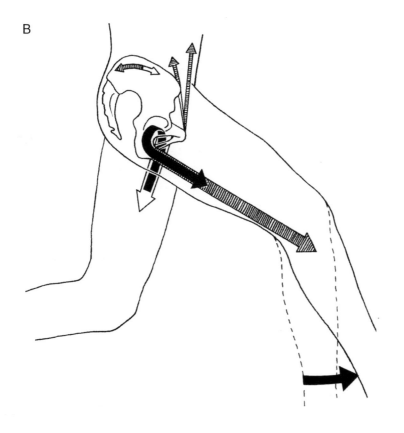

Figure 3.8   Build-up of pretension in the hamstrings

(A) During the scissor-like motion of the legs during the floating phase, developing forces tilt the pelvis backward and forward: the hamstrings (black arrow) and abdominal muscles (hatched arrow) tilt the pelvis backward, while the iliopsoas on the swing leg side (white arrow) tilts it forward.

(B) As the swing leg oscillates outward, the hamstrings (together with the abdominal muscles) exert a force that tilts the pelvis backward (hatched arrow). The iliopsoas can slow this backward tilt somewhat (white arrow), thus causing prestretch in the hamstrings of the front leg. In this way, the pelvis works like a lever so that energy can be transferred from the trailing to the leading leg (black arrows).

sary, certainly when running at speed, that the movement of the trailing swing leg 'chases' that of the leading leg involuntarily. This means that forward flexion in the trailing swing leg must be brought about as forcefully and rapidly as possible after toe-off. If the trailing swing leg is brought forward too slowly, the leading swing leg must 'wait', so to speak, with the consequence that tension can no longer be built up in the muscles optimally. The result will be a soft landing, with a loss of landing energy as it ebbs away. Moreover, backward flexion in the hip just before foot placement will be too slow and the foot will touch ground in front of the hip, which works to decrease speed. The outward pendular motion of the leading swing leg will slow, so that preloading the hamstrings with elastic energy will be less than optimal. The ability to preload the hamstrings counts as an important, if not the most important, limiting factor for reaching the highest speed feasible (Chapman & Caldwell et al 1983).

In order to avoid loss of energy (elastic) in the ankle during the landing, a lot of tension is needed in the muscles of the lower leg. Therefore, just before the moment of initial contact, the ankle should be in a neutral or slightly dorsiflexed position, so that it can build up sufficient pretension in the lower leg (see Section 1.3.3). Therefore, it is necessary to make a very powerful scissor movement directly after toe-off, which can best be achieved by keeping the motion of the trailing swing leg as linear as possible. When the movement is linear, the knee and hip will begin bending at the same time. A 'circular' movement (first bending the knee and then the hip) will slow the trailing leg as it moves forward, and therefore also the leading leg as it moves toward the rear. If the ankle remains in a strongly plantar-flexed position during the first part of the swing phase (after toe-off), the movement will generally be too circular. Keeping the ankle in either a neutral or dorsiflexed position and moving linearly appear to be mutually compatible processes. Forward flexion must also take place directly after the foot has left the ground. It is difficult to observe whether there is a moment of slight inertia during the transition from a closed chain or whether the transition flows without pause and with optimum speed. A trainer must be visually very well experienced or be able to make use of delayed video images in order to spot such frequently miniscule, but important, mistakes.

The speed at which the knee of the trailing swing leg is brought forward after toe-off is not determined only by the speed of change in the hip-joint angle (forward flexion) changes. The backward tilt of the pelvis that occurs immediately after toe-off can also contribute to accelerating the knee. This pelvic tilt is brought about not only by activity in the abdominal muscles (an upright trunk serves to tighten the abdominal muscles and thus contributes to the backward tilt), but also by tension in the hamstrings of the leading swing leg. (Hamstrings work as hip extensors and can therefore also tilt the pelvis backward.) By way of the hamstrings, knee extension in the leading swing leg can help to bring the knee of the trailing swing leg forward. However, the ability of the hamstrings to tilt backward will be used at the expense of tension in this muscle group. If the pelvis did not experience resistance from other muscles, then tension in the hamstrings would be converted almost totally into backward pelvic tilt.

Tilting the pelvis to the rear, however, cannot be done easily or without a great deal of force. In contrast to the abdominal muscles and hamstrings in the leading leg, which work to cause backward pelvic tilt, the iliopsoas in the trailing leg works to achieve forward pelvic tilt. Moreover, the iliopsoas not only has a function in relation to the femur (forward flexion), but also threatens to pull the pelvis forward. This counter-movement by the iliopsoas ensures that the outward pendular movement

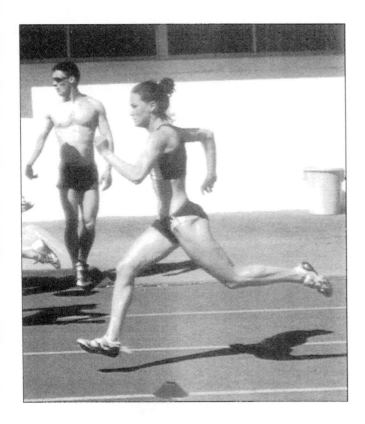

Figure 3.9 Circular backward pendular movement
After toe-off, the knee bends but there is no forward flexion in the hip. The swing therefore becomes circular and takes up too much time. The leading leg must then 'wait' for the trailing leg.

of the lower part of the leading leg not only results in backward pelvic tilt, but also is divided partly between backward pelvic tilt and elastic stretch of the hamstrings.

The scissor movement in the floating phase is thus highly coherent, allowing the pelvis to work as a lever (Chapman & Caldwell 1983, Ounpuu 1994). There is a relationship between pelvic tilt, the speed with which the lower leg swings outward, backward flexion in the leading leg, and forward flexion in the trailing leg. The energy that is generated in the trailing leg (by the iliopsoas) can be transferred to the leading leg (for pretension in the hamstrings). Therefore the energy of the scissor movement not only results in bringing the trailing swing leg to the front, but also allows a lot of energy to be stored, at the moment of foot placement, in the muscles responsible for thrust. When the running technique is good, exact coordination between all these important events that take place during landing result in an ideal posture for thrust, with optimum pretension present in the muscles (McMahon & Cheng 1990).

Ideal cooperation between forces and movements during the floating phase can provide a technically correct pattern of movement in a number of ways. One characteristic of a good running technique is that transition from the support to floating phase is always correct, rapid, and linear. In contrast, whether the knee bends much during its forward swing is of less concern. A good running technique can be achieved whether the angle of the knee is acute (i.e. the knee is greatly bent) or at 90°. An angle greater than 90° will slow down the pendular action too much and, therefore, is not to be recommended.

Not only is there much room for variation in how far the knee can be bent during the swing phase, but also for the ways in which backward flexion in the hip and outward pendular motion of the knee at the end of swing can be coordinated. Some runners tend to bend the knee first before swinging the leg toward the rear. Other runners start backward flexion in the hip earlier and then set the foot on the ground more vertically from above. As long as the various movements are well coordinated and result in the foot being placed on the projection of the body's center of mass on the ground, there will be no complaints.

As a measure of whether movements during the floating phase have been initiated with enough force, the following can be stated: at the moment when the total landing weight is resting on the foot of the stance leg, then the knees must at least be

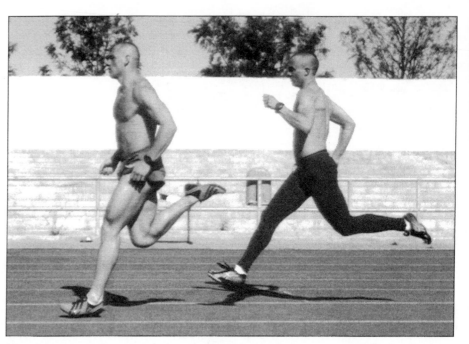

a

Figure 3.10a–c   Movements in the leading leg
The leading leg can move in various ways that are considered to be technically correct. The lower leg can oscillate completely outward before backward flexion in the hip is initiated (b), or the knee and hip can move more synchronously (c). Compare also the way in which the trailing leg is brought forward. The positions of the leading legs of the last runner in (a) and the runner in (b) are the same. The trailing leg in (b) (good neutral position for the ankle) has been moved much further ahead than in (a) (plantar flexion in the ankle). The runner in (b) has a far superior (scissor) technique.

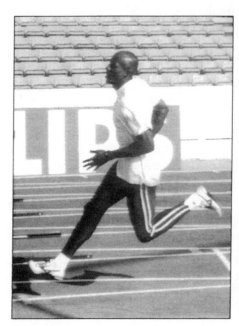

b

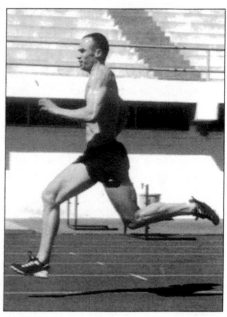

c

located side by side. It is a serious technical error if the shock of the landing must be absorbed while the knee of the swing leg is still behind that of the stance leg because, in this situation, much of the landing energy will be lost. In some athletes one can see that the knee of the swing leg is already clearly in front of the knee of the stance leg at the moment of foot placement. These runners generally make very good use of their reactive potential and are also nearly always categorized as talented.

The great degree of coherence between the movements in the trailing and leading legs during swing has important consequences when giving running instruction. Using isolated exercises for just one leg will prove meaningless. German methodologies are particularly known for focusing on 'grabbing' the front leg toward the rear without involving the other leg in the total movement. Using a hard foot strike in order to improve reactive running can best be carried out from the moment that forward flexion is initiated after toe-off (see Ch. 5). Furthermore, it will be helpful if the runner realizes that the floating phase lasts longer than the stance phase, and that an important part of the push-off impulse is generated during the floating phase. Many runners who have an incorrect view about how to run remain passive during the floating phase and only begin searching for tension and power during the support phase. Sprinting is what you do particularly when you are released from the ground.

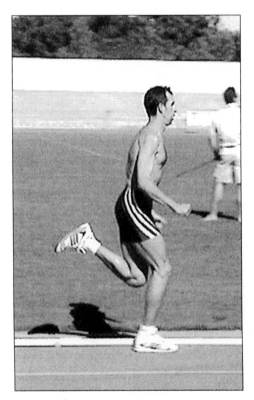

Figure 3.11 Example of a poor running technique
The weight of the body rests completely on the foot of the stance leg during the landing. Because the upper body is leaning forward and the pendular motion of the trailing leg is circular, the knee of the swing leg is still behind that of the stance leg. The running technique must therefore be considered poor.

Errors during the floating phase
- The swing phase is initiated too circularly: the knee lags behind before the forward swing begins. Thereby the ankle is frequently in a position of plantar flexion.

- Although the forward movement might indeed be linear, it is carried out with too little force.
- The knee is not bent far enough (<90°).

The following errors can force the leading leg to 'wait' for the trailing leg. In this way the landing becomes too passive and the foot too far in front of the projection of the body's center of gravity on the ground.

- During the outward swing there is too little tension present in the muscles (i.e. in the hamstrings) and they will not be optimally preloaded with elastic energy.
- There is too much plantar flexion in the ankle of the leading leg and too little tension in the muscles surrounding the ankle.

Foot placement: moment of initial contact

At the moment when the foot makes initial contact with the ground some amount of landing energy is transferred to the body. This energy must be stored as well as possible in the elastic components of the locomotor apparatus in order to be re-used during the thrust of push-off. As little energy as possible should be allowed to flow away or be converted into the heat of friction. In order to preload the tissues well, isometry is required in the muscle fibers (see Section 1.4). The following are requirements for the posture of the body at the moment of initial contact:

- There must not be too much plantar flexion in the ankle before the landing because in that position the muscles of the lower leg will not be able to tighten sufficiently. Just before initial contact, the leg causes powerful backward flexion in the hip, so that tightening the muscles around the ankle will result in a hard landing.
- Because the landing is hard, the foot must not be placed in front of the projection of the body's center of gravity on the ground. When running at speed, the foot does not carry through, but the pressure at foot placement is on the forefoot. During a sprint, the heel does not touch the ground. When the landing is hard, force is immediately applied to the ground, so that placing the foot too far forward will slow the body down.
- As already stated, at the moment of foot strike, the knees are located approximately side by side. The position of one knee in relation to the other at the moment of foot placement is a good indication of the quality of the running technique.
- The positions of the knee and hip at the moment of initial contact are closely related. Because the foot falls approximately on the projection of the body's center of gravity on the ground, an extended knee will be accompanied by an extended hip, while a bent knee will be accompanied by a bent hip (i.e. the athlete 'runs high' or 'sits low'). Running high (knee and hip nearly extended at initial contact) is frequently considered to be the standard. However, there are researchers who have demonstrated that good runners tend to sit somewhat deeper than athletes who run less well.
- The angles of the knee and hip at initial contact are directly related to how the hamstrings function. The gravitational moment with regard to the knee and hip, as well as the lever arm of the hamstrings with regard to the hip joint, vary according to the position of the knee and hip. Therefore, in order to make good use of the hamstrings, it is necessary for an athlete to find a position compatible with his own qualities. While one athlete will be able to convert a somewhat larger external force on the hamstrings into thrust (and thus must sit somewhat

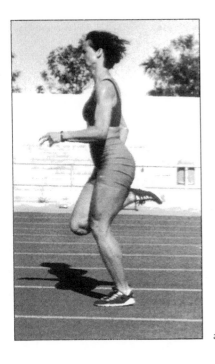
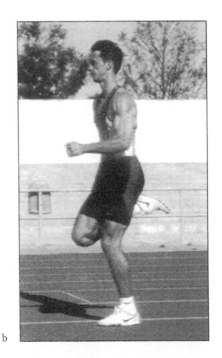

a b

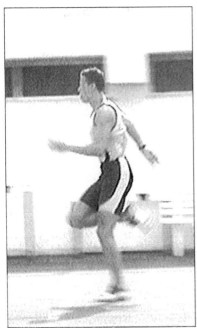
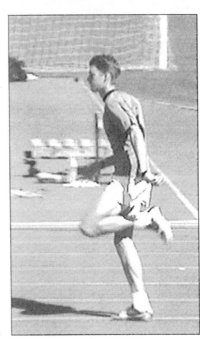

Figure 3.12a–d Correct body postures
Four very good body postures at the
moment the weight of the body comes to
rest completely on the foot of the stance
leg. The knee of the swing leg (c, d) has
already been moved quite high.

c d

deeper), another runner will use his hamstrings more effectively when there is
less prestretch during the landing and be able to unload energy earlier (and consequently running higher).

- The difference between running high and sitting deep is otherwise not that great.
  The position of the hips in both situations differs only by a few centimeters. The
  same is true for the position of the hips in a forward–backward direction. A difference of only a few centimeters can make a position either incorrect (hips too
  far to the rear) or correct. Being able to perfect this type of technical detail requires

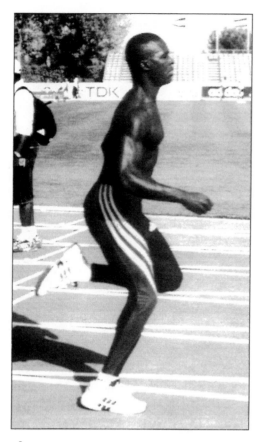

a

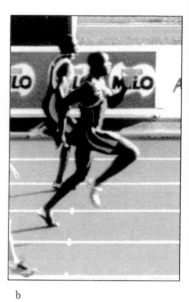

b

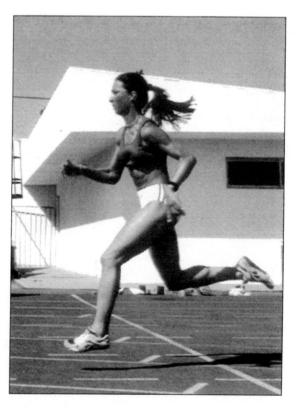

c

Figure 3.13 Body postures
(a, b) Top sprinters who sit relatively deep.
(c) The posture of this runner is incorrect.
The hips are held somewhat too far to
the rear. Therefore, during the landing,
reactivity will not be used optimally.

a lot of insight and belongs in the most advanced levels of technical instruction. During high-speed running, an athlete must never forget that the hamstrings work like a spider in the center of its web and that many of the qualities of an athlete can only become effective if the hamstrings are worked correctly.

The posture of the body at the initial moment of foot placement is therefore upright, with as much body mass possible in the vicinity of the long axis (i.e. knees together and arms held close to the trunk). In this position, the muscles can be tightened better, and thus are better able to absorb external forces and store elastic energy. This body posture is also seen when one jumps reactively on one leg. Thus when learning to understand how the forces of propulsion work, photographs taken exactly when all the body segments are grouped together close to the longitudinal axis will be more useful than photographs that have been taken during toe-off (as is the usual case).

Errors during initial contact

- At the moment of initial contact, the knee of the swing leg is still well behind that of the stance leg. At the same time, the foot is being placed in front of the projection of the body's center of gravity on the ground. The landing is consequently soft in order to keep the body from slowing down, so that the landing energy will be allowed to dissipate.
- There is too little tension around the ankle and too much dorsiflexion develops after the landing. As a result, the foot will leave the ground too late at the end of push-off.
- The knee and hip make angles that are not in agreement with the quality of the hamstrings. The thrusting action of the hamstrings therefore remains limited.

Thrust phase

Because backward flexion has already been initiated in the front leg during the floating phase, the thrust phase for the stance leg will already have begun at the moment of foot placement. The ground contact time, and thus the time during which thrust can be generated, is especially brief. A tendency to exert a lot of force at the beginning of the support phase can be observed more frequently in top runners. In sprinters, the ground contact time at speed is often considered to be a measure of quality in the runner. The ground contact time in good runners is 0.07–0.09 s. Even long-distance runners are beginning to attach more importance to keeping the ground contact time brief. Some runners even continue to land on the forefoot during an entire 10,000-m race. Muscles working reactively are most suited to such rapid loading and unloading of force. The hamstrings play a very important role during speed running, in directing the force of thrust toward the rear (see Section 1.6). The key to thrust during high-speed running can therefore be found in the reactivity of the hamstrings.

In addition to muscle reactivity (coupled with as much isometry possible in the muscle fibers), there is also important concentric activity, especially in the monoarticular backward flexors of the hip (i.e. the gluteus maximus).

Angular velocity in the hip joint in the direction of backward flexion during the support phase is particularly rapid during high-speed running. Being able to exert force when the angular velocity is rapid is one of the most limiting factors for achieving top speed. At the moment when the foot of the stance leg touches ground, its speed will be zero. At the same time, the forward velocity of the hip is high, so that the thigh is pulled to the rear.

Because the foot lags behind, backward flexion develops in the hip of the stance leg. The speed of the movement is determined by the velocity of the hip in relation to the ground. If during backward flexion the muscles need to exert extra force in the direction of the backward flexion, the speed of contraction will have to be in agreement with the angular velocity already present in the hip. The high speed of contraction that is 'prescribed' for speed running is not well suited to exerting a lot of force. After all, it can be concluded from the force–velocity diagram that speed and force are not mutually compatible for muscles (in this case particularly for the gluteus maximus).

The high speed of contraction imposed on the muscles when the stance leg is lagging behind can be partly compensated for by moving the pelvis. Such compensation during running is particularly important and effective. The ways in which the pelvis can move are discussed below, from the perspective of movement in the sagittal, transverse, and frontal planes, whereby movement in the sagittal and transverse planes is often compensated for by a high angular velocity in the hip (Ounpuu 1994).

Movement in the sagittal plane

Movement of the pelvis in the sagittal plane contributes the most when compensating for the 'imposed' speed of contraction of the hip-joint backward flexors during the stance phase. The pelvis is able to tilt forward, as well as to the rear. During the support phase, the pelvis tilts forward. The angular velocity in the hip joint in the direction of backward flexion therefore decreases because the range of movement for the leg allowed by the running speed can be spread over a number of joints: namely, the hip joint and the lumbar segment of the spinal column. The monoarticular muscles, which must create backward flexion (notably the gluteus maximus), need to shorten less quickly, and therefore can exert more force.

For the natural pattern of movement observed in man, backward flexion in the hip and forward pelvic tilt always occur together. The degree of hip movement possible for backward flexion is only 13° and is inhibited by strong ligaments on the front surface of the hip. Consequently, the leg can only be moved far to the back when the pelvis is tilted forward.

Forward pelvic tilt is brought about as the dorsal muscles (the erector spinae) and the iliopsoas work on the side of the swing leg. The erector spinae is particularly strong and has a large lever arm with regard to the hip joint. Research on how the erector spinae functions is always done during slow movement. It has been shown that the muscle fibers are not only capable of exerting a great deal of force, but that the passive structures also have an important function. One can conclude from this that the dorsal muscles are able to work reactively and contribute to the short powerful discharge of force during push-off.

The iliopsoas is responsible for forward flexion in the hip joint on the side of the swing leg, after it has left the ground. There is a particularly large increase in the velocity of the swing leg in a forward direction. The stance leg, however, lags behind during the support phase (the velocity of the foot is 0 m/s during the support phase) and halfway through the next swing its forward velocity is already much faster than the running speed. The large force exerted on the thigh by the iliopsoas in the swing leg is also exerted on the pelvis, which threatens to tilt forward.

Forward pelvic tilt also occurs when the above-mentioned muscles work even slightly, because the pelvis is pulled forward during support by the stance leg, which 'lags behind'. However, if these muscles function well, they will strengthen not only the pattern of movement mentioned, but also thrust.

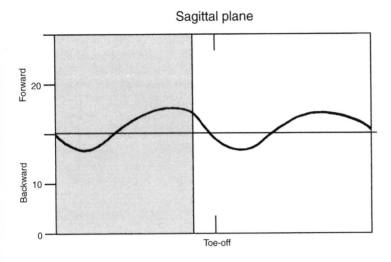

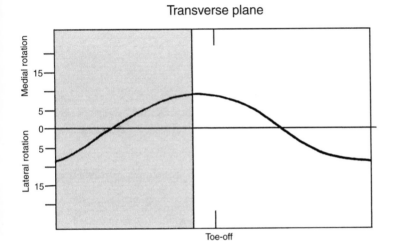

Figure 3.14 Movement of the pelvis during slow running
The pelvis moves in the sagittal and transverse planes during low-speed running. The characteristics of the movements vary between individuals and according to the speed.

Forward pelvic tilt also causes the hamstrings of the stance leg to stretch so that they can work more reactively. The powerful action of the iliopsoas in the swing leg and of the dorsal muscles strengthens hamstring reactivity in the stance leg. Forward pelvic tilt facilitates not only the gluteus maximus as it works concentrically, but also the hamstrings as they work reactively. Thrust during push-off is therefore brought about by an entire chain of muscles, not only those active in the stance leg, but also those in the swing leg and trunk. Just as during the floating phase, the pelvis functions as a lever, transferring a great deal of energy from one part of the body to another by means of small degrees of movement. In this context, it is interesting to compare the range over which the pelvis moves while running and the storage capacity per millimeter stretch in the series-linked elastic components (SEC) of muscle. The muscles attached to the pelvis often have a large lever arm with respect to the pivot of the pelvis. The pelvis need only move a few degrees to load the SEC segments of an attached muscle (if they are indeed located within this favorable range of stretch) with large amounts of elastic energy. The pretension that is needed to operate within this positive range is very high during high-speed running. Even small degrees of movement are important, and should certainly not be overlooked.

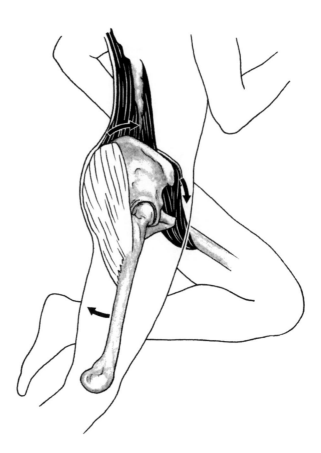

Figure 3.15 Facilitating the speed of contraction of the gluteus maximus
The dorsal muscles and the iliopsoas of the swing leg work to tilt the pelvis forward. The 'prescribed' angular velocity of the hip joint therefore decreases so that the gluteus maximus can exert force at a lower speed of contraction.

Movement in the transverse plane

Pelvic movement in the transverse plane can also compensate somewhat for the high speed of contraction 'prescribed' for the gluteus maximus. During the support phase, medial rotation develops in the hip joint of the stance leg. The hip on the side of the swing leg moves forward. This medial rotation is carried out actively, and results from the action of muscles (the front gluteus segments) causing medial rotation and from axial torsion that develops during the floating and support phases. Axial torsion will develop when the right leg takes a step, by which the left pelvic half moves forward while at the same time the right shoulder and arm move forward and the left shoulder and arm move towards the rear. If the upper body moves powerfully, the result will be strong medial rotation in the hip. This effect can develop in two ways:

- Torsion will develop because the oblique abdominal muscles are stressed reactively during each stride. At the end of the support phase, these muscles are repeatedly preloaded by stretch (during right-leg support, the diagonal runs upward from the right hip to the left). During the floating and support phases that follow, force is discharged from this diagonal stretch (the right hip and the left side of the trunk move forward). Subsequently, the other diagonal is pre-stretched. In this manner, both diagonals of the oblique abdominal muscles work in turn.

- Torsion, and therefore medial rotation in the hip, will develop due to the effect of pseudo-rotation. During pseudo-rotation, rotating one part of the body generates a counteractive rotation in another part of the body. Imagine someone sitting on a desk chair that can swivel in circles. He quickly moves his right arm forward and

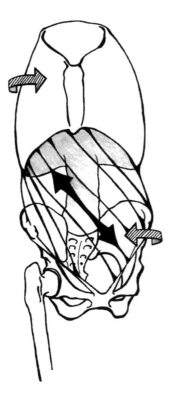

Figure 3.16 Movement of the pelvis in the transverse plane
The action of diagonally running abdominal muscles (black arrow) and pseudo-rotation (hatched arrows) cause the pelvis to move in the transverse plane (like medial rotation in the hip).

his left arm backward. As a reaction, his knees, and therefore the lower part of his body, will move toward the right. This movement toward the right can be compared with medial rotation in the hip joint when standing on the right leg (Cappozzo 1983).

By way of active medial rotation during running, the speed, necessary for rapid backward flexion in the hip joint, with which the gluteus maximus contracts, can be compensated for somewhat. Thus the position of the gluteus maximus can be both flexed backward as well as rotated laterally with respect to the hip joint. Consequently, medial rotation works eccentrically with regard to the gluteus maximus, so that this muscle need not shorten as rapidly and will be able to work more powerfully during medial rotation and backward flexion than during lateral rotation and backward flexion. To carry out this so-called 'hip swing', much force and good coordination is required in the muscle groups that bring about torsion in the trunk (i.e. the dorsal and abdominal muscles, the muscles surrounding the shoulder girdle, and the muscles around the hip). This movement of the pelvis possibly has less effect than forward pelvic tilt. The extent of hip swing in sprinters varies greatly, from being invisible to the naked eye, to being visibly manifest (e.g. in the sprinters Merlene Ottey and Donovan Bailey). However, when the level of running performance is high, it is worth the effort to pay attention to hip swing.

Movement in the frontal plane
Although pelvic movement in the frontal plane does not help facilitate the angular velocity in the hip, it is important for the vertical component during push-off. After foot placement, the free hip is moved upward by the action of the gluteal muscles in the stance leg and the dorsal muscles on the side of the swing leg. By increasing the vertical component, the floating phase lasts longer and the stride lengthens.

Movement takes place in the frontal plane, and is therefore relatively independent of other thrusting movements. The magnitude of this movement is substantially different from one runner to the next, ranging from being invisible to the naked eye to being expressed emphatically. Magnitude says nothing about whether a movement will be effective. A small but powerful motion can also result in a good vertical impulse. During running, pelvic movement in the frontal plane is linked to how well the inverse-extension reflex functions. A runner who moves his leg particularly forward after it leaves the ground (stumble reflex) and does not bend his knee too emphatically will frequently be passive when it comes to moving the pelvis in the frontal plane. In the most negative case, the free hip will continue to droop even during the support phase.

A runner who is able to use his pelvis as a lever quite well might give the impression of needing to move less at high speed. The push-off is a powerful well-aimed strike, unloading to the ground within 0.07–0.11 s a large amount of force originating in the trunk, arms, and pelvic girdle via groups of biarticular muscles (the hamstrings and the gastrocnemius) (see Section 1.6.1). The weakest link in the chain will determine the effectiveness of thrust. Because, in practice, the leverage effect of the pelvis is generally the weak link, teaching a runner more about this function is recommended.

The gastrocnemius and the hamstrings work simultaneously to an important degree during the support phase. They transfer to the hip and ankle energy resulting from the action of the monoarticular hip extenders with regard to the knee. How much of this energy is transferred to either the hip or knee must be well coor-

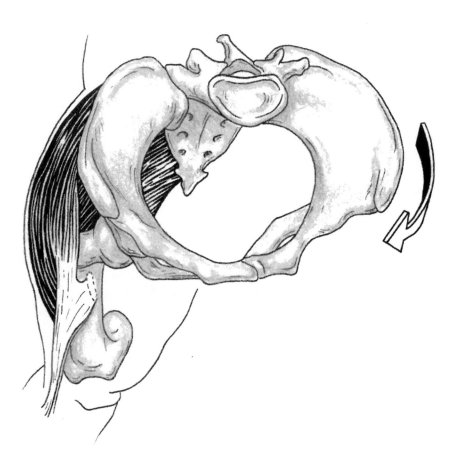

Figure 3.17   The pelvis, viewed laterally from above
The fibers of the gluteus maximus originate medially and run downward toward the side. This diagonal trajectory causes rotation in the hip (moving the free hip forward), so that it functions eccentrically with regard to the muscle.

dinated. If the action of the hamstrings becomes too dominant with regard to the gastrocnemius, then too much dorsiflexion will develop and last too long in the ankle. As a result, the transition between the support and swing phases will be slow, allowing axial rotation to develop (see the moment of toe-off, p. 174). One can learn to coordinate the gastrocnemius and the hamstrings to work well together by learning to control movement in the ankle (i.e. learning to hold the ankle stable).

After all the stored energy has been rapidly discharged, the support phase is kept brief, so that there is a rapid, linear transition to an open chain at the moment of toe-off.

Errors during thrust
- The athlete only runs with his legs, thus spreading push-off over a large part of the support phase. The trunk hangs, so to speak, passively from the spinal column. There is too little tension in the abdominal and gluteal muscles.
- The athlete has not built up enough tension in his calves so that force from the hip cannot be unloaded to the ground, but rather becomes invalidated, dissipating in the ankle. The system through which the gastrocnemius transfers force does not function correctly.
- By allowing the 'free' hip (on the side of the swing leg) to dangle during the support phase, the athlete will lose a lot of energy derived from the ground reactive force. The shoulder and hip on the side of the stance leg are closer together than those on the side of the swing leg. This 'invalidation' of energy makes it impossible to maintain a high running speed. Because the athlete must now run at a very high stride frequency, he can only maintain his speed for a short period.

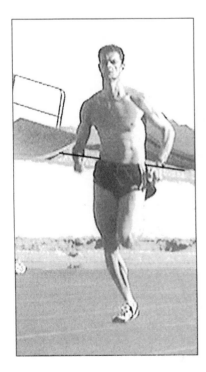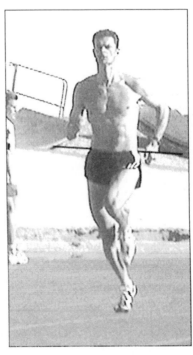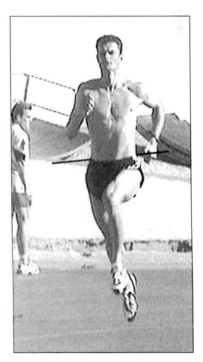

Figure 3.18 A runner demonstrating a large degree of pelvic movement in the frontal plane
Even a slight (perhaps difficult to observe) amount of movement might be sufficient to provide a vertical impulse for push-off.

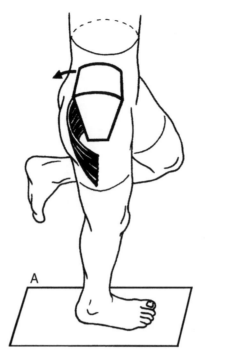
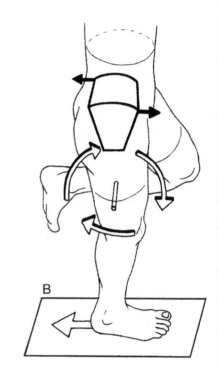

Figure 3.19   Pendular motion of the legs
If no forces are working to hold the pelvis stationary, the gluteus maximus will pull the free side of the pelvis toward the rear (A). At the same time, the backward pendular motion of the stance leg will push the ipsilateral half of the pelvis forward (B). In fact, this pendular oscillation is rotation of the leg, by which the axis of rotation tries to move in the direction of the center of mass of the leg. The swing leg oscillates in the opposite direction, attempting to push the free half of the pelvis backward. This threatens to cause powerful lateral rotation in the hip joint of the stance leg.

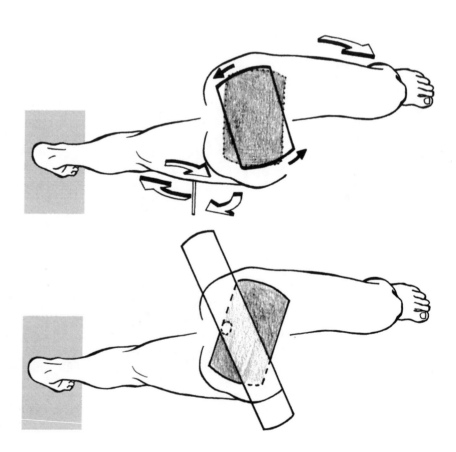

Figure 3.20   Medial rotation
The motion of the legs and the gluteus maximus is responsible for an lateral rotational moment in the hip joint of the stance leg (top). During running, however, medial rotation develops in the hip of the stance leg. A relatively large amount of power will be needed (from the abdominal muscles and pseudo-rotation) to achieve this medial rotation. Having a powerful upper body and wide shoulders will be particularly advantageous for a sprinter (bottom).

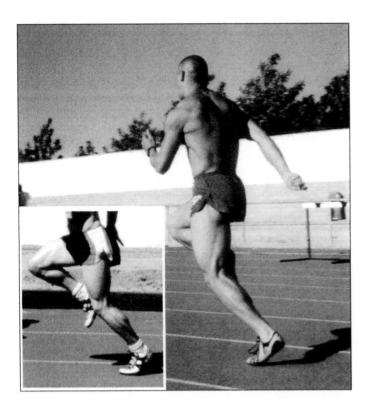

Figure 3.21   The way in which the hamstrings and gastrocnemius work
The hamstrings and gastrocnemius work at the same time halfway through the support phase. Both muscles slow knee extension. Energy is transferred to the hip by the hamstrings and to the ankle by the gastrocnemius. Both muscle groups must be well coordinated to function together.

- There is too little tension in the hamstrings. Although the runner demonstrates a high stride frequency and his body posture is correct, he has little forward thrust.

Arm action

When running at speed, it is necessary to move the arms powerfully (Cavanagh 1990, Bhowmick et al 1998). This is apparent from observing that a good sprinter always has a well-developed torso. Clearly the action of the arms has a greater function during running than merely maintaining balance or compensating for small disturbances in body posture. The action of the arms actually contributes in one of three ways to the amount of speed that a runner can develop:

- By increasing thrust in the direction of progression. When running at speed, the upper body is held erect. As a result, the forward force provided by one arm to support push-off is just as great as the counteractive force moving the other arm in the opposite direction. The net result in the forward direction is equal to zero. There is no direct contribution to forward thrust during speed running.
- By increasing the vertical component of push-off. After the arms have swung past the trunk, their impulse to swing is given a vertical component. This supports the vertical impulse of the entire body and contributes to the length of the stride. The order of magnitude of this contribution is about 7–10% of the total vertical impulse.
- By influencing movement around the long axis. The most important function of the arms is related to movements (rotation and torsion) occurring around the long axis. At the moment of greatest thrust, the arms are positioned alongside the body, with one arm directed to the front and the other arm directed to the

rear. When the runner is standing on his right leg, the coupled forces result in an impulse to rotate to the left, which can compensate for axial rotation and cause torsion around the long axis. When an athlete's technique is good, there will be either only slight or no axial rotation to be compensated for. In that case, arm action is chiefly used to increase the torsion, which will facilitate backward flexion in the stance leg. The force that is required to carry out medial rotation in the hip of the stance leg by means of torsion is very large. When the left leg is brought forward forcefully, the ipsilateral side of the pelvis threatens to twist backward. When backward flexion in the contralateral leg (at the end of the swing phase and during the support phase) is powerful, the right side of the

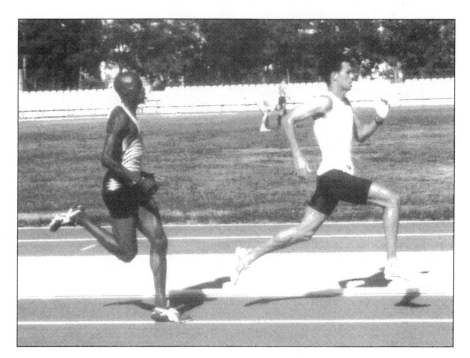

Figure 3.22a Arm movement during running
Torsion provides support when the arms work well. Arm movement is emphasized when the arms are positioned next to the body (left-hand runner). In particular, moving the arms to the rear should be carried out forcefully. Swinging the arms results in a posture in which the elbow of the back arm is raised high, while the elbow of the front arm is just in front of the trunk (right-hand runner).

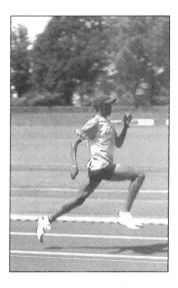
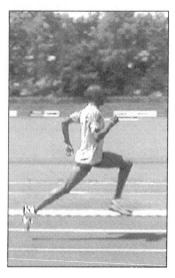

Figure 3.22b,c Arm movement during running
The runner tries to increase the vertical impulse by swinging his arms. The hand of the leading arm swings high, while the elbow of the trailing arm is rather low (left-hand runner). After a correction, the runner tries swinging his arms only to increase torsion (right-hand runner). Movement of the arms toward the rear is emphasized as the arms come alongside the body. The arms have changed position by the end of the swing, and the runner feels more tension in his body. He realizes that thrust is supported by movement of his arms.

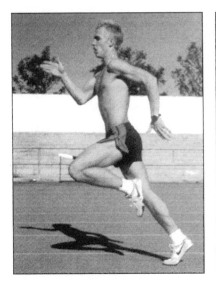

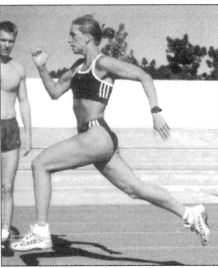

Figure 3.22d,e   Arm movement during running
The runner tries to increase the vertical impulse by swinging his arms, and therefore only creates slight torsion (left-hand runner: technically incorrect). A comparable degree of movement results, however, when an extreme degree of torsion (right-hand runner: technically correct) is induced.

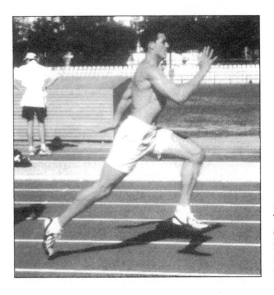

Figure 3.22f   Arm movement during running
The runner tries to support push-off in the direction of progression and swings his front arm up high. The trunk tends to lean forward so that rotation develops around the long axis.

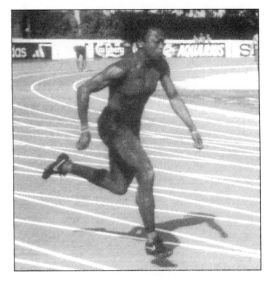

Figure 3.22g   Arm movement during running
The position of the elbow can change from being nearly extended to bent to about 90°. The sprinter is accelerating. Because the support phase lasts longer, there is enough time for arm movement to be circular rather than completely linear (favorable for torsion). Therefore the arms will be kept somewhat closer along side the body.

pelvis will threaten to move toward the front. The impulse transmitted to the pelvis as the legs make their scissor-like movement is thus opposite to the direction generated by the torsion. The counteractive force of torsion (together with the force from the muscles generating medial rotation around the hip) must therefore be much greater than what is simply needed to overcome the inertia of the pelvis. From this it follows that the force developed by the shoulder girdle must be large. For this reason, an athlete needs to develop strong muscles in the upper part of the body.

Conclusions regarding arm action

The linear support of push-off during speed running is slight (0% horizontal and 7–10% vertical). Torsion provides a lot of support for push-off. Being able to generate torsion powerfully is therefore the most important reason why a sprinter should develop strength in the upper body. Such torsion partly results from pseudo-rotation (action–reaction) and partly from the transfer of force by abdominal muscles. In order to execute torsion correctly, coordination between the muscles surrounding the shoulder girdle and the abdominal and small gluteal muscles is important.

During speed running, the action of the arms is kept within the sagittal plane as much as possible. The coupling of forces in order to generate rotation would be most advantageous if the arms could make a circular movement around the longitudinal axis. This is not possible, however, because the movement is so rapid. Therefore, the arm movement must be linear. When the arms oscillate linearly up and down in front of the body, the coupling of forces is less advantageous for torsion than if the motion takes place in the sagittal plane, which makes the former motion unadvisable.

Trainers place much emphasis on holding the elbows at an angle of 90° during speed running. In practice, however, it appears that good runners (e.g. Lynford Christie) frequently hold their arms more or less outstretched. Thus there is room for many variations in implementation. It is more important to be alert to whether the action of the arms results in good torsion, is carried out in the sagittal plane, and is synchronized well with the motion of the legs.

Errors during arm action

- The arms do not move correctly in the sagittal plane and torsion is not optimal.
- Arm movement is not well coordinated with the motion of the legs.
- There is too little tension in the abdominal muscles, so that the transfer of force is limited. The swinging motion of the arms lasts for a longer than optimal period of time, rather than being short and powerful.

3.2.4 Summary

One of the first requirements for speed running is to avoid rotation along the long axis. To accomplish this, it is quite important that the foot leaves the ground early and that the swing is started rapidly and remains linear. Sufficient tension in the ankle, a correct vertical posture for the trunk, and abdominal muscles that work reactively are required. During the swing phase that follows, the elastic components of the leading leg will be preloaded. Just before foot placement, the leading leg will make a powerful backward flexion. The moment of initial contact after the swing phase must be hard, followed immediately thereafter by the application of force. Push-off has already begun at the moment of initial contact, and the knees must at least be side by side. At that moment, the arms are positioned alongside the body and can thus support torsion, which is an active movement that facilitates push-off. The elastic energy is unloaded during thrust. The hamstrings have an important function in directing the force of push-off toward the rear. Sufficient tension in the dorsal muscles and the ankle of the stance leg is needed to control the action of the hamstrings. The gluteus maximus works concentrically and is the major motor driving the motion. The gastrocnemius has an important function in transporting energy to the push-off foot. At the moment of thrust, the pelvis works like a lever, transmitting forces from the trunk and swing leg to the stance leg. The pelvis can move in the sagittal, transverse, and frontal planes. When the push-off is carried out correctly, the total range of movement can thus be divided between a large number of joints, and the athlete will be able to unload a great deal of energy onto the ground surface within a very short time span. Consequently, the push-off will be brief and rotation around the long axis can be avoided.

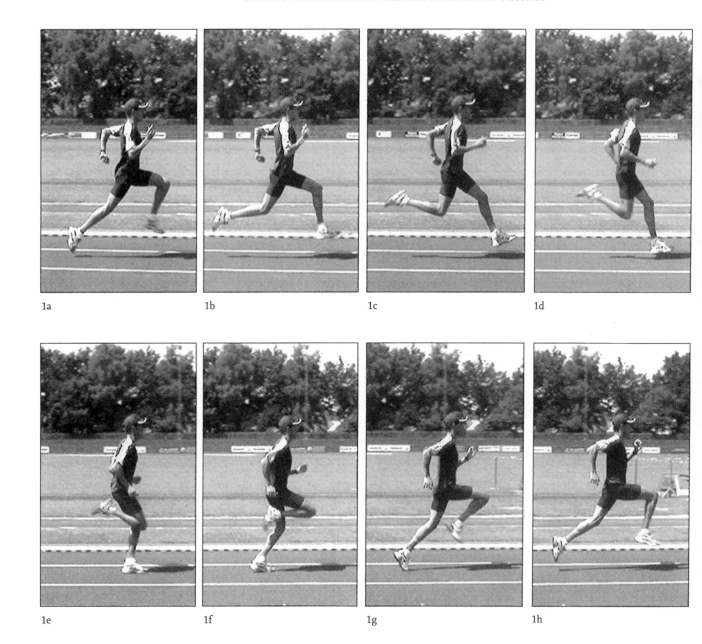

1a   1b   1c   1d

1e   1f   1g   1h

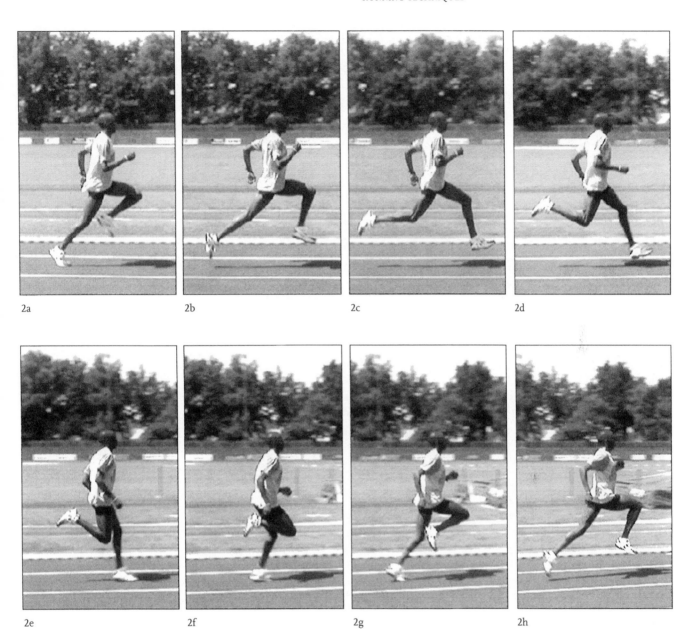

2a   2b   2c   2d

2e   2f   2g   2h

S3.1   Series 1a–h and 2a–h
Two top athletes (800 m) with very good techniques. The upper body is held well upright and long-axis
rotation is avoided. There is rather high vertical displacement of the body during the floating phase.
The large amount of landing energy which results can be re-used very well. Here running is very
reactive (regulated by good pendular motion by the swing leg). Torsion is not excessive and is very
well timed. Series 2 shows a stronger runner who tries to use more of this force. His body has
more spring during the support phase. There is also more torsion.

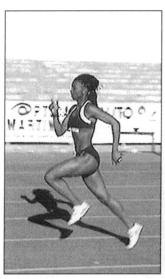
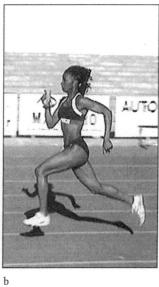
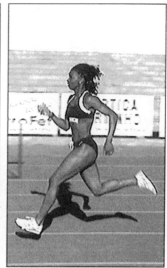
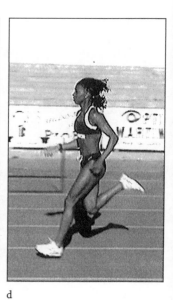

a   b   c   d

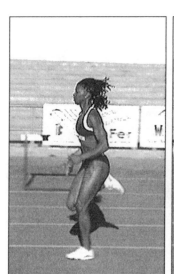
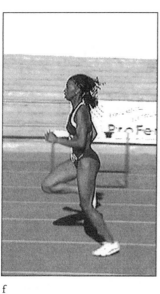
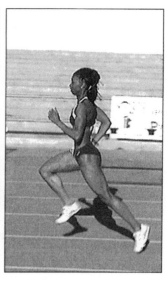

e   f   g

S3.2 Series a–g
The technique is good, with the trunk held upright (no long-axis rotation); torsion and arm movement are correct. In particular, foot placement is excellent (constantly close to a neutral position). Vertical displacement, however, is slight, so that the cadence must be very rapid. Improving the vertical impulse (pelvic movement in the frontal plane) would be a useful change in technique.

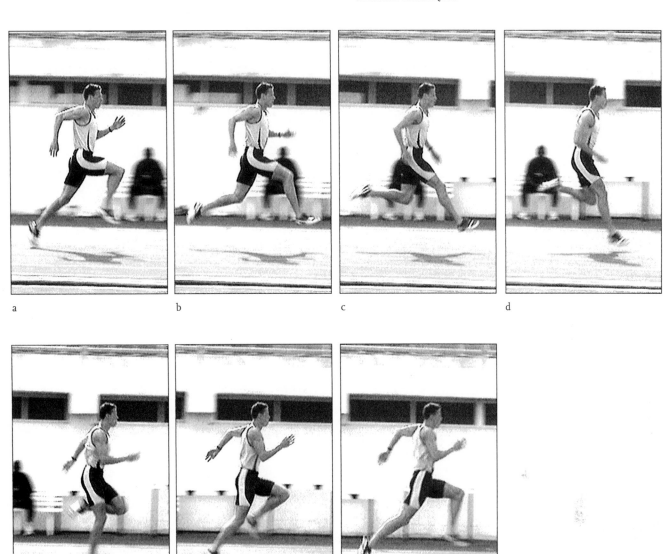

a b c d

e f g

S3.3 Series a–g
A very good sprint technique. The knee is not totally extended during push-off and the trunk is
held well upright. There is no long-axis rotation (a). Vertical displacement is quite high during the
floating phase (b). The trailing swing leg rapidly moves forward linearly (although there is somewhat
too much plantar flexion in the foot) (c–d). Consequently, the scissor-like movement is quite powerful,
and complete preparation for push-off has begun before landing (note arm movement). Foot strike is
hard, and the knee of the swing leg is positioned particularly far forward (e). In this way, energy from
the foot strike can quickly and correctly be returned. Push-off is brief, and torsion is limited but well
timed (f, g).

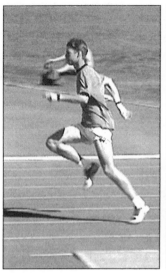
1a

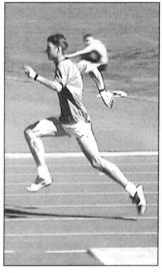
1b

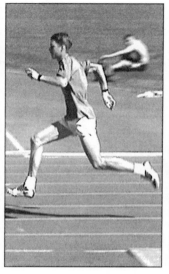
1c

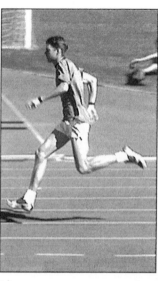
1d

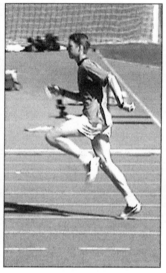
1e

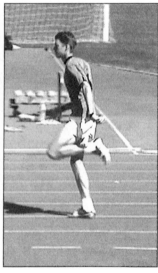
1f

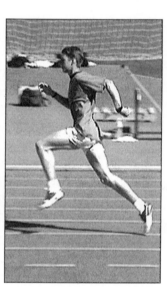
1g

1h

S3.4   Series 1a–h and 2a–h

Two young runners whose strength and training still need to be developed. Both runners are leaning forward, so that there is a threat of forward and long-axis rotation. The swing is initiated too late and the foot is placed in front of the ground projection of the hip (1a and 2a).

The runner (a natural talent) shown in series 1a–h has begun the swing before his knee is completely extended during push-off. Good linear swing begins directly after the foot has left the ground (1c). Consequently, the scissor-like movement is powerful and results in foot placement beneath (1f) the hip (no slowing down; in 1e the foot has not yet touched ground). The knee of the swing leg swings upward and far forward. The extra vertical impulse needed to compensate for forward rotation can be realized because of the position of the swing leg. Because of this runner's natural talent, the incorrect position of the trunk will not result in loss of landing energy. He can be instructed how to hold his upper body more erect and direct thrust more horizontally, making torsion more effective.

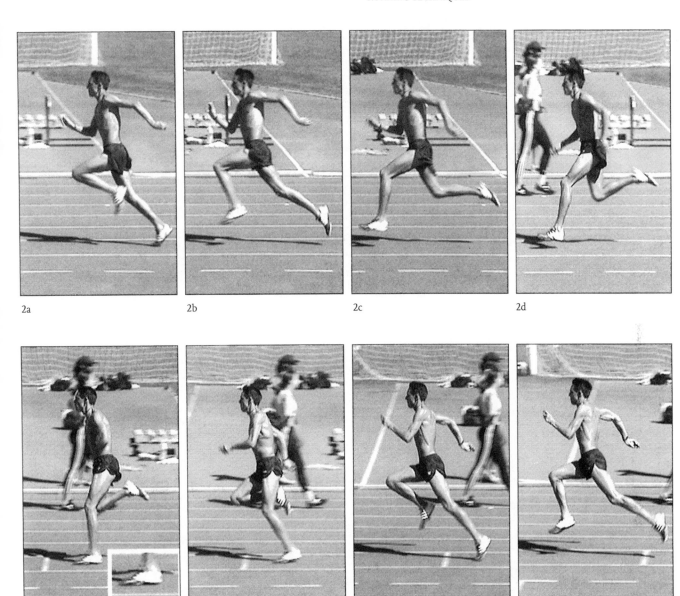

2a 2b 2c 2d

2e 2f 2g 2h

The runner shown in series 2a–h uses a technique resembling that shown in series 1a–h. However, there are a number of important differences in the details. Initiation of leg swing is somewhat slower and less linear (2c), resulting in a less powerful oscillation. The knee of the swing leg moves higher later in the support phase, leading to less vertical displacement during push-off. Therefore, the leading foot touches ground while it is still in front of the ground projection of the hip (2e; compare with 1e). Here foot strike must be softer than that shown in series 1a–h, and landing energy will be lost. The incorrect posture of the trunk will result in less reactivity. Reactivity can be improved by instructing a runner how to position the trunk and implement swing. Comparison of the two series shows that even very small differences in technique can have important consequences.

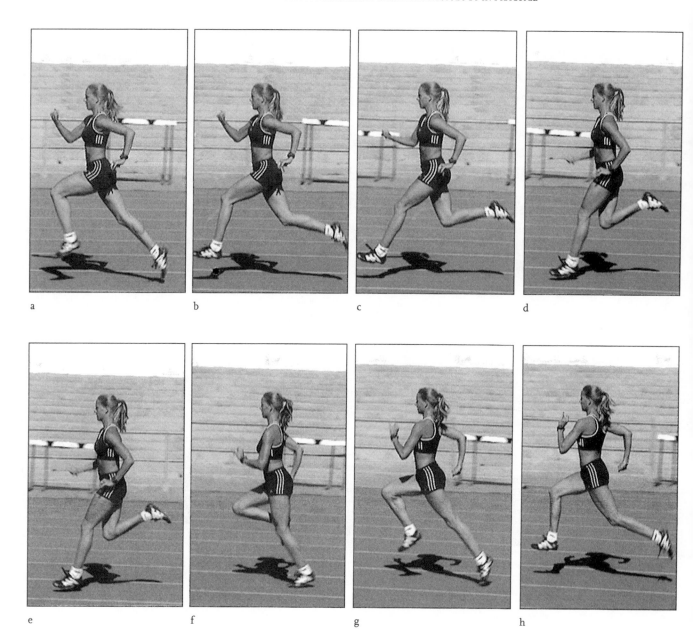

a   b   c   d

e   f   g   h

S3.5 Series a–h
The trailing leg swings linearly, beginning movement directly after push-off (the ankle returns to a neutral position correctly). Consequently, the legs are positioned well during the landing (e). The arms move too late with respect to the motion of the legs (e, f), causing too much torsion to develop too late (g, h). Leg movement can be supported effectively by initiating good arm movement somewhat earlier (alongside the body).

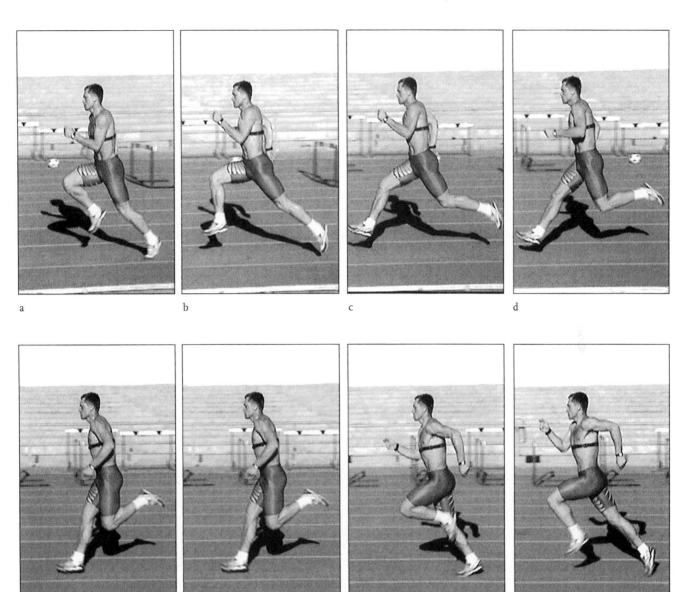

S3.6 *Series a–h*
A powerful runner whose outward swing of the leading leg is extreme and return of trailing swing leg to the front is delayed (c, d). A soft landing results, allowing energy to be lost (plantar flexion in the foot just before landing (e)).

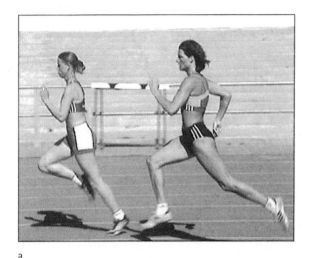

a

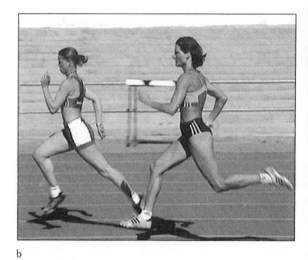

b

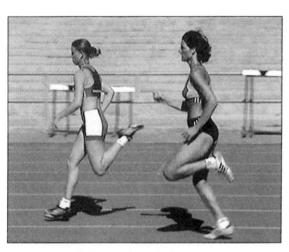

c

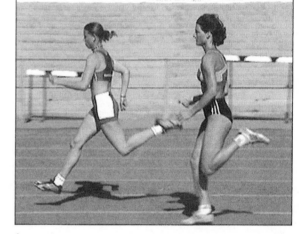

d

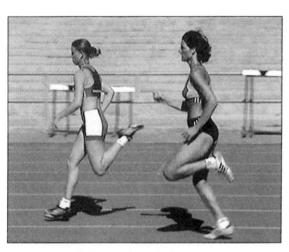

e

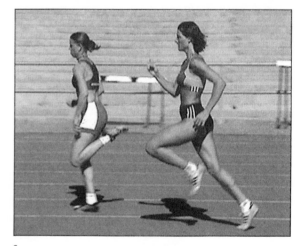

f

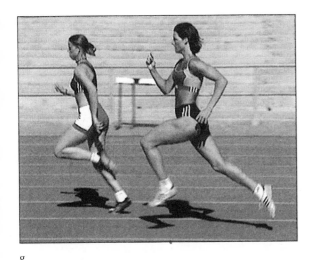

g

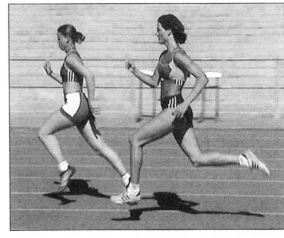

h

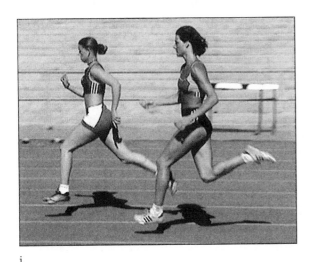

i

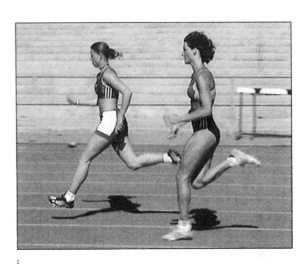

j

S3.7   Series a–j
The front runner combines late and 'circular' return of her trailing swing leg to the front with an extreme degree of plantar flexion in the ankle. The leading leg only swings slightly upward before backward flexion in the hip joint is initiated. Because the forward leg must 'wait' for the trailing leg, it has little time to accelerate backward during the oscillation. Therefore, the motion lacks power. Accordingly, the arms move within a small range, exhibiting little impulse. The last runner begins the swing phase much better, holding the foot in a correct neutral position (e). The oscillation that follows is nevertheless too passive and does not result in a powerful short push-off (compare (d) and (j) with Series S3.2). Correcting the movement of the arms (a powerful start alongside the body toward the rear) could rapidly help to improve push-off.

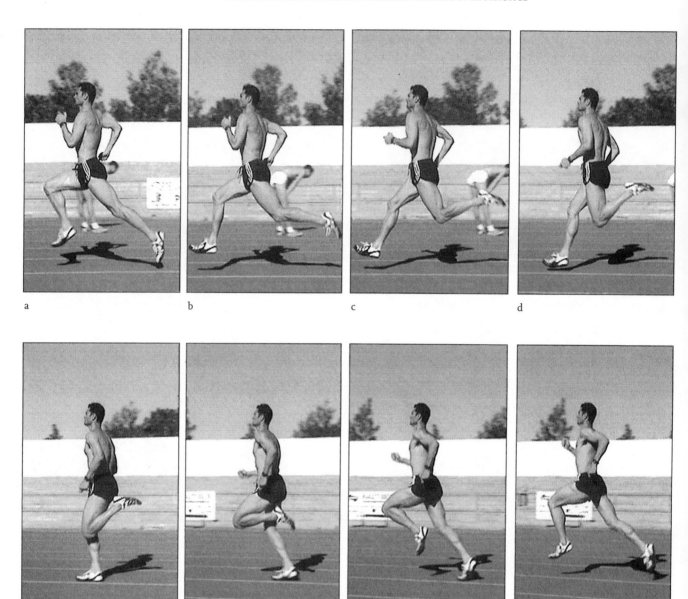

a b c d

e f g h

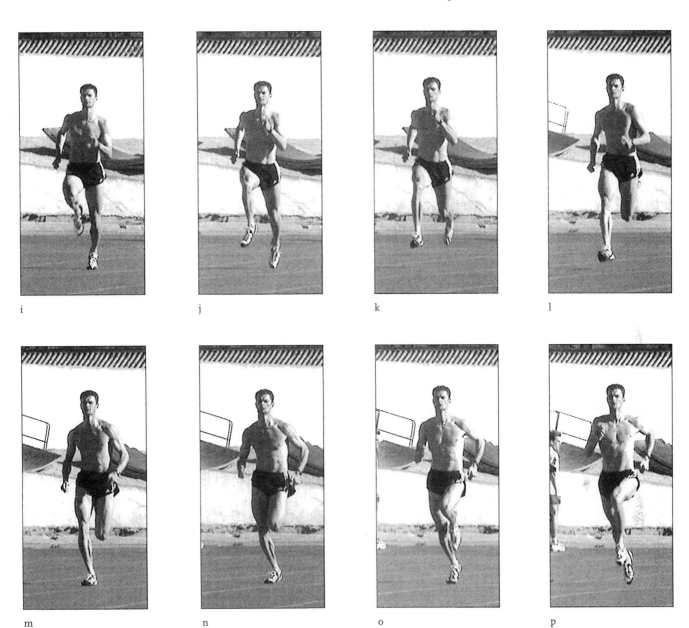

i   j   k   l

m   n   o   p

S3.8   Series a–p

The swing phase is too circular and not begun immediately after the foot has left the ground. The next foot strike cannot be optimally hard (braking moment). Furthermore, there is relatively little tension, so that during the support phase the body mass sags deeply (f) and push-off toward the back is lengthened. Both conditions will make the running cycle slower and decrease reactivity during push-off.

163

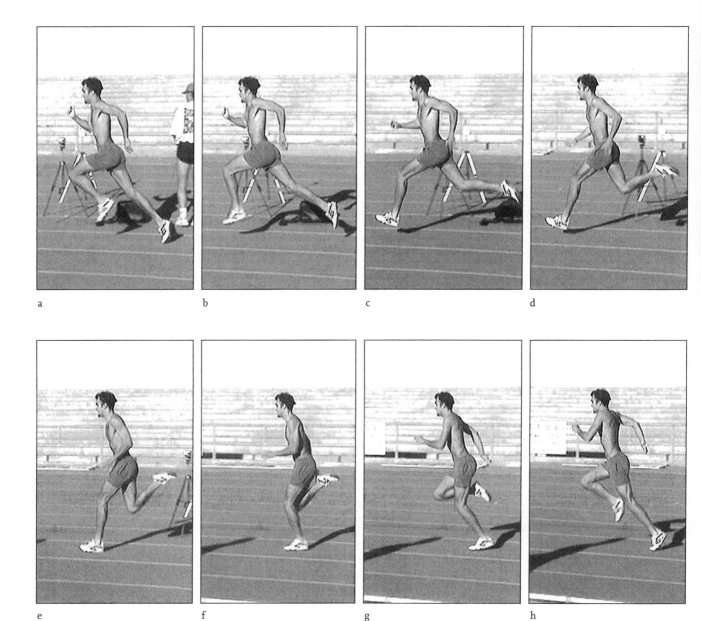

a   b   c   d

e   f   g   h

S3.9 Series a–h
The runner hangs forward, extending far to the back. The long-axis and forward rotations that develop must be compensated for. Therefore, the foot must be placed far in front of the ground projection of the hips (e). Foot strike decelerates the body, and much of the ground reaction force will be lost.

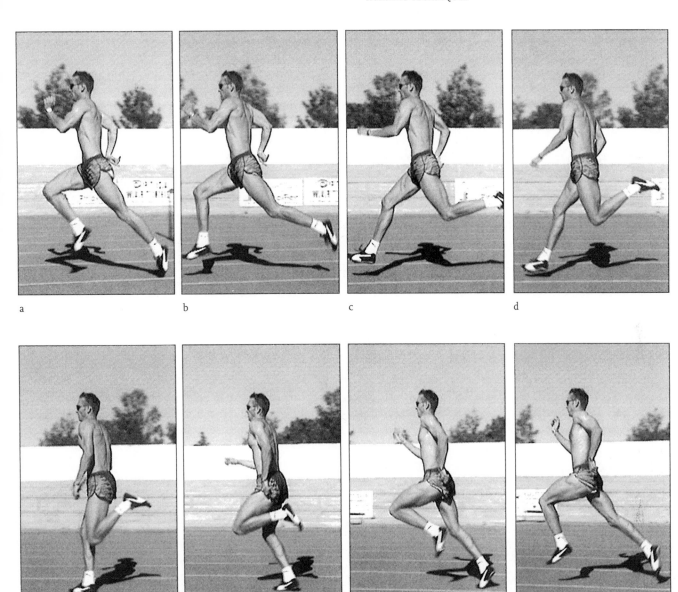

a b c d

e f g h

S3.10   Series a–h
The trunk is held well upright. The pendular oscillation of the trailing leg is reasonably good after
the foot has left the ground. However, because the runner tries to give extra thrust at the end of the
support phase, a lot of long-axis rotation develops, which must be compensated for during the next
support phase. To do this, backward flexion in the leading leg is slowed in order to place the foot in
front of the ground projection of the hip (which works to decelerate). Being aware of keeping ground
contact brief can dramatically improve running.

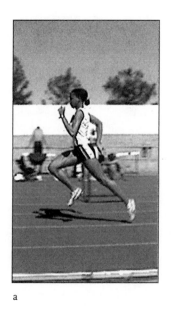

a

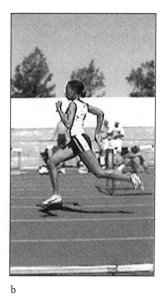

b

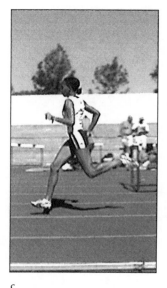

c

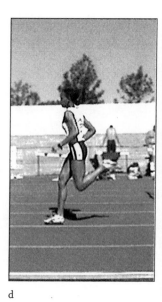

d

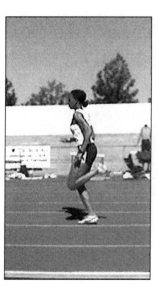

e

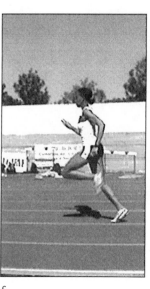

f

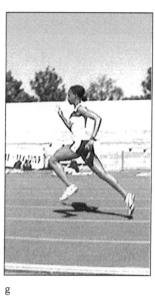

g

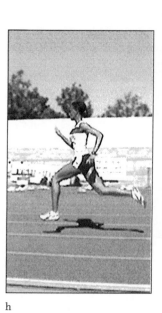

h

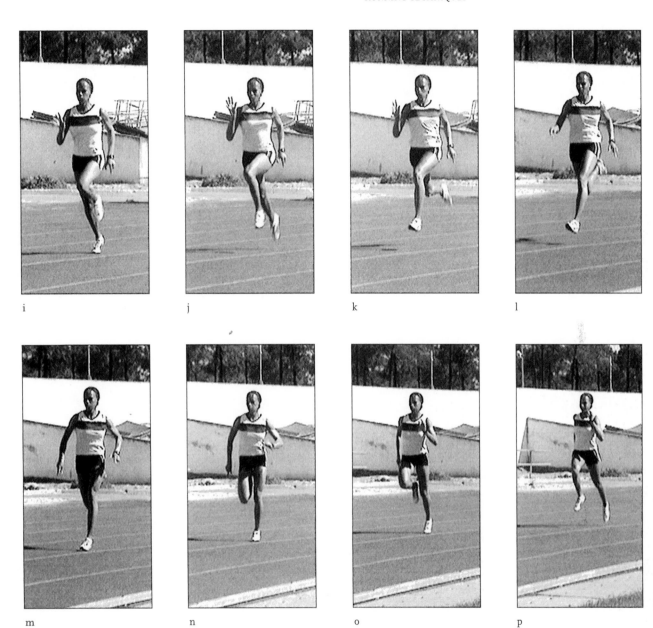

i j k l

m n o p

S3.11 Series a–p
This runner demonstrates a good neutral technique with no long-axis rotation and a good body posture
during the landing. The knee is not completely horizontal when brought forward. However, the legs
oscillate well. Compare with Series S3.2.

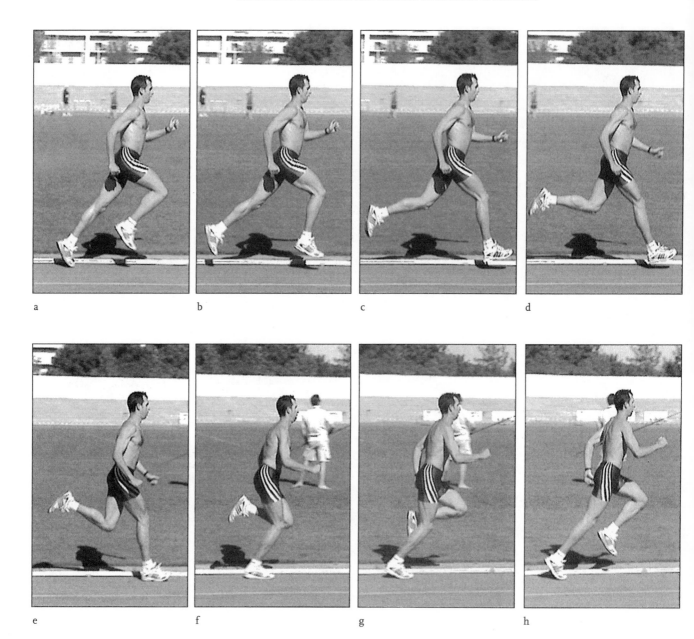

a b c d

e f g h

S3.12   Series a–h
The trunk leans forward, and the circular pendular oscillation of the trailing leg is delayed. There is long-axis rotation and too much dorsiflexion during the support phase. The legs cannot be oscillated forcefully and the runner uses the landing energy poorly.

3.3 START AND ACCELERATION

The posture and the way in which the body moves are clearly different during the start and acceleration phases than when running at speed. The runner hangs forward and places his stance leg on the surface with the knee strongly bent, while the range in which the joints can move is large and their power intense. The processes of starting and accelerating have their own qualities and follow certain patterns. For speed running, the pattern of movement is particularly determined by the need to avoid rotation and to unload elastic energy.

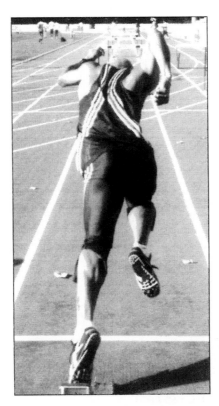

Figure 3.23   After leaving the starting block, the runner uses a great range of movement

3.3.1   The start phase

There are two factors that greatly affect the pattern of movement at the start: long ground-contact time and explosive concentric muscle action.

Long ground-contact time

At the start, the forward velocity is relatively low. Therefore the period for which the athlete makes contact with the ground (especially during his first strides, 0.12–0.18 s) is significantly longer at the start than when running at speed (0.07–0.09 s). The longer contact time with the ground makes it possible to compensate for the rotations that have developed during the previous push-off, without needing to reduce the force of push-off. Axial and forward rotations develop as 'by-products' at push-off, because the body must be positioned in order to ensure that the direction is most advantageous and that the magnitude of thrust is as great as possible. A runner can be observed to lean the furthest forward directly after the start, with the stance leg stretched the furthest from the position in which there is the most flexion in the knee. Therefore, the largest rotational moments will develop from that position. Because the support phase is long, these large rotational moments can be compensated for well. Later, during acceleration, the forward velocity is more rapid and, consequently, the ground contact time shorter. The runner is less successful in compensating for rotations, because he must hold his body more upright while running, making it impossible to exert much force at the end of the support phase. The body's posture appears less extreme and begins to resemble the position used for speed running.

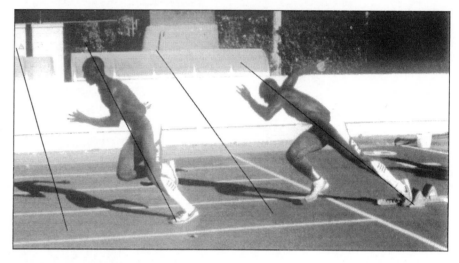

Figure 3.24 Body posture during the start
When the forward velocity is low, an athlete must hang far to the front to optimize thrust. This can be done because the ground contact time is long, giving enough time to compensate for a lot of forward rotation. When the forward velocity is higher, an athlete will need to run more upright because there is insufficient time to compensate for as much forward rotation.

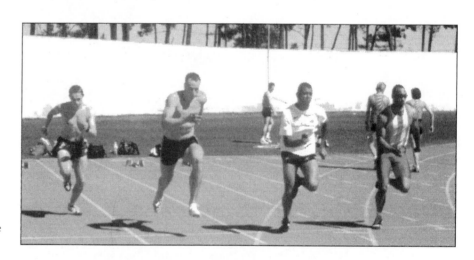

Figure 3.25 Body posture after the start
After 15 m, the velocity is already so high that the runner must avoid leaning forward, having little time to compensate for rotation.

Explosive concentric muscle action

When running at speed, how the muscles function in terms of reactivity will determine the pattern of movement. During the first strides at the start, a body posture is chosen that allows the strongly concentrically working muscle groups to function optimally. During this phase, reactivity plays a lesser role. On the one hand, this is because there is less drop (vertical relocation of the body's center of mass) during the start and acceleration than when running at speed. On the other hand, it is because the legs do not oscillate as rapidly at the start. Both these factors make it more difficult to preload the muscles so that they will work less reactively than during speed running. In particular, the outward pendular motion of the lower leg, and consequently preloading of the hamstrings, is absent during the start phase.

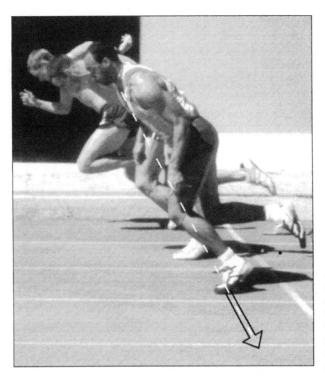

Figure 3.26   Placement of the foot during the start
At the start the foot is placed so that the ground reaction force runs behind the knee and in front of the hip. In this manner, the monoarticular knee and hip extensors can generate power optimally (see also Section 1.6).

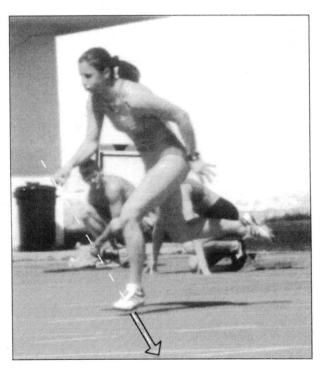

Figure 3.27   Incorrect foot placement
The runner continues to hang far forward. However, the forward velocity is already too high to compensate for a lot of forward rotation. Therefore, the foot must be placed in front of the ground projection of the hip. The ground reaction force passes in front of the hip and knee. The hamstrings must work to keep the knee flexed and to direct thrust backwards. Therefore, force from the knee extensors cannot be used optimally.

Because performance is determined by how much concentric 'power' is present at the start, it is important that the muscles generating this power are able to function optimally. In addition to the gluteal muscles, the quadriceps femoris is mainly involved. At the moment of initial contact, the knee is strongly bent during the first strides at the start, so that the thrust arising from the combined extension of the knee and hip will be optimal. The quadriceps femoris provides substantial power for extending the knee. As the speed subsequently increases, the knee becomes less bent at the moment of initial contact and the quadriceps will only be working on a very limited level after speed has been achieved.

During the transition from start to acceleration to speed, there is a progression from long to brief ground-contact times, from explosive to reactively working muscles, and from many to a minimum number of rotations for which the runner must compensate. These three variables are closely interrelated. The manner in which they can be coordinated to work together will determine the technical quality of the start and acceleration. For example, a runner who continues to hang forward too long in order to achieve extra thrust will find himself faced with a problem as the ground-contact time decreases, giving him insufficient time to compensate for rotation. He must learn to raise his body to an upright position earlier in the acceleration phase. One can observe a gradual transition in the body posture of good runners from the first strides at the start until the maximum speed has been reached. Body posture and thrust can be exactly attuned to the ground-contact time so that, as the ground contact time gradually decreases, the body also gradually changes position.

Nowadays, however, there is a tendency to make one abrupt transition, at the moment when the velocity is nearly maximum. The trunk is then directed more upright while the pelvis is pushed farther forward. At speed, there must be a great deal of tension present in the body, particularly at the front of the upper body. Such an abrupt transition makes it easier to increase tension in the body. When the transition is gradual, it takes some athletes too long to build up the necessary tension.

3.3.2   The acceleration phase

When analyzing the start and acceleration phases, attention should be paid to the first strides at the start. As has already been stated, at this point the power provided by the muscles is very high and the rotations created around the lateral and longitudinal axes are not a hindrance. The ground-contact time is long (0.12–0.18 s).

Posture influences how the body moves in different planes.

Posture and movement in the sagittal plane

Moment of initial contact

Because the body is leaning far forward, the body's center of gravity is projected onto the ground far in front of the point of support (i.e. a strong forward rotational moment will develop). Because the ground contact time is long, this forward rotation can be compensated for well during the support phase. At the moment of initial contact, the knee and hip of the stance leg are strongly flexed. The ground reaction force of thrust will pass behind the knee and in front of the hip, because the body is leaning forward and the hip and knee are bent. If the knee and hip are well coordinated, their extension can increase the ground reaction load without changing its direction. Muscles that are able to extend the hip and knee using a lot of concentric force (the gluteus maximus and the quadriceps femoris) are now active.

If at the start, knee extension occurs more rapidly than hip extension, the ground reaction force is directed more vertically (and is less favorable). Knee and hip extension must therefore be well coordinated if the direction of thrust is to remain advantageous. The rectus femoris plays a very important role in coordinating these movements more precisely (see Section 1.6.1). During the start, the rectus femoris is able to transfer energy from the hip to the knee. By varying the amount of energy transferred, the rectus femoris can coordinate movement in the knee precisely with that of the hip extension. As a rule of thumb, the hamstrings either work slightly or not at all in situations in which the rectus femoris plays a dominant role, such as during the start (knee extension + hip extension) (Jacobs & Ingen Schenau 1992). The opposite is also true: when the hamstrings have an important function, such as during speed running (extending the hip + keeping the knee bent), the rectus femoris works either partially or not at all.

The angle that the knee of the stance leg makes at the moment of initial contact is about 90° during the first strides after the start. The exact angle that the knee must make to achieve ideal acceleration varies between individuals. The same is true for how high or low the hips should be held and how far forward a runner should lean. Factors such as lever arms and amount of force that a runner can provide must be taken into consideration. Very strong runners, in contrast to their weaker colleagues, are able to hold their hips lower and make a more acute angle for the knee of the stance leg at the moment of initial contact. In this way, stronger runners are able to exert more thrust per stride compared to weaker runners.

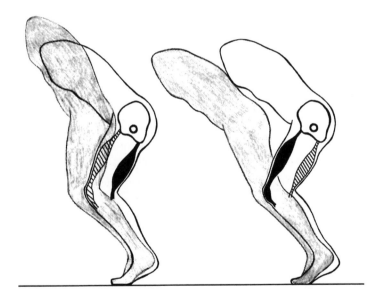

Figure 3.28 Biarticular action at the moment of initial contact
The hamstrings and rectus femoris are important muscles that regulate body posture during the start. The hamstrings transfer energy from the knee to the hip and help to hold the trunk erect (left). The rectus femoris transfers energy from the hip to knee and extends the knee, while the trunk continues to lean forward (right). During the start, the hamstrings gradually take on the work of the rectus femoris.

The back must be kept straight, because the dorsal muscles can work most effectively in that position, thus contributing to the force of push-off by way of forward pelvic tilt. If the back is too rounded, the dorsal muscles work less effectively, thus reducing their total contribution to the force of push-off.

Because, at the end of the swing phase, backward flexion is relatively limited in the leading leg, at the moment of initial contact the knee of the trailing leg will not yet have caught up with and passed the knee of the leading leg. This is not detrimental because the next support phase will be long and the thrust generated will be mostly concentric explosive and only to a small extent reactive.

The foot of the stance leg at the moment of initial contact is strongly dorsiflexed, particularly during the first strides after the start. Thereby, one must have a great deal of tension in the ankle.

Thrust phase

The knee of the stance leg is extended nearly completely during the thrust phase. Moreover, the runner will try to exert as much force as he can for as long as possible, especially at the end of extension. A complete knee extension is closely related to the action of the swing leg. When the swing leg is no longer causing forward flexion in the hip, the support leg will stop extending. These two movements are involuntarily coupled to one another. It is even true that the stance leg will straighten better and more rapidly when an indication is given to move the swing leg farther upward than when a direct order is issued to extend the stance leg itself. Moreover, the foot of the swing leg may not be held too far in a position of plantar flexion because there would then be insufficient tension in the muscles of the lower leg to support the next foot placement.

Many athletes do not extend the hip completely during the first strides after the start. This happens when the upper body is held quite far to the front. When the trunk is held more horizontally, the projection of the body's center of gravity onto the ground further in front of the point of support, thus resulting in a more favorable direction of the ground reaction force. To be able to extend the hip completely from such a position, the hips must remain quite low. However, when the hips are held low, an enormous amount of force is needed to raise the body out of the sharp angle of the knee at the moment of initial contact. Because the available force is frequently too low to achieve this, most athletes will choose to hold their hips somewhat higher. They will relinquish some thrust in the hip at the end of support in favor of a more economically directed reaction force during the entire support phase.

There is somewhat more dorsiflexion in the foot of the stance leg during the first strides after the start than when running at speed. This does not imply that tension in the lower-leg muscles may be allowed to dissipate. The transfer of force from the knee extension to the foot by way of the gastrocnemius is also extremely important during the start: having sufficient tension in the lower leg is therefore a requirement.

Moment of toe-off

The knee joint of the stance leg has achieved complete extension. Hip extension is dependent on the position of the trunk. The knee of the swing leg remains swung forward until the knee of the stance leg becomes completely extended. The knee is bent at least 90°, the pelvis is tilted forward, the back is erect, and the arms have been swung high.

Floating phase

The floating phase is relatively short because the vertical component of push-off is limited. This happens when the body is held far forward. Because the foot of the leading leg is already close to the ground at the moment of toe-off, it can subsequently be placed quickly on the ground surface. Foot strike takes place as hard as possible in order to preload the many elastic components, despite the fact that there is not much forward movement. The trailing swing leg is called into action as rapidly and linearly as possible.

Posture and movement in the frontal plane

During the first strides after the start the most notable movement in the frontal plane taking place occurs in the pelvis and trunk. At the moment of initial contact, the pelvis is lower in the frontal plane on the side of the swing leg than on the side of the stance leg. This position is in agreement with adduction in the hip joint of the stance leg. By turning the foot of the stance leg somewhat outward as it is placed upon the ground, it will be easier to keep the hip on the side of the swing leg lower. It is not clear whether the foot of the support leg is placed on the surface in this manner in order to push the free hip lower or whether there are other reasons for maintaining this typical stance at the start (e.g. to tighten the adductors better and thus exert more force). Nevertheless, at the moment of initial contact, the shoulder on the side of the stance leg is lower in the frontal plane than the shoulder on the side of the swing leg. In other words, at the moment of initial contact, the shoulder and hip are closer together on the side of the stance leg. At the moment of toe-off, the situation is simply reversed: the shoulder and hip are closer together on the side of the swing leg.

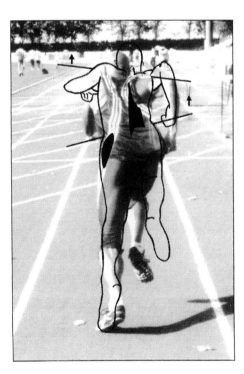

Figure 3.29 Movement in the frontal plane 1
During the start, movement in the frontal plane can contribute greatly to thrust.

The movements made by the pelvis and trunk are caused in particular by the action of the muscles that cause abduction on the side of the stance leg (gluteal muscles) and the dorsal muscles on the side of the swing leg. Moving the pelvis and trunk will intensify the push-off of the stance leg. The force required for these motions to be implemented is greater than that needed to overcome the mass inertia in the pelvis. Due to the force of push-off, the pelvis now threatens to move

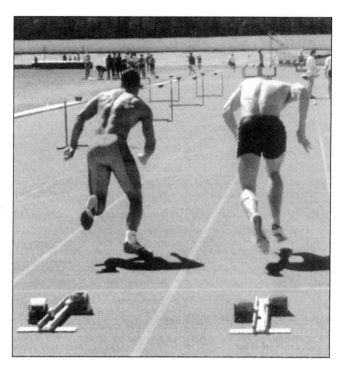

Figure 3.30 Movement in the frontal plane 2
The runner on the left makes good use
of his possibilities for movement in the
frontal plane. There is abduction (and
lateral rotation) in the stance leg as it
lands, so that the contralateral side of
the pelvis can be raised along a good
trajectory during push-off. The runner
on the right makes less use of such
possibilities and tends to round his back,
which will have a detrimental effect on
how the dorsal muscles work.

upward on the side of the stance leg, thus dropping further down on the side of the
swing leg. The force that the gluteal and dorsal muscles need to exert to overcome
this unfavorable motion is therefore rather large. Seen in reverse, this also means
that these groups of muscles are able to provide a great deal of force in support of
push-off.

During the floating phase, it is not necessary to make any major moves in the
frontal plane. At the moment of toe-off, the position of the pelvis with respect to the
trunk is identical to that required for the next moment of initial contact.

Later in the acceleration phase, the pelvis and trunk move less markedly. When
running at speed, however, the upward movement of the pelvis on the side of the
swing leg continues to be seen. This motion remains extremely important for development of the vertical component during the support phase.

Posture and movement in the transverse plane

Movements in the transverse plane during the first strides after the start can be
compared with those that occur in this plane during speed running. Typical of the
motion at the start is lateral rotation in the hip joint, which is frequently strong, and
lateral rotation in the lower leg at the moment of initial contact. It is not known why
such rotation occurs. The purpose of lateral rotation in the hip and lower leg might
be to facilitate medial rotation in the hip joint during the support phase. It might
also be true that the powerful adductors can be called upon to take part in thrust
because of this lateral rotation. Experience has shown that it is of little use to try to
change the lateral rotation in the stance leg. At first glance, placing the foot directly
in the line of progression would appear to be more advantageous from a mechanical
point of view. Nevertheless, there are so many additional factors that can affect the
force of push-off that the degree of lateral rotation can best be left to the intuition of
each individual runner.

3.3.3 Arm action during the start

There is a greater range in arm movement during the first strides after the start than when running at speed. Because the ground contact time is longer during the first strides than after speed has been achieved, the arms can offer assistance for a longer period. Because the trunk is held forward, the last part of the arm movement is of less help in supporting vertical motion, but offers greater assistance in supporting motion in the line of progression. Placing more emphasis on the end of the arm swing frequently causes a runner to keep his shoulder raised. This posture is quite often unjustly thought to be incorrect. Apart from giving extra support during the push-off, the function and implementation of the last part of the arm swing are identical to what are needed during speed running.

3.3.4 Errors during start and acceleration

- The posture of the body is incorrect for the speed being run and thus also for the ground contact time. The runner either raises his trunk upright too early, so that he is unable to produce optimum thrust, or he continues to lean forward for too long, so that rotations can develop that cannot be corrected because the ground contact time decreases as speed increases. Such rotations can only be compensated for if the runner places his foot in front of the projection line on the ground of the hip at the moment of initial contact.
- The hips are not held at the correct height. If they are held too high, the angle of the knee will be too obtuse at the moment of initial contact to make good use of the power provided by the knee extenders. If the hips are held too low, the angle of the knee is so acute that there will not be sufficient power to allow extension to take place fast enough.
- The hips are too far behind the foot of the stance leg at the moment of initial contact. Thrust can only be directed appropriately if knee extension is postponed. Extending the knee immediately after initial contact would slow the body down. Because hip extension is coupled to postponement of knee extension, a great deal of activity will be demanded of the hamstrings, which prefer to work reactively and are not well suited to providing power for concentric work.
- There is too little tension around the ankles and the start looks 'stealthy'.
- The knee of the swing leg does not remain mobilized until after the stance leg has been extended completely, and consequently extension will not be completed.
- There is not enough arm action occurring in the sagittal plane (too much in front) and torsion is not being optimally supported during the support phase.
- The back is too rounded and the upper body therefore reacts too passively during push-off.
- Not enough movement is made by the pelvis and shoulders in the frontal plane, so that some support for push-off is lost. Such a lack of movement between the pelvis and shoulder is frequently observed when the knees are held too close together halfway through the support phase. Such positioning of the knees limits movement in the frontal plane, particularly during the first strides after the start (i.e. the runner must try to start with his knees held wider apart).
- Because the runner tries to hold his knees facing forward in the line of progression during the first strides after the start, he cannot combine complete push-off with torsion around the long axis. Although the cadence (the combination of stride frequency and range of motion of the legs) is high, there is little force involved.

3.3.5 Summary

The start and first part of the acceleration phase are the only times during which power (concentric explosive) is the limiting factor. Moreover, because the ground contact time is long, there are no drawbacks to having to compensate for the rotations that develop. The body can therefore be positioned in such a way that the muscles providing concentric power can give optimum thrust in the line of progression. Slight abduction and lateral rotation in the hip joint (combined with lateral rotation in the lower leg) make optimum push-off by the stance leg possible. As soon as the velocity increases, and consequently the ground contact time decreases, then the amount of rotation that must be compensated for should also decrease. The body is raised more and more upright. Reactive muscle activity becomes increasingly important, while explosive muscle activity becomes less important. The quadriceps plays a lesser role as speed increases. The hamstrings only function to a small extent at the start, but their activity increases as the body becomes more upright.

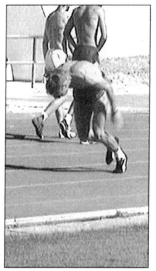 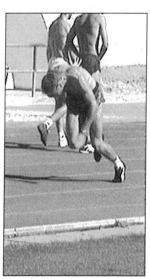 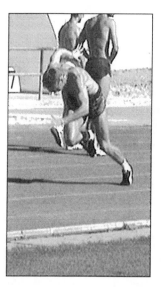 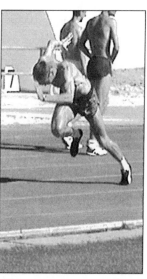

a   b   c   d

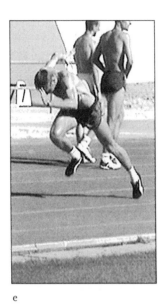

e

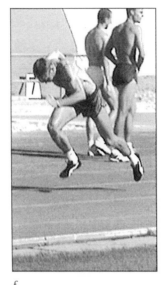

f

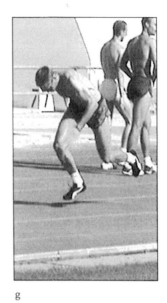

g

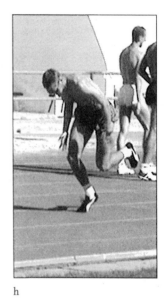

h

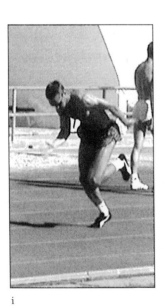

i

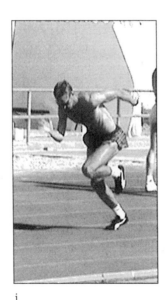

j

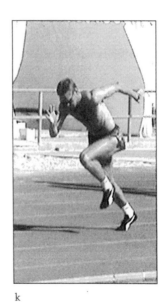

k

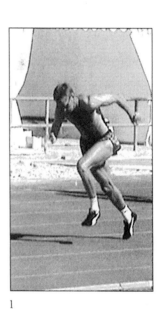

l

S3.13   Series a–l

During the start, the runner tries to make thrust effective by moving as well as possible (in the sagittal plane) in the direction of progression. He holds his hips quite low, trying to increase the force of push-off. As a result, he does not make use of other possibilities for thrust in other planes (notably the frontal plane) and he rounds his back (the dorsal muscles are used poorly). Because his ideas about how to start effectively are incorrect, the following push can no longer be executed correctly. Because his hip is quite low, the foot of the swing leg must be moved too rapidly. Consequently, the swing leg has already begun backward flexion in the hip before the push-off leg has been extended completely (k, l). Therefore, thrust will not be optimal.

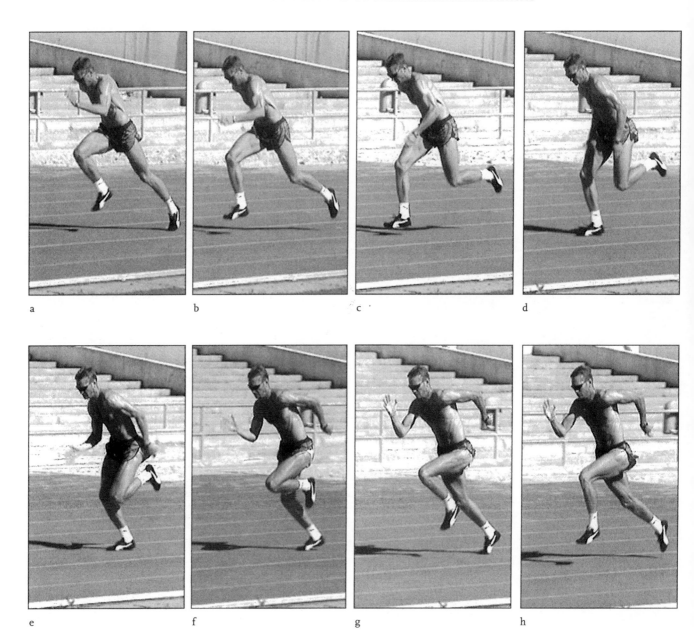

a b c d

e f g h

S3.14   Series a–h
At about 15 m after the start the forward velocity has increased. The runner still wants to exert a lot of force, and must continue leaning forward, although very little forward rotation can be compensated for in the time available. The foot must be placed in front of the ground projection of the hip (d). Foot strike must be soft and knee extension delayed.

3.4   CONSTANT LOW-SPEED RUNNING

Many trainers only observe how an athlete performs during endurance running from the perspective of energy expenditure. The athlete who is first to cross the finish line is thought to be in the best condition and therefore to be the most competent at maintaining the highest average production of energy across the entire distance. Many trainers consider technical skill to be only marginally important for using energy economically, and consider it satisfactory if the athlete can run in a manner that somehow imparts an impression of efficiency. Postures and movements that deviate from the norm are labeled as an athlete's 'personal style'. A runner must really deviate a long way from the norm before his running style will be called technically incorrect and his poor level of performance attributed to faulty technique. From this perspective, it is assumed that the metabolic capacity of an athlete is almost linearly related to his running speed, and that his performance is only marginally affected by the mechanics of movement. Therefore, training is chiefly aimed at the body's metabolic processes, with hardly any focus being placed on biomechanics.

In addition to the fact that one is frequently satisfied with only a rather vague insight into what actually defines a proper or an incorrect technique, it appears that the available ideas about technique are also frequently incorrect themselves. For example, some trainers attach too much importance to absorbing foot strike softly and to allowing much of the landing energy to ebb away. The circular movement of the wheel is seen as an ideal example. The stride should be rolling and circular, progressing silently and without shocks. From this point of view, it can be assumed that the fewer the peaks in the pattern of movement, the more economical locomotion will be.

3.4.1   Technique and performance

Many arguments can be introduced to support the idea that technique will have a major effect on performance during long-distance running. Technique can be so influential that the individual who wins the race may perhaps not be the runner with the highest stamina, but rather the runner who knows how to convert his (lower) endurance skillfully and most efficiently into speed.

There is almost no difference between the correct technique used for endurance running and that used for high-speed running. An upright posture, a (sufficiently) hard foot strike, and making good use of the landing energy are also crucial when running at an endurance speed. The similarities between the technique used for high-speed running and that used for endurance running are noteworthy. However, the aims are different: for high-speed running the aim is to convert as much energy possible into thrust, while for endurance running the aim is to use energy as economically as possible. The reasons why both techniques differ so little from each other is that reactivity and the avoidance of rotations that must be compensated for are crucial processes in both types of running. With respect to endurance running, the importance of reactivity and the avoidance of rotation can be defended as follows.

- Research data suggest that an endurance runner can take up only about half the amount of oxygen that would be required if all the movements that he made while running were brought about only by the generation of aerobic energy. The other half of the energy must therefore be obtained from other processes. One can assume that this energy must be obtained from energy stored in elastic tissues during foot strike (Cavagna et al 1964). Being able to perform with elasticity during foot placement will therefore be a major influence during performance.

It should be mentioned that quantifying the total power provided during running is extremely difficult. One can estimate how much power will be needed to carry out various movements (oscillation of the legs, vertical push-off, horizontal thrust, arm action, etc.) while running, but such estimates will be only partly accurate. Moreover, one cannot determine how much power will be needed to supply energy to the internal processes that do not contribute to positive work (e.g. stretching a muscle again after contraction).

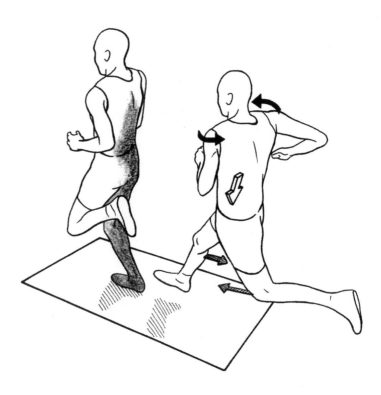

Figure 3.31 Economy of running
The economy of locomotion is determined, on the one hand, by how the degrees of movement are restricted and, on the other hand, by how energy is re-used during the running cycle. Energy derived from torsion, oscillation of the legs, and drop of the body's mass are converted as well as possible during the landing into elastic (stretching) energy.

- The upward and downward oscillation of the legs while running demands a great deal of energy, particularly in light of the fact that man is not a specialist in running and that there is a relatively large mass of tissue located in the distal segment of the leg. Therefore, running appears to be a rather inefficient way of moving forward. However, efficiency can be increased in two ways.
  - By 're-using' energy. The legs are constantly accelerating and slowing down. The kinetic energy that a moving leg has at one particular moment can be stored as elastic energy in muscle tissue during deceleration, and thereafter be 're-used' (reactively) to initiate the next movement. This kinetic energy is not then converted to (unusable) frictional heat. By storing in muscle (in the hamstrings during the outward swing of the leading leg) the energy generated by the scissor motion during the floating phase, the energy is not lost but re-used (reactive) for thrust during the next push-off.

- The amount of energy needed to oscillate the legs up and down can be decreased by limiting the degree of movement of the entire pendular action. The best way to do this is by keeping the support phase short and pushing off reactively. Reactive use of muscles allows energy to be 're-used' to oscillate the legs up and down. Oscillating the legs in such a way is more energy efficient; in total, less energy is needed and part of this energy is 'free' because elastic energy is cheap (Williams & Cavanagh 1987, Simon & Mendoza 1998).

- The absence of forward and axial rotations during speed running offers the runner the possibility to push off more forcefully and therefore to achieve a higher speed. During endurance running, the advantage of avoiding rotation is that the movements repeatedly needed to be made for compensation can be omitted, thus saving energy.

Points to consider

During competitions, one will often observe, even in good athletes, that the running speed decreases rather suddenly instead of decelerating gradually. This cannot be explained by a sudden decline in the production of energy. Rather, it is explained by an inability to maintain the reactive running technique, so that there is a much greater demand for energy in order to maintain the same speed. Because the aerobic capacity cannot be infinitely improved through training, but reaches a plateau at a given point, it is in the interests of endurance runners to train also those factors (coordination, power, etc.) that might affect their technical skill and use of reactivity. Technical factors are of great influence during the entire endurance run, but are possibly decisive during the final sprint and determine whether a runner will win or lose the race.

3.4.2   Some aspects of running techniques

Running at an endurance tempo resembles speed running in many ways. Thus when analyzing techniques for endurance running one can begin with those for speed running. The differences between the two types of running are fewer and the degree to which these differences occur is less than one might first assume.

Reactivity of push-off and foot placement

For endurance running, landing on the heel is frequently considered to be one of the most important characteristics. Heel strike, together with pronation, which develops in the foot, have the important function of absorbing the shock of landing. In addition, attention is frequently paid to the detail of how the foot completes its move after heel strike. The standard motion is from behind laterally toward the front medially. Completion of this movement is considered very important because it is associated with the rolling and ergonomic progression of the stride.

One can ask oneself whether these ideas are in accordance with the actual situation and whether standardization is possible with regard to foot placement and the completion of its movement. In practice, there appears (from measurements using a force platform) to be a variety of ways in which pressure under the foot can shift during the support phase. These pressure differences are observed not only between individuals but also between the left and right sides of an individual runner (Hinrichs 1990, McClay et al 1990, Miller 1990). The exact way in which pressure shifts within the foot appears not to be a relevant factor when transferring the force of push-off to the ground.

That the heel is the first part of the foot to touch ground and is actually of relatively little importance. The body posture at the moment when all the weight of landing rests upon the foot is much more influential for the entire progression of movement. At that moment, the entire foot is on the ground, and the distance between the projection of the body's center of gravity on the ground and the foot is different from that during heel strike. Photographs taken at the moment when the heel strikes the ground surface have offered no decisive answer about what exactly is happening. If, at that moment, there is still no backward flexion in the hip, then when the entire weight of the body comes to rest on the foot of the 'landing' leg, the foot will still be far in front of the hip, causing the forward velocity to decrease greatly. If there is sufficient backward flexion in the hip joint at the moment of heel strike, then when the entire weight of the body comes to rest on the foot it will either be less far in front or exactly beneath the hip, i.e. a better position for good reactive muscle activity. Heel strike will therefore not necessarily result in the ebbing away of energy or opposition to reactivity. Good runners execute backward flexion so rapidly before foot placement that one can almost no longer, if at all, speak of heel strike. In such runners, the foot is directly under the hip at the moment when the entire weight of the body comes to rest on the foot of the stance leg. There are even long-distance runners who are able to carry out backward flexion so quickly that they actually land on the forefoot without making any heel contact, which is an even greater benefit for reactivity. In such runners, the pattern of movement is actually identical to that used by sprinters.

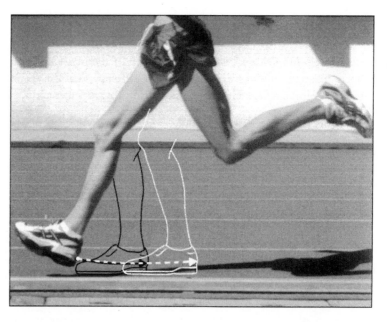

Figure 3.32 Reactive running
Just before foot strike, the weight of the body appears as though it will be fully absorbed by the heel. When backward flexion in the hip joint (white) is sufficiently rapid, however, the foot will be located directly beneath the hip, and the total weight of the body comes to rest on the foot. When backward flexion, and therefore oscillation of the legs, is too slow (black), the foot will be in front of the hip, so that it will be impossible to run well reactively.

Knee and hip angles and hamstring function during thrust

Endurance runners frequently sit somewhat deeper than short-distance runners. Because the rhythm of movement is slower, backward flexion in the hip joint just before foot strike occurs more slowly. As a result, less energy is stored in the elastic tissues. The control of discharge of this energy also proceeds in a different manner than for speed running. The moment of discharge and the direction of thrust can

184

be regulated by keeping the knee in a somewhat more acute or more obtuse angle during the support phase, and therefore by running somewhat higher or lower. Keeping the hips low while running should not necessarily be seen as an error. However, the mechanism for storing energy at the moment of initial contact and then unloading that energy for thrust must remain intact. A moment of inertia must not be allowed to develop during the process of storing and unloading energy, because any loss of tension will result in the loss of a great deal of energy. Sitting low and loss of tension between storage and discharge of energy are particularly seen in athletes whose level of power is too low or whose coordination in the muscle groups working reactively (i.e. the hamstrings) is too faulty.

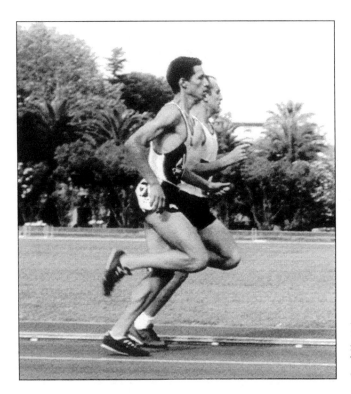

Figure 3.33 Endurance tempo running
Sitting deeply during endurance running is not necessarily technically incorrect. The determining factor is that landing energy must be re-used.

Position of the knee at toe-off

In most good runners the knee has not yet been extended at the moment of toe-off, but rather is at an angle of significantly less that 180°. This shows that the hamstrings have important work to do with regard to the knee and thus for directing thrust to the rear. At the same time, adjusting the action of the hamstrings to that of the rectus femoris helps to control the vertical component of push-off. The more active the rectus femoris, the larger the vertical component, while the more active the hamstrings, the smaller the vertical component (see Section 1.6). A knee that is bent during the support phase is related to hamstring activity, and thus with limiting the vertical component of push-off. This limitation has a favorable aspect because a great deal of energy is needed to oscillate the body's center of mass vertically. There must be a minimum amount of vertical displacement for the body's center of mass. If there is less displacement than this minimum, at a certain velocity the stride will have to decrease and the cadence increase. The legs will need to oscillate up and down more frequently in order to cover a certain distance, which is unfavorable for energy expenditure. The correct amount of vertical displacement for the body's center of mass is therefore a compromise. Because the hamstrings must work to direct thrust in an advantageous direction, it is worthwhile to generate vertical displacement less through movement in the sagittal plane (i.e. by adjusting the hamstrings and the rectus femoris) and more through movement in the frontal plane (i.e. by using the small gluteal muscles on the side of the stance leg and the dorsal muscles on the side of the swing leg). Developing power and coordination in these muscle groups will therefore contribute to helping the hamstrings function well during running. When an athlete is running, one can see whether these muscle groups are being used correctly by observing the upward undulation of the pelvis on the side of the swing leg during the support phase. If this side of the pelvis continues to drop during the support phase, the hamstrings will not be able to work optimally because the vertical component of push-off will have to be generated in the sagittal plane, which will demand a lot of work from the rectus femoris.

A knee that is still bent at toe-off will help the runner avoid rotation around the long axis, as well as keep the vertical component within limits. Moreover, after the support phase, it will not be necessary to bring the thigh as far forward from the rear. Both effects of such hamstring activity are favorable for energy expenditure.

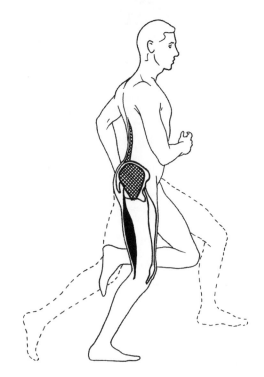

Figure 3.34　Position of the knee during toe-off
The hamstrings direct the force of push-off toward the rear and keep the knee flexed. The small gluteal and dorsal muscles function in the frontal plane and provide for a vertical impulse without slowing down the forward velocity.

Rotation and torsion

Running upright impedes the development of a forward rotational moment. Because the runner has enough time, compensation can be achieved by placing the foot on the ground in front of the hips. However, this demands more from the hamstrings (backward flexion in the hip must be carried out using yet more flexion in the knee). Moreover, it is difficult for running to remain reactive in this position. If the upper body continues to lean forward, the hamstrings will become the limiting factor on the performance of an endurance runner.

The arms are no longer active in the sagittal plane, but rather move along the front of the body. Because the arms move less rapidly in endurance running than in speed running, their motion need not be strictly linear. The torsion that pushes the free side of the pelvis forward can now take place via a circular motion of the trunk around the long axis. Because there is sufficient time to carry out the movement, the trunk is able to rotate further than during speed running. Thereby, the shoulder on the side of the stance leg moves forward. As for speed running, in endurance running the arm and trunk movements should serve as little as possible to compensate for rotation around the long axis, but rather should be used to generate as much torsion as possible in the spinal column. The arms often remain quite far bent to avoid rapid development of fatigue in the muscles around the shoulder girdle. Muscles between the shoulder girdle and trunk probably assume an important part of the task, while muscles between the shoulder girdle and arm are somewhat less active.

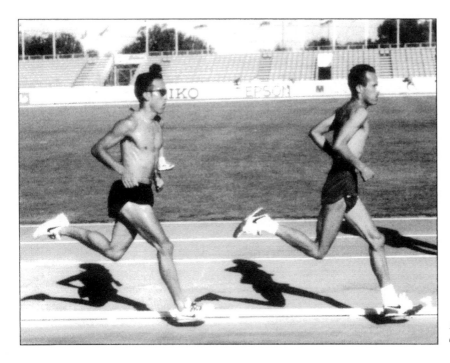

Figure 3.35 Arm movement for an endurance tempo

3.4.3 Summary

A good technique for endurance running must comply with a number of clear-cut demands, although there are also more variations possible than when running at speed. The techniques for both endurance and speed running are similar. Central issues are to avoid rotations and to optimally re-use the energy from the landing and the pendular motion by making the muscles work reactively. Whether the heel is the first point to touch the ground during foot placement is not relevant. Good runners often do not use heel strike. The magnitude of the vertical component of push-off is a compromise: on the one hand, one strives to limit vertical motion to help conserve energy; while, on the other hand, one strives to maintain a low cadence by having sufficient vertical displacement. This compromise works optimally if vertical displacement is brought about mainly by movement in the frontal plane and if the hamstrings are able to function well when directing force. The knee will then remain well bent during the support phase and the vertical component of push-off will be powerful enough to permit the stride to be long. Because the knee is bent during support, the hips will be held somewhat lower in endurance running than when running at speed. Torsion will mainly develop due to the rotation of the trunk and the arm around the longitudinal axis.

4
Training and adaptation

4.1 INTRODUCTION

The essence of training is to improve performance and to learn to produce top performance at just the right moment. In addition to scientific knowledge about training, the years of experience gained by coaches and trainers have led to the formulation of a number of training principles. With the help of such principles, one can design a plan of how to train a runner. These training principles are based on three important biological patterns (overload, specificity, and reversibility), which in turn are derived from the laws of diminishing returns, optimum workload, and individuality. Further training principles that can be derived are progressive, continuous, and specific workloads, as well as periodic and cyclic organization of the training process, and variations in the type of training (Swinkels 1980).

The origin of all the biological laws of nature eventually can be found in the concept of 'adaptation'. The human body has the ability to adapt to various forms of stress. The physical exercise due to running is a stressor that sets up the process of adaptation in terms of motion. The starting point during training is to use an optimum stimulus to disrupt the homeostasis of the body's internal environment. Disturbing the homeostasis initiates processes for recovery. After a period of recovery the body adapts, and is therefore better able to regulate homeostasis if subjected to an identical stimulus again. In other words, the athlete becomes better trained.

Depending on the type of stimulus used, adaptation can refer to how the heart, blood vessels, and lungs function, to processes providing energy, or to muscles. In addition to discussing the principles of training, and the means and methods for training to which they have given rise, ample attention is given in this chapter to the cardiorespiratory and metabolic adaptation resulting from training. In the study of adaptation, a prominent place is given to the alternating processes of physical exercise and recovery. There is a lot of room for error when training an athlete to run. For example, if the next stimulus is applied too soon and several times in succession, the result can be overreaching or even overtraining (see Section 4.5.3).

4.2 PRINCIPLES OF TRAINING

4.2.1 Background
The principles for training have been developed mainly as a result of trial and error. Trainers applied stress to the bodies of the athletes whom they were training, and later judged what the effects might be. In particular, the way in which good runners were trained was followed with more than average interest. It was the individual experiences of trainers and their athletes that formed the first step on the scientific path to training. This step toward understanding is known as the knowledge or skill of training. The next step was formed by compiling the personal experiences of trainers and their athletes. If common characteristics could be found, these could be used to formulate a theory of training, i.e. to principles of

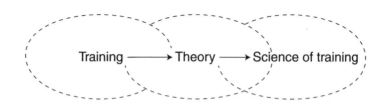

Figure 4.1   Various phases in the development of the science of training

training. The next step was to gather knowledge about training in a scientific manner. During the past decades, the human capacity to perform has increasingly been the object of scientific inquiry. Sciences such as psychology, sociology, and physiology have been devoting more resources within their research programs to the study of sports.

In today's world of sports, it appears that running must be bolstered by scientific inquiry if one wishes to achieve top performance. However, training runners will never be a completely scientifically based process. The experiences of trainers and their athletes are indispensable to an individual's process of adaptation due to training. Although the practice of sports and science appear to be mutually complementary, contradictions still remain between them, and various areas (Table 4.1) can be named that are still in dispute. While science strives to generalize, in the world of sports one is concerned with the athlete as an individual. The scientist tries to understand a specific problem, which he then wants to report in as many publications possible, while the trainer is interested only in athletic performance, and training is generally surrounded by a cloud of secrecy regarding the means and methods that are applied. The trainer faces a wide spectrum of problems when teaching athletes how to perform. However, the trainer may never give the impression that he is in doubt, while the scientist may give the impression that he is never actually certain what he knows. The final difference between the two areas of study is that, in practice, the scientist feels misunderstood, while the trainer feels threatened by science. Despite the areas of tension between science and training practice, there is consensus on a number of biological laws.

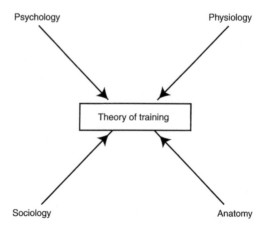

Figure 4.2   Sciences that play a role in the theory of training
The theory of training is fed by various sciences, four of which are mentioned here for illustration.

190

Science	Sports
Generalizations	Individuals
Knowledge	Performance
Never knows for certain	May never appear doubtful
Publish	Maintain secrecy
Misunderstood in practice	Threatened by science
Specific problems	Wide spectrum of problems

Table 4.1   Areas of tension between science and the practice of sports training

4.2.2   Biological laws

Overload

When an optimum stimulus is applied during training, homeostasis is disturbed. Here the word 'optimum' means that the stimulus used in training complies with the requirements of overloading. The term 'overloading' means that the stimulus requires greater physical effort than the body's momentary capacity for carrying a load (Roovers 1999). Because the state of equilibrium has been disturbed, many kinds of recovery process are initiated. For example, the supply of glycogen, which has been depleted, is replenished during the period of recovery. It is known that the supply of glycogen in muscle and the liver will be replenished to above the initial level. In this example, at the end of the recovery phase, the athlete's ability to cope with a challenge is improved because there is more glycogen stored in the liver and muscle.

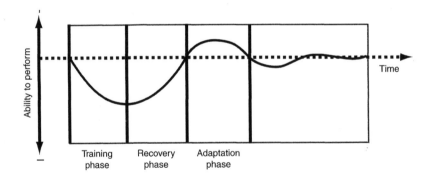

Figure 4.3   Supercompensation or one-factor model
The ability to perform is modeled over time from the moment when homeostasis (equilibrium) is disturbed by the application of a training stimulus.

Recovery of muscle tissue that has been damaged by strength training follows a similar pattern. For example, during strength training the rate of breakdown (catabolism) of muscle proteins exceeds the rate of their build-up (anabolism), but during recovery the anabolic phase predominates. This results in a build-up of muscle proteins to above the original level (for the strength training): the muscle involved shows hypertrophy. These examples of adaptation are described in the theory of training as supercompensation. The *supercompensation model* is also called the *one-factor model*. In time, one is concerned only with the immediate effect of training on the extent to which the body can undergo stress through exhaustion of certain biochemical parameters (Zatsiorsky 1995).

The above-mentioned supply of glycogen is the best known example of super-compensation. However, the existence of supercompensation for many other biochemical parameters has never been demonstrated experimentally. Moreover, according to the supercondensation model, it appears that the metabolism of various substances will require different periods of time before recovering to the initial level. This phenomenon has been described as asynchrony of recovery processes. This concept has led to the idea that there are a variety of ways in which to train (Swinkels & Goolberg 1994). It is thought that supercompensation should occur more rapidly for speed and technique after strength training than after training for stamina. Because of the asynchrony of recovery processes, one could plan to use different types of training stimuli in such a way as to optimize supercompensation. For example, the day after applying a strength-training stimulus, one could work through a training session aimed at increasing stamina.

This extremely simplified representation of adaptation processes does not take into account the multitude of biochemical parameters, which all have different speeds of recovery. Thus it is impossible to establish criteria for determining the ideal period of rest between two training sessions. In general, one can state that the supercompensation model is too simple to be correct (Zatsiorsky 1995). Indeed, the term 'supercompensation' itself is actually incorrect, because it suggests that physiological processes other than those taxed by the training stimulus must be responsible for restoring the state of equilibrium (Roovers 1999). Another principle of training, i.e. specificity, is thus violated (see pp. 195–196).

The *two-factor model* makes the process of adaptation appear more subtle than described by the supercompensation model. The two-factor model includes the factors physical fitness and fatigue when modeling the course of performance over time (Morgan et al 1987). As a component of an individual's ability to perform, physical fitness is seen as a parameter that changes slowly, in contrast to the component of fatigue, which can change rapidly. In this model, training is considered to be a form of input that can give rise to two physiological responses: (1) an increase in physical fitness and (2) an increase in fatigue. Summation of these two responses gives the output, i.e. the actual ability to perform. Directly after completing a training session, a gain may be realized in the area of physical fitness, while the individual's ability to perform has been negatively affected by the component of fatigue. During the ensuing period of recovery, fatigue rapidly fades and a gain in physical fitness is slowly realized.

At first glance, there are no large differences between using one or the other of these two models when planning training based on the variables physical exercise and recovery. The trainer who adheres to the one-factor model will try to plan the following training session during the phase of supercompensation. The trainer who prefers the two-factor model will try to lengthen the period of rest between two training sessions sufficiently that the athlete has time to recover from fatigue without forfeiting too much physical fitness.

The differences between the two models become especially clear when planning training for an important competition. The supporters of the one-factor model will try to reduce greatly the number of training sessions during the final week before the race, while maintaining the relatively heavy strain that the planned sessions must deliver. Supercompensation must be optimized by alternating a heavy training session with sufficient periods of rest. Using the two-factor model, however, the frequency of training will not be reduced much, but the physical exercise involved in individual training sessions will be greatly reduced. The aim of this system is to

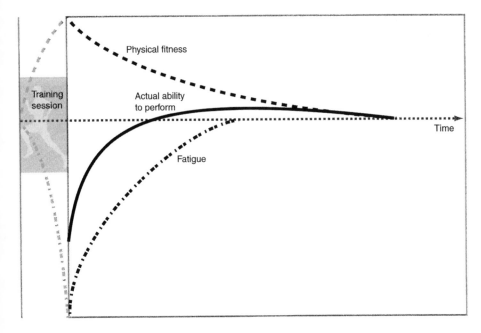

Figure 4.4   The two-factor model
The change over time is illustrated for the factors physical fitness and fatigue after ending a training session. Together, physical fitness and fatigue will decide a runner's actual ability to perform.

avoid fatigue during the week preceding the race and to sustain the physical fitness already achieved (Zatsiorsky 1995).

Application of the training principle called overload requires insight into how the physiological processes of adaptation proceed. In particular, the time required for physiological processes to recover will determine when the next training stimulus can be applied. In addition to ascertaining the optimum period of rest between two training sessions, it is also important that one understands how the ability to carry a load develops, so that the degree of physical exercise can be adapted accordingly. The training principle called 'reversibility' plays an important role here.

Reversibility

The principle of training called reversibility often conveys a negative connotation because it is associated with injury. Injury forces an athlete to adapt or even discontinue his training. Reversibility implies that organic and functional changes that can improve performance as a result of training will revert to their original level in the absence of training stimuli (Swinkels 1980). In the modern theory of training, the concept of reversibility is applied with full awareness when setting up a training program, rather than being seen merely as an inevitable principle of training that will begin to take effect after an injured athlete has been compelled to stop training. Comparison between conventional and modern training programs clearly demonstrates why the concept of reversibility imparts a much less negative connotation in the present-day theory of training.

Using a conventional set-up for training, the methods are applied during the first period of preparation are non-specific and low-intensity in character (Matveyev 1972). The arsenal of methods available for training is highly diverse. During the first period of preparation, stimuli are presented that focus on strength, speed, stamina, and technique. Such a period of training, called a *complex-parallel training plan*, will last from 4 to 6 months (Verchoshansky 1992). Generally, the scope is widened as the period of training progresses, while the intensity remains relatively low. During the next period of training, the scope is narrowed, while the intensity is increased. Thus in this period, specific training methods are given a more prominent place within the program. The role played by reversibility is of little significance. Using a modern training set-up, the situation is quite different. A training program consists of a number of periods of 4–12 weeks, in each of which a certain basic motor property is emphasized. The underlying idea here is that the various processes of adaptation, which would occur simultaneously in a complex-parallel training plan, should not interfere with each other. Adaptation thus proceeds more optimally in such a *successively linked training plan* (Verchoshansky 1992). In other words, the effect of training with regard to the basic motor property being accentuated is greater than when using a conventional training set-up.

The concept of reversibility can be applied when determining the length of the *accent period*. During the next accent period, one must take into account the fact that the effect of training achieved during the preceding accent periods will decay. The central question is how rapidly the previously achieved effects will decay after training. During a training program one must determine to what degree it is permissible for the effect of training for a certain basic motor property to retrace its course. In some situations it is impossible to ignore a certain basic motor property, and one will be compelled to carry out maintenance training.

Factors that influence the speed with which the progress achieved may revert are the age of the athlete, the length of the training period, and the type of basic motor property being trained. For the basic property of strength, it is known that, when an increased level of strength is the result of a long period of training, it will only decline slowly when training is stopped. Conversely, there is rapid decline in the strength gained from short-term power training (Hettinger 1966). In American literature, this effect has been described by the saying 'soon ripe, soon rotten'. Therefore, in athletics, when the periods of preparation are long and those of competition relatively brief, certain forms of strength training can be greatly reduced. The loss of adaptation in strength will only be slight because the period of no training was brief. Moreover, the basic motor property of strength adapts according to

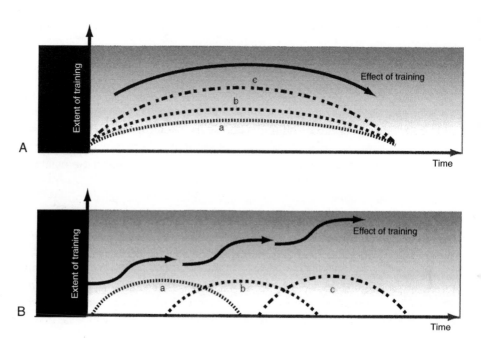

Figure 4.5A,B Effects of training over time
The change in magnitude over time of the effects of complex-parallel (A) and successively linked (B) training.

the principle of delayed effect (Verchoshansky 1987). During an intense period of strength training, the capacity to perform declines temporarily because of accumulated fatigue and the time needed to adapt to the strength stimuli applied. If this period is followed by a training period in which strength-training stimuli are greatly reduced, then adaptation will proceed toward a higher level of strength. Although it depends on the length and intensity of the strength-training period, positive adaptation will, on an average, become manifest after a 4-week recovery period (Zatsiorsky 1995).

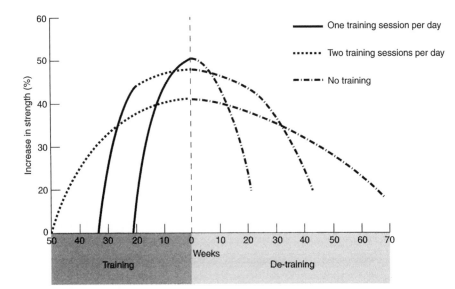

Figure 4.6 Relationship between training and detraining
The effects of detraining (period without strength training) on the increase in strength gained during the previous period while training once daily and twice weekly for about 20 weeks. Compare this to the loss of increased strength gained after a longer training period of about 50 weeks.

Athletes who have been training longer will lose the adaptations they have achieved less rapidly than individuals who have been training for a shorter period of time. The former are characterized by their ability to perform consistently despite not training. This statement must be somewhat qualified by adding that losing the effects of training depends also on the type of basic motor property concerned. Anaerobic endurance diminishes rapidly, while velocity, maximum strength, and aerobic endurance decline less quickly. Aerobic endurance is prominent in the list of consistent training effects. However, this depends on how aerobic endurance is evaluated. When maximum oxygen uptake is used as the criterion, aerobic endurance appears to remain stable over a 6-week period of no training (Viru 1995). However, when the activity of aerobic muscle enzymes is used as the criterion, a marked decline is seen within 2 weeks of no training.

Specificity

The adaptations that occur in the various tissues and organs as a result of training are specific, in that adaptation occurs only in muscles that have been stressed. However, the manner in which muscles undergo exertion is what actually determines the degree of specificity of the training load.

When the training load is specific, a number of criteria must be met with which one can measure how closely the load matches that which will be experienced during competition. (1) A specific training load, with regard to the structure of the movement, must resemble that which will be present during competition. (2) It is necessary that the types of muscle contraction are similar. Criteria (1) and (2) are the external and internal structures of movement, respectively. (3) The load can also be described as specific when it calls upon the energy system that will be dominant during competition.

It has become a cliche that many trainers call the race itself the best form of training. While the race is the most specific load that can be applied, the cliche is only partly true. Naturally it is valuable to include build-up competitions in a training program so that an impression can be gained about an athlete's strong and weak points. In addition, such competitions can be used to test certain competitive tactics. However, physiological adaptation diminishes rapidly after several races, contradicting the archaic notion that by running many (training) races training can be optimized. The major limitation of this approach is that after a certain number of races the training lacks overload. If an 800-m runner regularly runs 800 m keeping close to the speed that will be run during competition, he will rapidly stop improving. The factors that determine his performance will not be challenged in such a way that they can continue to adapt positively.

When setting up a training program, it is a better strategy to discover which factors will determine performance for a certain type of running. Next it must be decided how to put together a training load in such a way that one performance-determining factor can be brought into a condition of overload. Depending on the periodization (complex–parallel or successively linked) method chosen, one or more performance-determining factors will be emphasized simultaneously during training. The degree of specificity is now made equal to the extent to which transfer of training takes place. In other words, how can a specific training exercise contribute to increasing an individual's level of performance? Does improvement pay off in faster times when doing an exercise such as squatting on one leg? Which other performance parameters will also be positively affected as the runner learns to perform this exercise more adroitly? These are questions that a trainer must continuously ask himself and which will be quite difficult to answer. Determining the effectiveness of a training load is complicated still further by the fact that several months have usually passed before the effects of training are manifested as an increase in physical capacity or competitive results (Viru 1995). Therefore, when giving running instruction, a trainer only has access to information derived from delayed feedback. Moreover, changes in form and function reflect the integrated effect of the various means and methods used during training.

Central–peripheral model

As already stated, training will benefit from overload and specificity. Therefore, ideal forms of training are those that combine a large overload with a high specificity. Thus an ideal form of training should be able to provide a greater workload than an athlete's current stress-handling capacity can deal with, while also complying with the criteria that must be met for an optimum transfer of training. However, overload and specificity are not mutually compatible. If one wants to include a large overload in the training, then one must always deviate from some of the characteristics of goal- or competition-oriented forms of training. Conversely, if one wants to maintain high specificity of training, then a sizeable overload will not be possible. The incompatibility between overload and specificity can be represented using the central–peripheral model. The movement targeted, e.g. being able to run 800 m as

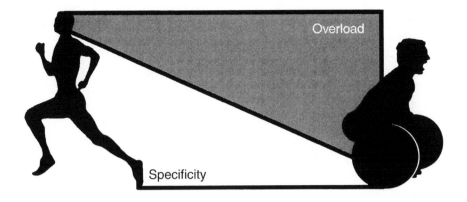

Figure 4.7 The central–peripheral model
The specificity of the exercises declines from the center to the periphery, while one or more partial aspects of performance-determining factors can be given a heavier overload.

quickly as possible on an athletic track as would be expected during a competition, stands central in this model. Somewhat off this center, the runner would be asked to run 800 m up a slight incline in the shortest possible time. Still further from the center, the runner would have to run 200 m as rapidly as possible. Still further from the center, he would have to rebound reactively across hurdles, and on the periphery would be lifting dead weights to train for maximum strength. Thus in the central–peripheral model the specificity of the exercises decreases from the center toward the periphery, while the potential to overload one or more aspects of the performance-determining factors increases. The negative influences of overload and specificity are compelling in both directions. In Section 5.1.5, examples are given of coordination exercises that at first appear to combine a large overload with a large specificity; but this proves not to be the case after further analysis. An example of this illusion of compatibility from the perspective of physiology are ideas about endurance training in which achieving resistance to fatigue is the most important criterion. Exhausting a runner during training, which is naturally accompanied by a large overload, could be seen as specific training. However, the demands made by specificity on a training directed toward improving stamina go much further than just disrupting homeostasis.

The reason for using the central–peripheral model to see whether a type of training will be efficient and energy-saving is that the question can be encapsulated in terms of the relationship between specificity and overload. It is not difficult to achieve an enormous overload during training if one does not take specificity into consideration. Countless practical examples can be found to illustrate this point, such as the unlimited potential increase in the number of kilometers run during a mild endurance training for a 5000-m runner. The art of training is simply to choose a type of training by which the product of specificity and overload becomes as high as possible. It is also quite important that the specificity of a particular type of training is assessed accurately, and that vague descriptions and collective terms (e.g. 'stamina', tempo severity, endurance strength) are not used. A good analysis of the degree and the way in which a form of training is specific will permit one to decide whether overload is sufficiently large to make the training efficient.

Individuality

Each runner is a unique individual. For example, everyone differs physiologically, anatomically, and psychologically (Bon 1998), and thus the same type of training can bring about very different results in two athletes performing at a similar level. The point of departure must always be based on the individual characteristics of each

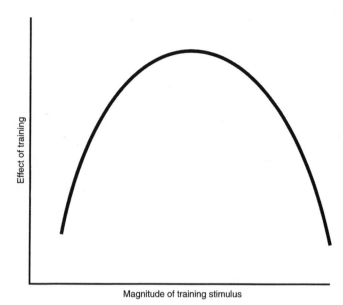

Figure 4.8 Relationship between the weight of the training load and the magnitude of its effect

athlete. In differentiating between types of workload for each individual during training, factors such as age, talent, and speed of adaptation play important roles.

Law of diminishing returns

The longer an athlete has been training, the more difficult it is to improve his level of performance through practice. The first improvement made at the of beginning a goal-oriented training program will be tremendous. Thereafter, it is necessary to increase the intensity and scope of the training if one is to continue recording gains. Such progress will continually diminish as the length of training increases, despite the fact that the training regimen is being made more difficult. For this reason, top runners must work much harder while training in order to achieve only a minimal advance in their performance level than will 'lesser' runners. Furthermore, an extra burden is placed on the athlete, because increasing the running speed demands exponentially more energy. In other words, a small gain in speed requires a disproportionate increase in the amount of energy generated.

Optimum workload

It is the aim of training to generate positive adaptation. The stimulus used must be neither too strenuous nor too easy. The relationship between the magnitude of the workload and the magnitude of the effect of training resembles an inverse letter 'U'. When the workload has barely disturbed homeostasis, the effect of training will be null and void. This is likewise the case when the body has been stressed too heavily. The range in which a workload can function optimally is quite narrow. In order to keep training within such boundaries, it is important that one discovers which factors will determine the training load.

The workload can be set up based on the components intensity, duration, and scope of training. Furthermore, when using an interval or other training method in which periods of stress and recovery are frequently alternated, the component called stimulus density must also be included. In general, the frequency with which a training takes places is also a factor that must be taken into account when deciding the intensity of a training period.

4.3 DERIVED PRINCIPLES OF TRAINING

4.3.1 Types of workloads

Progressive workloads

The biological laws of overload and optimum exercise and the law of diminishing returns form the basis of the principle that the body should be stressed progressively through training. The runner should be overtaxed during training, and the supposition that this method should be avoided is incorrect. From the perspective of overload, overexerting the body is a principle of training. However, if the wrong stressors are applied, the body will be stressed incorrectly. The stressor used to work the body during training must be weighed against a runner's ability to withstand the load. The biological law of 'optimum exercise' states the relationship between the magnitude of the load and magnitude of the effect of training. A prerequisite for adaptation is that any training stimulus applied must disturb homeostasis. The stressor that can disrupt the body's homeostasis on one day may fail to do so on another, because the human body is able to adapt and thus increase its ability to withstand stress. From this one can deduce that practice must be intensified over the course of training in order to guarantee an improvement in performance.

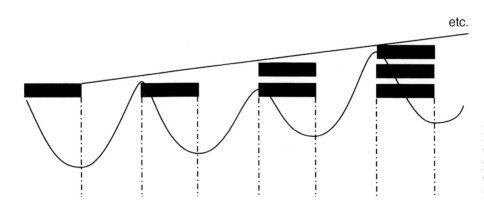

Figure 4.9 Creating a situation of overload
Because the body continuously adapts to training stimuli, it must be stressed progressively in order to create a situation of overload. The number of black boxes shows the severity of the training.

Continuous workloads

In his book *Lore of Running*, which has since become a classic, Noakes (1992) has spoken of the first law of training being the consistency of training. Today it is impossible for top runners to maintain their levels of performance when their training periods are interrupted by periods in which they either stop training or hardly train at all. The program for a top runner can be characterized by training that lasts an entire year, with 3- to 6-week rest intervals, the so-called relative rest periods. However, it is customary for middle- and long-distance runners to continue working through these relative rest periods, undertaking three mild endurance sessions.

Specific workloads

See the section on specificity (pp. 195–196).

4.3.2 Variations in types of training

All training principles derived from biological laws have as their final goal the optimization of the workload during training. The type of training chosen should place the runner in a situation of overload. Moreover, a certain type of training should bring about a specific effect. Earlier it was stated that a large overload and a high degree of specificity are mutually incompatible, a fact that restricts one's choice when considering suitable types of training. A choice that is too limited will quickly lead to unbalanced training. In that case, the law of diminishing returns quickly comes into operation. In order to guarantee that the effect of training is optimal within the narrow range available, it is necessary to vary the forms of training chosen. Such variation can be achieved by altering the means and methods used to train, and the magnitude of the workload applied in one particular training period. The means of achieving variation can be applied within a short training cycle (up to 4 weeks). In other words, within individual sessions, the components used to exert the body (e.g. scope, duration, and magnitude of workload) can be varied while the means of training remain unchanged. Other ways and methods of training can be applied for longer successive cycles (4–12 weeks) within a training program.

4.3.3 Periodization and cyclic organization

In order to provide top performance on a predetermined day, both periodization and cyclic organization of the training process are necessary. The ultimate success of a well-planned training program is demonstrated when an athlete actually performs at his best at a predetermined time, such as during a national championship or the Olympic Games. Even at lower levels of performance, runners are concerned with trying to peak at just the right moment. For example, a runner training for a large city marathon will hope to record a good running time on that specific day. However, things often go wrong, and an athlete may achieve his top performance just prior to or just after the desired moment (Os 1999). It appears that periodization and the resulting cyclic organization of the training process is no guarantee of success. It is nearly impossible for a runner to maintain a high level of performance throughout an entire year. During the year that an athlete is training, space must be created for periods of mental and physical relaxation.

Periodization implies that a year can be subdivided into training periods (Swinkels 1980, Bompa 1999). Cyclic organization of the training process refers to the characteristic training phases that are repeated throughout the year of training. Application of specific means of training or accentuation of certain motor properties are examples of such characteristic training phases. The concept of competitive form, as used by Matveyev (1972), who laid the foundation for periodization, is central in this. Matveyev analyzed the preparation of Russian sportsmen for the Olympic Games in Helsinki in 1952, where the Russians were especially successful (69 medals, including 21 gold) in various sports. Based on questionnaires filled in by athletes about their training for the Olympic Games, Matveyev was able to design a theoretical system that came to be known as the periodization model. This classic model, which is still frequently used today, states that the competitive form behaves in a certain manner under the influence of training and that it can be manipulated in such a way that it reaches its highest level during period(s) of competition. Adaptations and variations of Matveyev's basic model have been constructed (Tschiene 1989). In addition, critics of Matveyev have proposed other periodization models based more on biological processes of adaptation (Verchoshansky 1987) than on experiential data.

Periodization and cyclic organization of the training process aim not only for a climax in performance, but also for optimum increase in an athlete's ability to perform (Swinkels 1980). Such an optimum increase in the direction of a climax in performance is made possible by, among other things, running in practice races during the period near to competition.

Periodization of the training process can take place on various levels. On a macro-level, plans may be set up that span 1 year or even longer. On a meso-level, attention is directed globally to establishing training cycles that last for 4–26 weeks. Finally, on a micro-level, concrete plans are made regarding which ways and methods should be used during cycles that do not exceed 4 weeks. In addition, on a micro-level, attention must be placed on how to alternate optimally periods of exercise and recovery. The periodization models of Matveyev, Tschiene, and Verchoshansky are discussed in the following sections.

Matveyev's model

The two most important factors that determine how the body should be stressed during training, and which run as a thread throughout Matveyev's model, are the scope and intensity of the load (see optimum workload, p. 198). The relationship between the variables scope and intensity is inverse. During the first period of preparation, the trainer strives for a high scope, while the intensity is kept low. During the second period of preparation, the intensity is increased rapidly, while the scope is decreased equally rapidly. It is during this period, in which the lines for scope and intensity intersect, that a competition runner will usually plan a training camp abroad. During the period from March to May, track athletes from the northern hemisphere go looking for warmer climates in order to complete successfully their training with high intensity and relatively high scope. In The Netherlands, at this time of year it is often still too cold to carry out this type of physical training, thus greatly increasing the chance for injury. During the period in which competitions are being held, the scope of training is decreased further, while the intensity is raised to its highest level.

The variables scope and intensity are directly related to the concept specificity. The first period of preparation, which can be described as having a high scope and

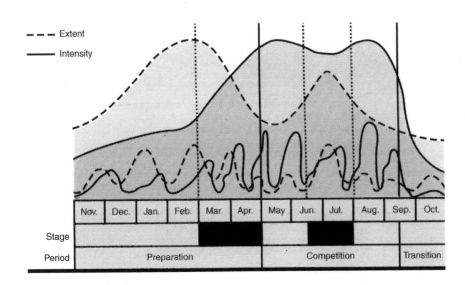

Figure 4.10 *The classic periodization model* Single periodization according to Matveyev.

low intensity, is non-specific in character, while the period of competition is highly specific due to its accent on high intensity and low scope.

In his classic periodization model, Matveyev differentiates between several periods: one or two for preparation, one for competition, and one for transition. In the case of two preparatory periods, the first period, which usually lasts for 3–4 months, can be characterized as having a strong focus on non-specific condition training, with little attention being paid to technique. In this period the ratio of non-specific condition training to technique training is approximately 80:20. Only 35% of the effort put into training is specific in character. During the second period of preparation, more emphasis is placed on technique, and 65% of the condition training is specific in character. The duration of this specific period of preparation varies between 6 and 12 weeks, and the ratio of condition training to technique training is 60:40. During the competition period, there is even less condition training, comprising no more than half the total amount of work put into training during the preceding period. Much of the training comprises competition-specific work and practice matches. In athletics, the season in which outdoor track competitions can be held is from May through September. Because it is impossible for an athlete to maintain such a high competitive level of physical preparedness for such a long time, the competition period is divided into two parts. A mini-period of preparation, lasting from 3 to 4 weeks, is inserted in the program between the two periods of competition. In this brief interim period, the focus of training is on the physical

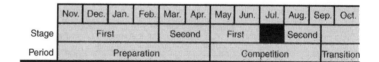

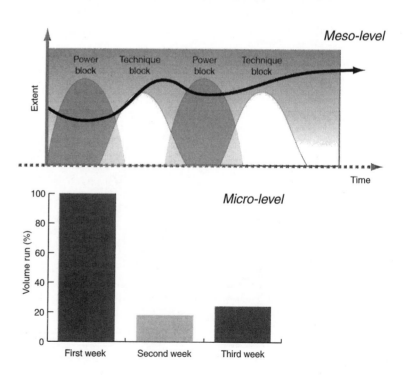

Figure 4.11 Examples of periodization
Periodization can take place on different levels. Three examples are given for periodization on a macro-, meso- and micro-level.

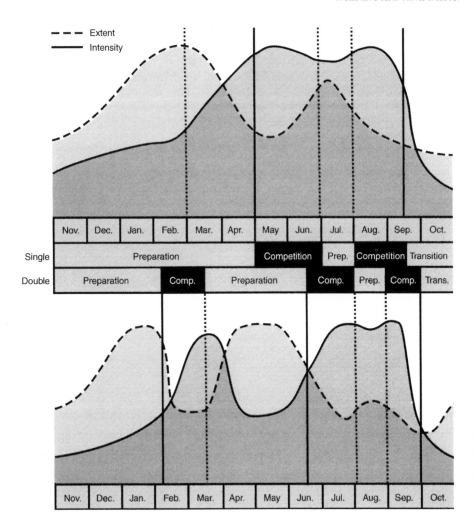

Figure 4.12 Single and double periodization model according to Matveyev
In a single periodization there is one period of competition, while in a double periodization there are two periods of competition.

stress that will be applied during the second preparatory period. In other words, the scope is increased and the intensity decreased in comparison to the first phase of the competition period.

In addition to the fact that it is impossible to maintain the ability to perform at a high level during the entire competition period, the mini-period of preparation is also used to make some adjustments to the training program on the basis of negative results in the first phase of competition. Various mental and physical aspects can be used to explain why an athlete's ability to perform diminishes over a long period of competition. The mental aspect relates to the absence of 'staying power', or the mental stamina to mobilize 100% of the body's physical potential. The physical aspect relates to parameters that can be trained, such as aerobic endurance, which are somewhat neglected during the competition period, and those specific parameters that offer only slight room for adaptation. The latter parameters are very heavily taxed during the second period of preparation and the first phase of competition, so that they will be in need of a period of recovery. The first-mentioned parameters will have regressed so far that they will have a negative effect on the results of the competition. During a 4-week training period with an increasing scope, for example, it will be possible to regain an acceptable level of aerobic endurance.

During the transition period, the scope of the training declines to about 15% of that commonly applied during the competition period. For 3–5 weeks the emphasis is on active recovery. During this period, in addition to gentle running, an athlete also takes part in other sports in order to refresh himself mentally for a new period of preparation.

Matveyev's model as described above is a single periodization model. One can speak of single periodization when there is one period of competition, even when it has been divided into two phases with an interim mini-period of preparation. If the performance of an athlete must climax twice within 1 year, and the climaxes are separated by an interim period of several months, then it is better to apply a double periodization. Examples of this are when a runner tries to combine both indoor and outdoor seasons or tries to run spring as well as autumn marathons. The advantage of using a double periodization, when observed over a number of years of training, is the greater improvement in performance in comparison to using a single periodization. Matveyev demonstrated that this is particularly true for aspects of running in which maximum strength and fast energy supply are the factors determining performance. Based on experience, the double-periodization model can be applied successfully for middle- and long-distance running. The explanation for this must be sought in the increase, on a yearly basis, of specific physical exercise that will probably bring about a greater effect from training.

Tschiene's model

Tschiene found Matveyev's classic model to be unsuitable for top athletes. The rather large variations in the scope and intensity used by Matveyev are only suitable for a specific type of training during brief periods. If training top athletes is to have any effect, particular emphasis must be placed on high-intensity, specific forms of workload. Matveyev's model was therefore considered to be suitable for training young athletes and beginners, but not top athletes.

Tschiene constructed a periodization model in which, with the exception of the transition period, a slightly alternating scope and high intensity is applied over an entire year of training. This results in an exceptionally heavy training program that can only be completed when a wide range of measures is applied for recovery. The speed of recovery between training sessions is the limiting factor in Tschiene's model.

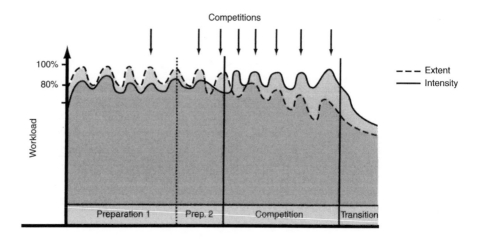

Figure 4.13 Periodization model according to Tschiene
Intensity is kept high and the scope only changed slightly when a runner trains according to the characteristics of this model.

On a micro-level, Tschiene is an advocate of complex training, i.e. that a training session should consist of both general physical exercise and exercise specific to the movements used in the competition itself. For example, a sprinter will first undergo a knee-bending session in the power gym, followed by a series of jumps, before completing the training session with acceleration running on an athletic track.

Tschiene's periodization model demands much more from an athlete because during training his body is continuously being placed under intensive, specific stress. In comparison to Matveyev's model, physical exercise and recovery are frequently alternated within the shorter training cycle. Within the limited choice of intensive, specific workloads, the ways and methods used for training are frequently varied.

Verchoshansky's model

In the periodization model proposed by Verchoshansky, the processes of physical adaptation are used as the point of departure. Verchoshansky discovered a pattern in the development of explosive strength and fast energy supply when extensive strength training was applied over the entire year of training. After an initial slight increase, the development of explosive strength and fast energy supply leveled off. However, there was a strong increase in the strength parameters during the period after the extensive strength training had ended. Verchoshansky called this phenomenon the 'delayed effect of long-term training'. The explanation for this adaptive mechanism lies in the amount of time needed for the strength parameters to adjust to the training stimuli imposed during a period of heavy training. In addition, extensive strength training causes fatigue to accumulate, which leads to a temporarily lower level of performance. In order for the effect of training to be optimal, it is necessary that the subsequent training period is composed of less strenuous workloads.

By separating concentrated periods of strength training from periods of technique and speed training, one can profit optimally from the delayed effect of long-term training. This manner of periodization is better known as 'block organization' of strength and technique training. Within a strength block there are relatively many non-specific strength-training sessions and almost no sessions for training technique or speed. The concentrated strength training causes negative 'transfer of training' to technique, and through that to speed, leading to a temporarily lowered level of explosive strength. When the strength block has been set up well, there is

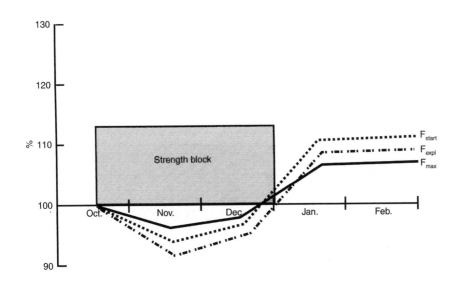

Figure 4.14 Delayed effect of strength training
Three different force parameters followed over time: F_{start}, starting force; F_{expl}, explosive force; F_{max}, maximum force.

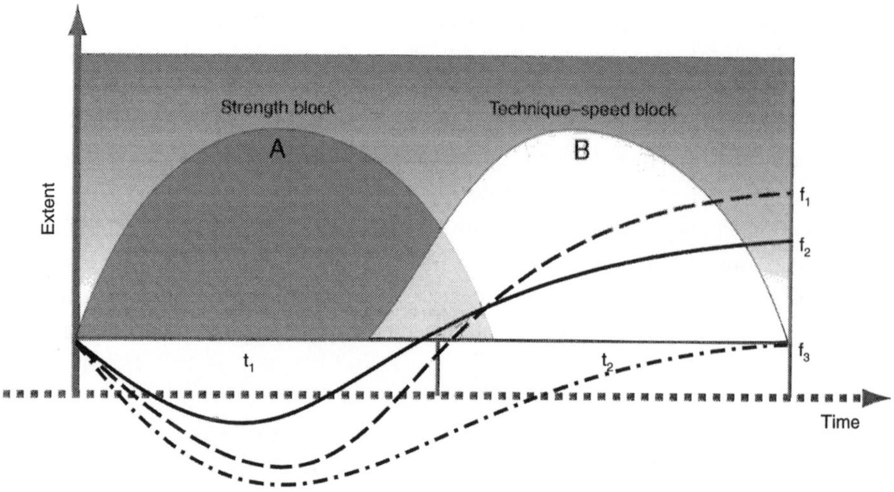

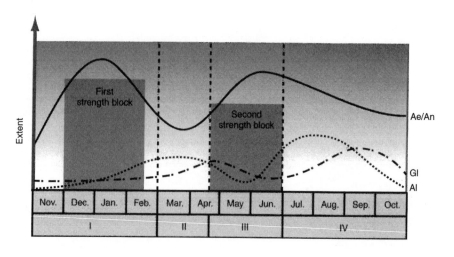

Figure 4.15 Long-term effect of training
An example where a period of strength training is followed by a period with only slight emphasis on strength (technique and speed training). Adaptation for a certain force parameter (f) is dependent on the weight of the previous strength block. The f_1 curve is optimal, while for curves f_2 and f_3 the strength block was too easy and too strenuous, respectively.

an optimum increase in explosive strength parameters. However, these parameters, which are followed up both during and after a period of strength training, are difficult to define (see Section 6.1). The tests employed to evaluate how the strength parameters develop are therefore also dubious. The duration of a strength block varies between 4 and 12 weeks. The maximum effect of training becomes manifest after a period of at least 4 weeks. During the period following the concentrated strength block, the athlete undergoes specific strength training as well as training for technique and speed. The reason for this is that the higher level of strength must be inserted into the technique. Correct integration of power and technique guarantees an increased level of performance. Depending on the number of competition periods, approximately three concentrated periods of strength training are planned within one training year. The methods for training strength within the various strength blocks should be alternated in order to encourage a beneficial effect.

Verchoshansky, trusting his own periodization model, is a fierce opponent of the complex training method proposed by Tschiene. Verchoshansky also views

Figure 4.16 Example of periodization
Periodization for a middle-distance runner for whom strength training has been organized in blocks. Ae/An, intensive endurance load; Gl, training directed at improving the generation of energy by way of 'fast' glycolysis; Al, training directed at improving the generation of energy by way of the creatine-kinase reaction.

206

Matveyev's complex-parallel organization of workloads as being less than ideal for optimum adaptation. From his perspective, Matveyev's model is not based on biological laws, but merely describes general plans for training successful athletes (Verchoshansky 1998).

Verchoshansky has designed a periodization model in which the singularly directed workloads are linked in succession. Verchoshansky's periodization model is not limited by being a model only for the explosive areas of athletics; it can also be applied when training middle-distance runners. Concentrated strength blocks combined with workloads directed toward increasing the aerobic potential are followed by periods in which the athlete is trained for the sprint and given workloads directed at improving 'fast' glycolysis. Application of this type of planning gave rise to a significant improvement in running performance of a group of middle-distance (800, 1500, and 3000 m) runners.

4.4 Adaptation

An individual workload that exceeds the minimum stimulus threshold can be seen as the trigger for acute adaptation processes. Each cell in the human body is sensitive to the stress caused by strain, and will react to the situation with a specific response. The acute adaptation that results after a training stimulus has been applied involves in particular the adaptation of physiological processes to increased energy metabolism (Viru 1984). Such adaptation is necessary in order to prevent undesirable changes in the internal environment of the body. Acute adaptation is also directed at maintaining or repairing homeostasis; Cannon (1929) described this as regulation of homeostasis.

The repeated application of stress in a structured manner leads to stable adaptation over the long term. Homeostasis should chiefly be regulated in order to maintain optimum enzyme activity. For example, by keeping the temperature and pH constant, the speed of various biochemical processes is guaranteed. The human body has a balanced system of dynamic and invariable parameters in its

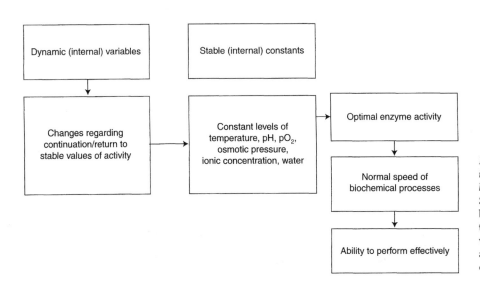

Figure 4.17 Relationship between the internal environment and maintaining homeostasis
Schematic illustration of the role played by dynamic and constant variables within the internal environment of the body when trying to maintain homeostasis and to guarantee that the activity of enzymes remains optimal.

internal environment that make it possible to maintain homeostasis. In addition to temperature and pH, other constant factors within the body are, for example, pO_2, the concentration of ions, water content, and osmotic pressure. Dynamic internal factors can fluctuate widely within certain limits in order to keep the factors that must remain constant as invariable as possible. For example, one dynamic factor might be the change in blood flow because of local vasodilatation.

In addition, hormones play an important role in regulating homeostasis. Hormones can determine the extent of adaptation, while the workload itself will determine the direction in which adaptation will proceed (Bon 1998). For example, the degree of hypertrophy in muscle tissue is strongly influenced by the presence of anabolic hormones during the recovery phase.

4.4.1 Cardiovascular adaptation

Cardiovascular adaptation is caused by both strength and endurance training. Adaptations in the heart and blood circulation are generally only seen in relation to training aerobic endurance. In any case, it is the well-trained long-distance runner who is regularly diagnosed as being the proud owner of an 'athlete's heart' due to training. At first, doctors were greatly concerned when finding hypertrophied heart muscle in such athletes. Now this type of heart is seen as a normal phenomenon in long-distance runners, resulting from adaptation (Costill & Wilmore 1994). Less is known about whether cardiovascular adaptation will likewise result from strength training.

Adaptation through strength training

Because muscle contractions must be generated in order to overcome high resistance, which is common in strength training, the heart muscle experiences high peripheral resistance during the discharge of blood from the left ventricle. This high afterload can only be overcome by an increase in the contractile force of the heart. The heart muscle reacts just like skeletal muscle to this increased strain by becoming hypertrophied. The wall of the left ventricle becomes thicker and stronger. This has been demonstrated in bodybuilders by using echocardiography (Urhausen & Kindermann 1989).

In comparison to endurance training, for example, a lower heart rate has been recorded during for strength training. The heart rate during power training increases in proportion to the amount of muscle mass and to the percentage of the maximum contractile force applied (Brooks et al 1996).

Adaptation through aerobic workloads

Here we consider the physiological adaptation of the ability of the cardiovascular system to transport oxygen after the application aerobic workloads. Cardiovascular adaptation in athletes trained for endurance running is usually seen in relation to the development of maximum oxygen uptake. This relationship is self-evident, because the cardiovascular system is responsible for transporting oxygen. Oxygen uptake ($\dot{V}O_2$) can be defined as the product of the circulating blood volume (V_{circ}) and the arteriovenous difference in oxygen ($_{a-v}\dot{V}O_2$).

$$\dot{V}O_2 = V_{circ} \times {}_{a-v}\dot{V}O_2$$

The parameters that determine oxygen uptake are discussed below. In particular, attention is given to how these parameters adapt as a result of training directed at increasing the aerobic potential.

Circulating blood volume (V$_{circ}$)

The concept of circulating blood volume has already been mentioned in Chapter 2. As shown there, V$_{circ}$ can be determined using the heart rate (HR) and stroke volume (V$_{stroke}$):

$$V_{circ} = HR \times V_{stroke}$$

V$_{circ}$ is a measure of the quantity of oxygen-rich blood that is pumped through the heart each minute. Adaptations in V$_{circ}$ can be seen in relation to adaptations in heart rate and stroke volume. The relationship between heart rate and running speed for a runner who is at first less well trained and then has run regularly for 3 months is shown in Figure 4.18. This athlete underwent extensive interval training and various types of endurance training. What is striking is that his resting heart rate (HR$_{rest}$) and heart rate at submaximum exercise (HR$_{submax}$) are lower in the trained situation. The maximum heart rate (HR$_{max}$) shows no difference.

Adaptation of V$_{stroke}$ is mainly responsible for the changes seen in HR$_{rest}$ and HR$_{submax}$. In Figure 4.18 it can be seen that preloading (i.e. the measure to which the cavities of the heart are enlarged when filled with blood) has increased due to the training applied. When the return of venous blood is increased, more blood flows into the right atrium. When a larger quantity of blood is pumped through to the right ventricle, it too becomes enlarged. The response of the right ventricle, described earlier as the Frank–Starling mechanism, is to contract with more force. An increased flow of blood from the right ventricle is immediately answered by a larger stroke volume in the left ventricle. An increase in the end-diastolic volume can be attributed to an increase in the volume of blood plasma.

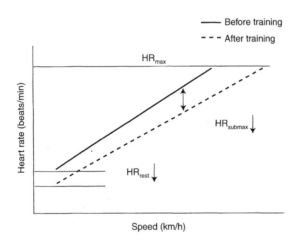

Figure 4.18 *Relationship between heart rate and running speed before and after 3 months of regular training*
HR$_{max}$, maximum heart rate; HR$_{submax}$, submaximum heart rate; HR$_{rest}$, resting heart rate.

There are two physiological mechanisms that lead to an increase in the volume of blood plasma as a consequence of training. First, after a period of extensive interval and endurance training, more aldosterone and antidiuretic hormones are secreted. An increase in these hormones in the blood results in more water being retained by the kidneys, thus increasing the volume of blood plasma. Second, more proteins are found in blood plasma, which will cause the osmotic pressure of blood to rise. Increasing the concentration of protein in plasma also causes the volume of blood plasma to increase (Costill & Wilmore 1994). Approximately 55–60% of the total volume of blood consists of plasma. Using the types of training mentioned above, the volume of blood plasma in a runner can be increased by about 10%. When the volume of blood is 5 l, the quantity of plasma increases by about 300 ml. In addition, there are more erythrocytes in the blood, although they increase less than the volume of blood plasma. The result is a decreased ratio between erythrocytes and total blood volume, also known as the hematocrit. An example can be used to illustrate this: a runner's total blood volume of 5.2 l has increased to 6 l after a period of training. His blood plasma has risen from 3.1 to 3.6 l, while the volume of erythrocytes has increased from 2.3 to 2.5 l. The final result is a decrease in the hematocrit value from 44.0 to 41.6% (Table 4.2).

Measurement	Volume (l)			Hematocrit (%)
	Total blood	Blood plasma	Erythrocytes	
Before training period	5.2	3.1	2.3	44.0
After training period	6.0	3.6	2.5	41.6

Table 4.2   Adaptation as a result of training: changes in blood volume, blood plasma, erythrocytes and hematocrit

As erythrocytes are responsible for transporting oxygen in blood, at first glance it would appear that the percentage reduction in the volume of erythrocytes should have a detrimental effect on a runner's ability to perform. However, due to the increase in the volume of blood plasma, the blood is less viscous. The blood is thus less sticky and its flow encounters less resistance, resulting in an improved circulation of blood to active masses of muscle. The flow of blood through capillaries is

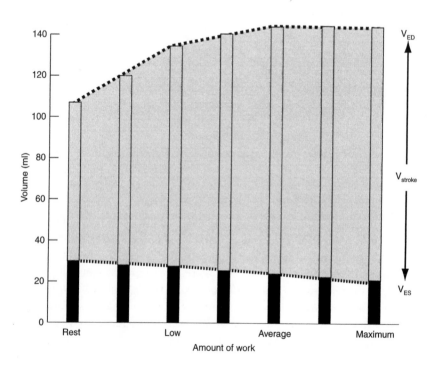

Figure 4.19   Relationship between stroke volume and running intensity
Changes in the stroke volume and the end-diastolic and end-systolic volumes of the left ventricle for various running intensities.

facilitated, and oxygen is transported better to muscles. When the hematocrit value is high, the viscosity of the blood will increase, and the flow of capillary blood becomes more restricted.

The primary factor responsible for enlarging the stroke volume, due to the workloads described, is an increase in the volume of blood plasma. Anatomically, the heart adapts by enlarging the cavity of the left ventricle. Another factor that determines the stroke volume is the force of contraction in the left ventricle. Just like the case of cardiovascular adaptation due to strength training, hypertrophy of the left ventricle has also been found to result from training aimed at increasing the aerobic potential. The muscle mass of the left ventricle increases and thus it can pump blood into the aorta with a greater contractile force. These two factors reinforce each other by increasing the stroke volume. In other words, an increase in V_{stroke} can be attributed to an increase in the end-diastolic volume (V_{ED}) and a decrease in end-systolic volume (V_{ES}):

$$V_{stroke} = V_{ED} - V_{ES}$$

The effects of training, using strongly aerobic running workloads, on HR_{rest} cannot be attributed only to a greater stroke volume. The autonomic nervous system, which regulates internal body processes that cannot be controlled by one's will, is also influential here. The autonomic nervous system includes the parasympathetic and sympathetic nervous systems. While the parasympathetic nervous system is responsible for most body processes that can take place during rest (e.g. digestion), the sympathetic nervous system starts up various processes that prepare the body for action (e.g. heart rate).

In most cases, the two parts of the autonomic nervous system function to bring about opposing effects. The final effect on physical processes is a balance of the activities of the sympathetic and parasympathetic nervous systems. This is also true for the effect that the two systems have on HR_{rest}. That HR_{rest} decreases during training, as has been described, can be attributed to the increased activity of the parasympathetic nervous system and the lower activity of the sympathetic nervous system. Even when the running workload is submaximum, down to 50% of the maximum capacity, the autonomic nervous system still influences the heart rate in this manner.

The interaction between V_{stroke} and heart rate during the development of resting V_{circ} for submaximum and maximum workloads remains a dilemma in the physiology of exercise. It is difficult to separate cause and effect. Does an increase in V_{stroke} cause a decline in heart rate or does a lower heart rate allow V_{stroke} to increase? Nonetheless, one should always strive to meet the demands that are made for optimization of V_{circ} with an eye to the best possible way to use energy. In general, V_{circ} is more efficient when an increased V_{stroke} is accompanied by a lower heart rate. Even when the running workload is maximum, a slight decline in HR_{max} can be found in runners with a high untrained HR_{max} (>180 beats/min), in order to optimize V_{stroke} and therefore also V_{circ}. For such high HR_{max}, the time needed to fill the ventricles is too brief for them to be filled optimally with blood. Because the supply of blood is lower, V_{stroke} decreases. A further increase in heart rate to maintain V_{circ} will result in still less time available to fill the ventricle with blood, and is moreover unfavorable from the perspective of energy efficiency. It is actually a decrease in heart rate that can return to its former level and thus allow V_{circ} to reach its optimum value. The increase in V_{stroke} achieved when an athlete is better trained will result in a substantial increase in the maximum V_{circ}. Maximum V_{circ} values measured in untrained individuals are about 20 l/min, while those found in top marathon runners can be as high as 40 l/min. The V_{stroke} during maximum exercise for well-trained long-distance runners is about 200 ml, while that for untrained individuals is about 100 ml.

In addition to the influence of an increased blood-plasma volume and the autonomic nervous system on V_{circ}, there are a large number of other factors that can indirectly affect V_{circ} by way of preloading, afterloading, force of cardiac contraction, and heart rate. Because of the complexity and diversity of these factors, they are not discussed further here.

Arteriovenous oxygen difference

After a period of training using workloads that focus mainly on increasing the aerobic capacity, an increase in arteriovenous oxygen difference is found, especially after using maximum running loads. An explanation for this increase can be given after comparing the concentrations of oxygen in arterial and venous blood before and after the training period.

Arterial blood is almost 100% saturated with oxygen, both at rest and during a maximum load. Thus alveolar ventilation at sea level is not the factor that limits transport of oxygen, because even under maximum demand arterial blood can become almost completely saturated with oxygen. However, after a period of training, venous blood will contain less oxygen. This means that muscle tissue is better able to extract oxygen from the blood. In addition, active tissues are more generously provided with blood.

4.4.2   Respiratory adaptation using aerobic workloads

The effect that aerobic workloads have on respiratory parameters is limited. Only the vital and maximum ventilatory capacities appear to adapt as a result of training. In long-distance runners, the vital capacity (i.e. the volume of air that can be maximally exhaled after deep inhalation) will increase with the number of years of training (Costill 1986). This is also true for the strength and stamina of the respiratory muscles. Because of this, there will be an increase in the maximum ventilatory capacity (i.e. the volume of air that can be maximally inhaled and exhaled at rest).

In contrast to the cardiovascular system, however, the respiratory system has large functional reserves at its disposal. The pertinent question that must be asked is whether the respiratory system is indeed a limiting factor for the performance of middle- and long-distance runners. In Section 2.4.2, it became clear that ventilation is not the limiting factor because arterial blood is nearly 100% saturated with oxygen during maximum exercise. The partial pressure of oxygen in the alveoli can be maintained, or even increased, by alveolar ventilation during maximum exercise. Furthermore, the passage of erythrocytes through the capillaries supplying the lungs with blood lasts long enough to supply them with sufficient oxygen from the alveoli. The exchange surface for gases in the lungs (i.e. the total surface of the alveoli) is estimated to be 50 m² for a man with a normal build who weighs about 70 kg. During maximum exercise, about 200 ml of blood is present at each moment in the capillaries supplying the lungs with blood. The relationship between the total gas-exchange surface and the volume of blood in the pulmonary capillaries guarantees a large overcapacity in order to take up oxygen across the alveolocapillary membrane.

In addition, a runner is also able to increase ventilation relative to oxygen uptake, from a resting state up to the point of maximum exercise. In a resting state, about 5 l/min is being ventilated and oxygen uptake is 0.25 l/min. In well-trained runners weighing 70 kg, the maximum values for ventilation and oxygen uptake have been measured to be 200 and 5 l/min, respectively. The aerobic metabolism increases comparatively less than ventilation. The value of 200 l/min that ventilation may reach can be further increased on purpose. Runners who have been tested for the maximum volume of air that they can consciously exhale during rest can achieve values that are clearly higher than those measured at maximum exercise. Nevertheless, in spite of these data, which show that ventilation is not the limiting factor, well-trained runners still experience limitations during maximum ventilation. In particular, when ventilation is high, around 200 l/min, and must be maintained for longer periods of time, it can be assumed that the respiratory muscles (notably the diaphragm) can experience fatigue just like skeletal muscles. Moreover, during maximum exercise almost 10% of the total energy will be utilized by the respiratory muscles. The extra energy that is provided by a further increase in ventilation will be completely used up by the respiratory muscles as they perform extra work. Therefore, it appears that expanding the strength, stamina, and efficiency of the respiratory muscles through training will prove useful. It is possible to train at high altitudes for this purpose. At higher altitudes, a runner's respiration will be limited at a lower running intensity, but it is possible that his respiratory muscles will become better trained. In contrast to training at sea level, at high altitude the respiratory muscles will more frequently be confronted with a situation of overload.

4.4.3 Metabolic adaptation using aerobic workloads

Increasing the capacity of the cardiovascular system to transport oxygen, in order to increase aerobic endurance, is always considered to be an important goal of training. Because of the strong relationship between cardiovascular adaptation and the development of oxygen uptake, this appears to be a logical line of thought (Fallowfield & Wilkinson 1999). Untrained runners can quickly improve their stamina through regular practice. For a long time it was thought that such an improvement only resulted from cardiorespiratory adaptation by training with aerobic workloads. In particular, an increased capacity to transport oxygen to working muscles was thought to be responsible for the strong rise in $\dot{V}O_{2\,max}$. The improved pumping function of the heart must play a greater role here. When $\dot{V}O_{2\,max}$ is measured in previously untrained runners after 3–4 weeks of training, it appears that the rise in the value of $\dot{V}O_{2\,max}$ keeps step with performance. Thereafter, the value of $\dot{V}O_{2\,max}$ levels off, even though performance continues to reach higher levels (Viru 1995). An increase in the value of $\dot{V}O_{2\,max}$ can only be found in previously untrained runners after 3–4 weeks of training and in well-trained runners after a long, perhaps even an obligatory, period of rest after which training recommences. Particularly in very well-trained runners, improvement in running performance cannot be attributed to an increase in $\dot{V}O_{2\,max}$ (Verchoshansky 1992). Furthermore, historically it has been shown that $\dot{V}O_{2\,max}$ does not mirror the level of running performance. The running times recorded during various middle- and long-distance events have shown great improvement internationally, while the value of $\dot{V}O_{2\,max}$ measured in top runners is still about 80 ml/kg/min. Moreover, the value of $\dot{V}O_{2\,max}$ measured in trained middle- and long-distance runners during the competition period actually decreases slightly (Verchoshansky 1992).

On the basis of these data, it must be concluded that no close relationship exists between $\dot{V}O_{2\,max}$ measured in trained runners and their levels of performance. It is therefore surprising that some trainers still set as their goal increasing the value of $\dot{V}O_{2\,max}$ in this category of runners. The theory of training today views the role of

$\dot{V}O_{2\,max}$ in evaluating the possible effects of training in a radically different way in comparison with earlier ideas. The reason for this change in course can be described using the analogy of a gasoline motor, where oxygen uptake is equated with the supply of gasoline. While the fuel supply can be increased (through training), the maximum power that the motor (muscles) can generate remains the limiting factor. In other words, the limiting factors lie not in the area of energy supply, but rather at muscle level. This implies that $\dot{V}O_{2\,max}$ must not be seen as a limiting factor and that striving to increase $\dot{V}O_{2\,max}$ will not be relevant for training process. In practice, it has frequently been demonstrated that good runners appear to have muscles that can generate a great deal of power. Such an observation is justified by the fact that runners who perform well over short distances (800 and 1500 m) likewise show exceptionally good performance when running longer distances (3000, 5000, and 10,000 m). That they also can be characterized as having a high $\dot{V}O_{2\,max}$ is because their 'motors' have more horsepower. The solution that must be found when training is how to increase the power that the muscles are able to generate. Unfortunately, no criterion that can easily be applied for evaluation has yet been discovered.

Anaerobic threshold as a topic for discussion

Placing an emphasis on increasing the $\dot{V}O_{2\,max}$ as an important goal when training has often resulted from drawing some wrong conclusions based on underlying physiological mechanisms. An incorrect theory about training has been linked to the relationship between oxygen uptake and running speed. It is generally known that oxygen uptake increases proportionally with an increase in running speed (Åstrand & Rodahl 1986). As speed increases, more muscle mass is required to work and contraction becomes stronger, so that an increase in energy is needed. This demand for more energy is satisfied by an increase in oxygen uptake. Many tests for exercise have shown that as $\dot{V}O_{2\,max}$ is reached, the linear relationship between oxygen uptake and running speed disappears (i.e. the uptake of oxygen levels off). One criterion that has been used to measure when $\dot{V}O_{2\,max}$ has been reached is that the uptake of oxygen must remain constant during further increase in intensity. On this basis $\dot{V}O_{2\,max}$ is measured using a protocol in which the workload is made more strenuous in increments.

Figure 4.20 The relationship between oxygen uptake and running speed
The characteristic change in oxygen uptake as speed increases. At high intensities the relationship is no longer linear: oxygen uptake ($\dot{V}O_{2\,max}$) then reaches a plateau. In many laboratories where physical exercise is studied, the formation of such a plateau for $\dot{V}O_2$ is used as the criterion for calculating maximum oxygen uptake.

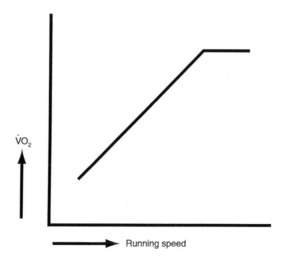

$\dot{V}O_2$

Running speed

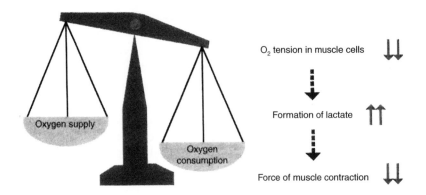

O₂ tension in muscle cells ⇓⇓

Formation of lactate ⇑⇑

Force of muscle contraction ⇓⇓

Figure 4.21   The anaerobic threshold
A seductively simple model for explaining the existence of an anaerobic threshold: the oxygen supply is insufficient so that an oxygen deficiency develops in the muscle cells; generation of energy from anaerobic processes must be increased; and more lactate is formed, causing muscles to contract less powerfully.

The plateau in oxygen uptake was first discovered in 1927 by the physiologists Hill and Lupton (Noakes 1988). They found from their research that a plateau in oxygen uptake always occurs when the running speed is increased in increments, and they proposed a simple explanatory model. As the speed of running becomes faster, at a certain point oxygen becomes deficient (hypoxia) in the working muscles. Thus the energy that can be supplied by oxygen is insufficient and must be supplemented anaerobic (without oxygen) energy supplies, which quickly produce lactate. This concept is still frequently used to explain the phenomenon 'anaerobic threshold'. Simple reasoning shows, however, that this concept can never be proof for the existence of an anaerobic threshold, as discussed below.

Using such reasoning, improving the body's ability to transport oxygen through training would lead to an increase in oxygen uptake at similar submaximum running speeds. However, in both trained and untrained individuals the uptake of oxygen at submaximum workloads either remains constant or even decreases. It appears that the explanation for the increase in aerobic endurance and the lower production of lactate due to training should probably be sought in changes in metabolism resulting from biochemical adaptation in muscle.

Moreover, recent studies have shown a plateau in oxygen uptake occurs in less than 50% of people tested when the workload is increased in discrete steps. Although the uptake of oxygen did not plateau, these runners also had to end their tests due to exhaustion. This discovery offers very little support for the theory that oxygen deficiency in muscle arises when the running intensity is high.

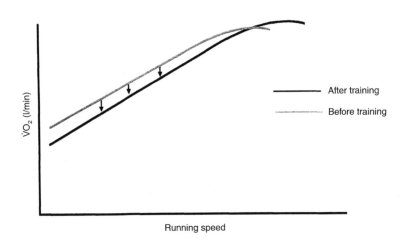

Figure 4.22   The relationship between $\dot{V}O_2$, running speed and the influence of training
As a result of training, the $\dot{V}O_2$ either declines or remains the same at submaximum running intensities.

There has been much discussion within the field of exercise physiology about the existence of an anaerobic threshold. A sudden increase in the concentration of lactate in the blood during physical exercise has long been associated with oxygen insufficiency in muscle (Wasserman & McElroy 1964, Myers 1996). The term 'anaerobic threshold' finds its origin here, i.e. that energy must be generated anaerobically due to hypoxia in the muscle. That a non-linear increase in the concentration of blood lactate is characteristic of the existence of an anaerobic threshold can be found in various definitions. According to Viru (1995), the anaerobic threshold represents the highest intensity of exercise at which the formation of pyruvate does not exceed the maximum speed of oxidative phosphorylation. In this case, the lactate produced can either be oxidized or used for gluconeogenesis by less active muscles, the heart, and liver. Up to this point, the production and elimination of lactate has remained in equilibrium.

According to Davis (1985), when the effort reaches a certain intensity, which differs between individuals, the anaerobic threshold represents the point at which the concentration of blood lactate begins to increase. When the intensity of exercise is increased further, the concentration of blood lactate also rises progressively. The consequence of the last two definitions is that, when the workload is only slightly intensified, from the moment that the rate production of lactate exceeds the rate of its elimination, an athlete's endurance time will fall from about 1 h to 15 min (Åstrand & Rodahl 1986). In various pieces of research, therefore, endurance time has been included in the definition of an anaerobic threshold. In the area of training, there has been much interest in the concept of an anaerobic threshold in relation to regulating the optimum intensity applied in training and competitions. However, criticism has been directed in particular at the assumption of a causal relationship between the sudden increase in lactate concentration, oxygen insufficiency in muscle, and changes in ventilation.

In other descriptions of the anaerobic threshold, these factors have been equated with the point at which ventilation suddenly increases, i.e. the ventilatory threshold (Simon et al 1986). Various parameters are involved in detecting the ventilatory threshold (Wasserman et al 1997). These parameters have their origins in the buffering action of bicarbonate, which maintains the pH of the blood and reg-

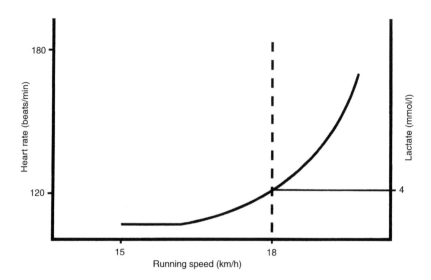

Figure 4.23   The concentration of lactate in the blood
The point where the concentration of lactate starts to increase exponentially is generally considered to be the anaerobic threshold.

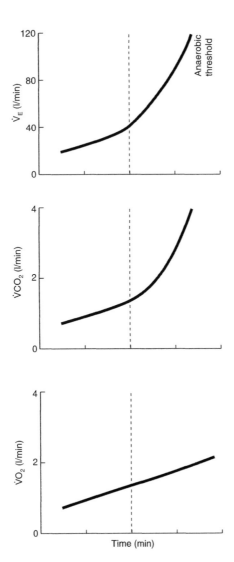

Figure 4.24 Detection of the anaerobic threshold
Use of ventilatory parameters to detect the anaerobic threshold: $\dot{V}_E$, ventilation (expiratory); $\dot{V}O_2$, oxygen uptake; $\dot{V}CO_2$, emission of carbon dioxide gas.

ulates the production of carbon dioxide. Ventilation is increased not only by the additional production of carbon dioxide from the bicarbonate buffer, but also by the formation of lactate, and therefore protons (H^+), when anaerobic metabolism increases.

Proof that no anaerobic threshold exists

Proof that there is no anaerobic threshold that can possibly be detected on the basis of ventilatory parameters was provided by a group of patients suffering from McArdle's disease. These patients are not able to break glycogen down into lactate because they do not have the phosphorylase enzyme. However, as exercise intensity increases, at a certain point ventilation will show an exponential increase similar to the pattern found in individuals who do have this enzyme. Furthermore, various studies have demonstrated that the ventilatory threshold frequently does not coincide with an exponential increase in the concentration of lactate in the blood (Gaesser et al 1984, Gaesser & Poole 1986). For that matter, an exponential increase in the blood lactate concentration is not clearly seen when exercise intensity is increased in discrete steps (Myers 1996), and thus an anaerobic threshold becomes difficult to

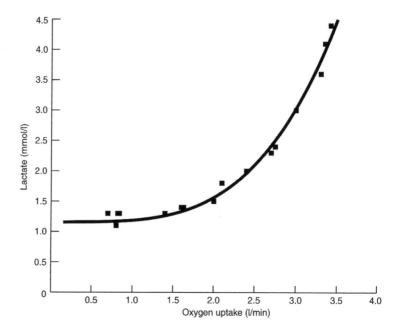

Figure 4.25 The relationship between the concentration of lactate and $\dot{V}O_2$
The relationship between the concentration of blood lactate and $\dot{V}O_2$ as the running speed increases. When the speed is increased incrementally, there is no clear kink in the curve at the start of the exponential rise in the concentration of blood lactate.

determine. Moreover, the sudden rise in the concentration of lactate appears to be highly dependent on the experimental protocol employed, the surrounding temperature, and the individual's nutritional state (Brooks et al 1996).

Furthermore, it can be stated that the concentration of lactate in the blood does not correctly reflect what is happening within the muscle. First, the lactate concentration measured in the blood is a result of the production of lactate in the muscle and its elimination by less active muscles, the heart, and the liver. Although the blood lactate concentration was found to be 4 mmol/l, values measured by means of muscle biopsy were 2.5–9 mmol/l. In addition, there is always a delay in the transport of lactate produced in muscle to the blood. Therefore one can conclude that the concentration of lactate in the blood cannot provide explicit information about anaerobic metabolism (Brooks et al 1996). Therefore, in the discussion of the means and methods of training given later in this chapter (see Section 4.5), exercise intensity is not assessed in terms of the anaerobic threshold. One must note, however, that a running intensity near an alleged anaerobic threshold does reflect a training-sensitive zone for middle- and long-distance runners. A training-sensitive zone implies that training carried out close to such a running intensity can produce a considerable effect. However, one must nevertheless conclude that any concept of an anaerobic threshold based on physiological mechanisms will prove weak.

Types of metabolic adaptation

The degree of training will influence the percentage of $\dot{V}O_{2\,max}$ that can be maintained for a certain workload. Trained runners can maintain 80–90% of $\dot{V}O_{2\,max}$, while untrained runners achieve their alleged anaerobic thresholds near 50–80% of $\dot{V}O_{2\,max}$. The shift toward a higher percentage of $\dot{V}O_{2\,max}$ when the body is better trained is called 'metabolic adaptation' (Bunc & Leso 1993). The most important adaptations that result from the use of aerobic workloads are an increase in the size and number of mitochondria (Holloszy & Coyle 1984) and an increase in capillarization of stressed muscle tissue. In addition to increases in mitochondrial density and muscle capillarization, an increase in key enzymes involved in fatty-acid oxida-

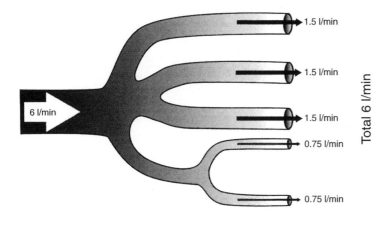

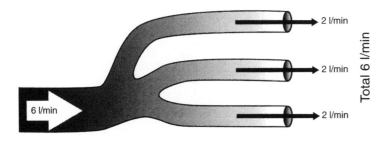

Figure 4.26   The influence of training on the capillary density of a muscle
Because the surface area of the total capillary cross-section increases as a result of training, the rate of capillary blood flow will decline, thus facilitating a better exchange.

tion, the Krebs cycle, and the respiratory chain has also been demonstrated in runners trained for endurance. The resulting consequence for metabolism is that the rates at which glycogen and blood glucose are used are slower, when the running workload is aerobic in character, because the contribution to the total delivery of energy of fatty-acid oxidation is greater and the production of lactate is lower at the same submaximum running load.

It has been determined at the muscle-fiber level that, particularly in type-II (fast twitch (FT)) muscle fibers, there is an increase in mitochondrial density. By their nature, type-I (slow twitch (ST)) muscle fibers have the most mitochondria, but after intensive endurance and interval training the difference in the mitochondrial densities of type-IIa and type-I muscle fibers levels off. The result is that homeostasis is more greatly disturbed in untrained individuals than in trained runners, when the running intensity is constant. Trained runners are better able to regulate their production and use of energy. In particular, the increase in mitochondrial density causes a lower flux of substrate per enzyme in the respiratory chain at submaximum running speeds. The result is that, in contrast to untrained individuals, in trained runners there is less need to change the substrate and enzyme concentrations in order to attain a certain speed for the resynthesis of adenosine triphosphate (ATP) (Holloszy & Coyle 1984).

In Chapter 2 it was stated that the presence of adenosine diphosphate (ADP) is required to initiate mitochondrial respiration. Because trained runners have more mitochondria per gram of muscle tissue, oxygen uptake per respiratory chain decreases when the running load is submaximal. As noted previously, oxygen uptake at a submaximum running load is identical in trained and untrained runners. The consequence is that the concentration of ADP need not increase as much

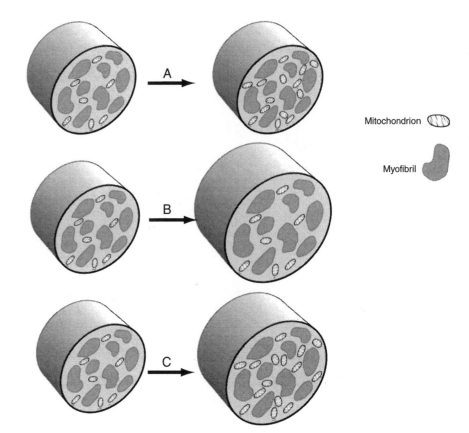

Mitochondrion

Myofibril

Figure 4.27a   Metabolic adaptation in runners
When training middle- and long-distance runners, one must strive to achieve an optimum balance between adaptations resulting from changes in metabolism and from strength training.
(A) Mitochondrial density increases while the diameter of the muscle fiber remains constant.
(B) The diameter of the muscle fiber increases, leading to a decrease in density when the number of mitochondria remains constant.
(C) The optimum balance between both types of adaptation: slightly hypertrophied muscle fiber with increased mitochondrial density.

in trained individuals in order to achieve a certain level of oxygen uptake. An incidental advantage is that keeping the concentration of ATP high while ADP does not have to increase as much, as in trained runners, has an inhibitory effect on phosphofructokinase, the key enzyme in glycolysis. This might possibly explain why trained athletes use less glycogen and produce less lactate when running at submaximum speeds. This inhibition of phosphofructokinase is further supported by the fact that the contribution of fatty-acid oxidation increases as a fraction of the same the total delivery of energy through an increase in the enzymes involved in the metabolism of fat. In addition, when the body is trained, fat metabolism is stimulated by an increase in the supply of intracellular triglycerides as well as an increased release of free fatty acids from fatty tissue into the circulation.

Eventually such metabolic adaptations will result in increased aerobic stamina. Trained athletes are thus able to run longer at a higher percentage of $\dot{V}O_{2\,max}$, while the rate of glycogen depletion is reduced and less lactate is produced. In contrast to the untrained runner, this difference becomes even more obvious because the supply of glycogen in the liver and muscle has increased in the trained runner, whose body has adapted to types of training, such as tempo endurance, which exhaust the glycogen supply.

Influence of the capillary flow rate

Another adaptation to a chiefly aerobic running workload that has not yet been discussed is the increase in capillarization in stressed muscle tissue. In particular, the exchange of oxygen and carbon dioxide is improved because blood can flow more

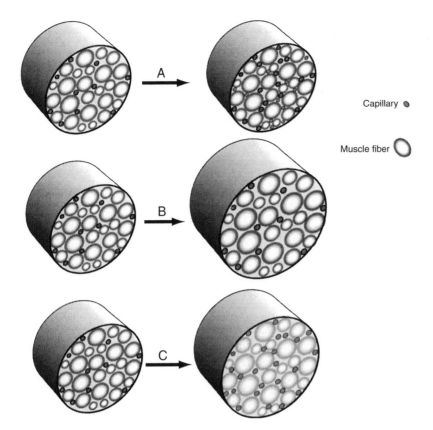

Capillary ●

Muscle fiber ○

Figure 4.27b   Metabolic adaptation in runners
When training middle- and long-distance runners, one must strive to achieve an optimum balance between adaptations resulting from changes in metabolism and from strength training.
(A) Capillary density increases while the diameter of the muscle fiber remains constant.
(B) The diameter of the muscle fiber increases, leading to a decrease in density when the number of capillaries remains constant.
(C) The optimum balance between both types of adaptation: slightly hypertrophied muscle with increased capillary density.

slowly through the capillaries when the capillary density is higher. At first glance, it is tempting to think that the capillary flow rate will be higher due to the smaller diameter of such blood vessels in comparison to those blood vessels situated closer to the heart. However, the rate of flow is determined by the total cross-sectional area, which is larger at the level of the capillaries than that of any other blood vessels, including the veins (Silverthorn 1998). An aerobic running load can contribute to an increase in capillary density in stressed muscle tissue and thus to a reduction in the flow rate of capillary blood. Furthermore, capillaries can open more completely in a trained runner, thus resulting in a more effective circulation of blood. The latter applies to the arterioles lying before the capillaries, which are able to restrict the supply of blood to certain capillaries but allow it freely to others. Because of such an adaptation, the erythrocytes take more time to pass through the capillaries and blood gases are exchanged more optimally.

Summary

The metabolic adaptations thus far described cannot be considered independently of those adaptations that occur as a consequence of strength training in middle- and long-distance runners (see Ch. 6). If the output of power from the muscle groups involved in locomotion can be increased together with an increase in capillary and mitochondrial density, there will be a desirable adaptation in middle- and long-distance runners. Furthermore, the increase in power output from those muscle groups should occur without the development of too much hypertrophy in the muscles concerned (see Ch. 6).

4.5 MEANS AND METHODS OF TRAINING

It has already been stated that if a runner wishes to improve through practice, the training must always be directed at increasing speed over a certain distance. This is valid for both the sprinter and the long-distance runner. Therefore, when a training program is being set up and definite plans made, one will always begin with the central question: In what manner can a moving body increase its speed? In order to answer this question, it is first necessary to analyze which factors will limit performance. An analysis based on the relative contribution of various basic motor properties has too many limitations. It is better to approach the problem of how to increase speed, which is closely related to increasing the mechanical power generated (see Ch. 2), from a number of perspectives. Using a biomechanical approach, one can cause more mechanical power to be generated by using specific types of technique and strength training. This is described in detail in Chapters 5 and 6.

The question can also be approached from the perspective of the physiology of physical exercise. Here the emphasis lies particularly on the adaptations that occur in the body's metabolic and vegetative systems. When, through training, an athlete increases the amount of energy generated metabolically in his body, he also increases his mechanical power and therefore his running speed. Vegetative systems exert a large influence on how the energy-delivering systems function. One example is the role played by the cardiorespiratory system during the generation of aerobic energy. The heart and lungs are responsible for providing the oxygen necessary for the respiratory chain to function. In this section we discuss the means and methods of training that are especially directed at metabolic and cardiorespiratory adaptations. Little attention is given to the way in which a runner can train for the sprint in athletics, as it is much more appropriate to approach this topic from a biomechanical perspective. Training that is aimed at high-speed running (sprinting) involves training the body to become coordinated. Technique and strength training can also be applied here. The definite choice of specific running workloads that can be applied for the sprint are dictated by the degree to which an athlete can maintain his coordination. Processes that generate energy and the role played by the cardiorespiratory system are almost never included when setting up or adjusting a sprint training program. Even the effects of training can be evaluated according to criteria associated with coordination. For a description of the means used to train for the sprint, see Chapters 5 and 6.

It is impossible to achieve an optimum effect if only one type of practice or method is used during training. When discussing the training principles, which have been derived from biological patterns, the importance of providing variation in order to achieve an optimum effect is underlined. Training in different ways will yield the highest adaptation. For example, when only an endurance workload is employed, then after the first period of adaptation no further increase in running performance will be observed. After some time, endurance training will no longer bring about a disturbance in homeostasis and the effect of training will disappear. There is a narrow range within which the ways of training can be varied because the principle of specificity must be adhered to to achieve an optimum effect. Within the stipulations demanded, one can differentiate 15 different ways of training, which can be grouped under five training methods. These five methods can be differentiated on the basis of how certain characteristics of the running workloads are categorized, in that each running workload has five separate characteristics for stress.

4.5.1 Workload characteristics

Intensity

Intensity refers to the severity of a running load and can be defined as either absolute or relative. The word 'absolute' implies that the intensity is independent of the athlete, while the word 'relative' implies that the intensity is related to an individual. An example of absolute intensity is the running speed given in meters per second or kilometers per hour. The relative intensity, for example, can be expressed as the running speed at a certain percentage of the individual's maximum heart rate or maximum oxygen uptake, or at a certain concentration of blood lactate. The intensity of a running load is a factor that determines whether the training will have an effect. In much of the literature on training, intensity is the criterion used to categorize the various types of training (Zintl 1995).

Being able to pinpoint an optimum intensity for training, so that an athlete can most rapidly improve his performance, appears to be a factor that determines whether a training program will prove to be successful. Although long-distance runners, in particular, focus strongly on the total volume of their weekly training, the intensity of the training is probably a more important factor (Foster et al 1999). In practice, it can be observed that middle- and long-distance runners can only complete a large volume of intensive running loads with difficulty. Data based on the experience of trainers clearly show that 5–20% of the total volume may consist of intensive running loads (Daniels 1998). However, results of experiments in which the number of intensive training sessions was increased or in which the existing intensive training was extended, showed that running performance improves (Lehmann et al 1991). The limitation of such studies is the duration of the intervention. As a rule, this was no longer than 8 weeks, and so the results of these studies cannot be applied to longer periods of training. In practice, it is generally known that a relatively intense period of training must precede any improvement in the level of running performance. A runner must make time to adjust to the specific intensity required for the distance that he will run during competition. This requires a period of 4–12 weeks during which training sessions are at an intensity similar to the distance which will be run during the competition.

Duration

Here one is speaking of the duration or distance of a single repetition within a running workload. For example, in an interval training session in which the athlete runs 10×1 min with 2-min pauses, the duration of the workload is 1 min.

Volume

The workload characteristic of volume is related to the total distance covered in one training session. Usually this is expressed in meters, kilometers, or units of time. For example, the volume of an interval training session of 3×2 km with pauses of 500 m, is 7 km: $(3 \times 2 \text{ km}) + (2 \times 500 \text{ m}) = 7$ km.

When long-distance runners are asked if they have been training rigorously, they usually reply by specifying their weekly volume of training. The number of kilometers run each week is the central issue, while the intensity of the training is seen to be a means of perfecting one's form (Foster 1998). This is a perfect starting point for a recreational runner when he must make a 2–3 h effort for a competition. According to the 'collapse point hypothesis', introduced by Young (1973), the optimum preparation for a competition lasting 2–3 h requires a weekly training volume that is greater by a factor of 2.5. Thus the weekly workload for a recreational runner training to run a marathon successfully must be at least 105 km. If fewer kilometers have been covered during the preparatory period, there is a high chance that the runner will not be able to maintain the tempo during the last leg of the marathon. It appears that there is a strong relationship between training volume and performance level for recreational marathon runners. However, this relationship becomes less precise when the weekly training workload exceeds 140 km. From this point onward, an unrestricted increase in the number of kilometers run weekly does not lead to improved performance and may even prove to be counterproductive. Many scientific studies have shown that increasing the training volume can actually lead to overtraining (Lehmann et al 1991) (see Section 4.5.3).

Density

The term 'density' refers to the relationship between exercise and recovery. For example, when the exercise/recovery ratio is 1:1, the duration of an individual repetition will be the same length as the pause that follows (e.g. 10×2 min with 2-min pauses).

Frequency

This component of exercise stands somewhat apart because, in contrast to the above-mentioned relationships, it relates to more than one training session within a certain period of time (generally 1 week). Here frequency can be defined as the number of training sessions per period of time, and is used to determine the magnitude of the workload, as viewed over a longer period of time. Some top middle- and long-distance runners with long training experience find themselves required to work through 10–14 training sessions each week. The law of diminishing returns will prevail here. These athletes will throw themselves into a strenuous training program with the hope that their bodies will adapt in a manner that can be translated into a slight improvement in performance. During such high-frequency training, it becomes imperative that exercise and recovery are alternated correctly.

4.5.2 Training methods

Training methods can be differentiated on the basis of five characteristics:

- endurance methods
- interval methods
- repetition methods
- competition or control methods
- other methods.

Each of these is described below.

Endurance training

When undertaking endurance training, an athlete will run without stopping for periods of rest. The way in which this type of training is conducted is by running continuously. Based on intensity, one can differentiate three tempos of endurance running:

- endurance tempo-1
- endurance tempo-2
- endurance tempo-3.

The subdivision into three tempos is based on the type of substrate used in the aerobic pathway. As the intensity of the endurance training increases, comparatively more glycogen will be used to resynthesize ATP. When the endurance load is highest, the share of free fatty acids serving as substrate for the resynthesis of ATP will be greater. Furthermore, one can differentiate between different forms of endurance running in which the three running tempos are alternated.

Endurance tempo-1

Endurance tempo-1 is the slowest. The intensity of endurance tempo-1, expressed as the heart rate for which the runner strives, is 65–75% of the maximum heart rate (HR_{max}) or 60–70% of the heart rate reserve (HRR). When using maximum oxygen uptake as the criterion for intensity, the running intensity can be scaled at 60–70% of $\dot{V}O_{2\,max}$ or 65–75% $_v\dot{V}O_{2\,max}$ (see Section 2.5).

Distances can vary between 5 and 40 km. This wide range in the duration of the workload is due to whether endurance tempo-1 is used in the short-term (e.g. after a strenuous training or a competition on the previous day) or long-term (e.g. in preparation for running a marathon). In the first case, the purpose of endurance tempo-1 is active recovery. In the second case, one is aiming more for specific training before running a marathon. The percentage share of fatty-acid oxidation in the total delivery of energy is high in long-term endurance tempo-1. A marathon runner who has chosen to include such endurance training as part of his preparation is aiming to stimulate fatty-acid oxidation in such a manner that it will contribute a greater share of the total energy generated. In the end, increased fatty-acid oxidation will have a glycogen-saving effect. Glycogen supplies in muscle will then become exhausted less rapidly. During long-term endurance tempo-1, the supply of glycogen in ST muscle fibers decreases strongly because it is impossible to pump only free fatty acids into the Krebs cycle (see Section 2.2.3). Moreover, the intensity of endurance tempo-1 is high enough that glycogen must also be used as substrate for the aerobic pathway. A spirometer can be used to measure the uptake of oxygen and the emission of carbon dioxide gas at various running speeds. The relationship between the emission of carbon dioxide gas and oxygen uptake can be expressed as a ratio and used to estimate to what extent glycogen and free fatty acids are involved as substrate for the aerobic generation of energy. This ratio, which is called the respiratory exchange ratio (RER), can be determined from the composition of exhaled breath and reflects the uptake of oxygen and emission of carbon dioxide gas at muscle level:

$$RER = \dot{V}CO_2/\dot{V}O_2$$

The value of RER is 0.7 when only free fatty acids are oxidized. The following calculation illustrates how this value of 0.7 has been obtained. The oxidation of palmitic acid, which is a free fatty acid that occurs frequently in the body, requires 23 molecules of oxygen, thereby releasing 16 molecules of carbon dioxide:

$$C_{16}H_{32}O_2 + 23\,O_2 \rightarrow 16\,H_2O + 16\,CO_2$$

$$RER = \dot{V}CO_2/\dot{V}O_2 = 16/23 = 0.7$$

The oxidation of free fatty acids uses more oxygen than the processing of glycogen in the aerobic pathway. During oxidation of glucose or glycogen, the ratio of oxygen uptake to emission of carbon dioxide gas is 1:1:

$$C_6H_{12}O_6 + 6\,O_2 \rightarrow 6\,H_2O + 6\,CO_2$$

$$RER = \dot{V}CO_2/\dot{V}O_2 = 6/6 = 1.0$$

When the value of RER is 0.85, the contributions of free fatty acids and glucose or glycogen in the generation of energy are identical. At endurance tempo-1, the value of RER is quickly reached. When the substrate is fatty acids, 4.69 kilocalories (kcal) of energy per liter of oxygen is generated, while 5.05 kcal/l is generated when either glucose or glycogen is the substrate. Oxidation of glycogen or glucose therefore provides 6.4% more energy per liter of oxygen than oxidation of free fatty acids. However, 1 g of fat contains 2.3 times more energy than 1 g of carbohydrate. The practical consequence of this is that when the running load is intensive, but not too lengthy (2–45 min), glycogen and glucose are the preferred substrates because the degree of oxygen uptake will play a limiting role. When the workload is lengthy, the glycogen-saving effect is positive because of the increased share of fatty-acid oxidation when applying long-term endurance tempo-1 during training. Coupling endurance tempo-1 with the aim of the training, i.e. increasing the percentage by which fatty-acid oxidation contributes to aerobic metabolism, is only relevant if the glycogen supply is expected to be more of a limiting factor than is oxygen uptake for the distance that will be run during the competition.

The physiological method used for measurement is called indirect calorimetry. A number of assumptions are made here. First, the contribution of 'fast' glycolysis must be negligible. Measuring the emission of carbon dioxide gas and oxygen uptake in exhaled breath is a correct indicator of aerobic metabolism if the workload during running is submaximal and is steady-state in character. The contribution from 'fast' glycolysis will increase the concentration of H^+, and thus the bicarbonate buffer will release extra carbon dioxide, which arises from the supply of bicarbonate that is already present and is not a direct product of aerobic metabolism. When the value of RER is approximately 1, the contribution of glycogen and glucose tend to be overestimated for aerobic metabolism. Second, it is assumed that the contribution of protein oxidation is negligible in terms of the total amount of energy generated. When the running load is lengthy, however, the contribution of protein oxidation can be estimated at 10%. In summary, the RER can be used to estimate what type of substrate will be used for steady-state running loads that are not too lengthy.

Endurance tempo-2

Endurance tempo-2 is the middle tempo. The running intensity is 70–80% of HRR or 75–85% of HR_{max}. Because it is related to maximum oxygen uptake, the intensity is 70–80% of $\dot{V}O_{2\,max}$ or 75–85% of $_v\dot{V}O_{2\,max}$.

Depending on the aim and degree of training, endurance tempo-2, can be maintained between 5 and 30 km. It is the tempo most frequently used to train long-distance runners and is an important way to build up the volume of training, particularly by increasing the individual training sessions planned or by applying them more frequently. Because its intensity is higher than that of endurance tempo-1, free fatty acids contribute less and glycogen more as substrate for the aerobic pathway.

Endurance tempo-3

This tempo is the fastest. Another frequently used name for this tempo or intensive endurance training, while endurance tempo-1 and -2 are also called extensive endurance training. In better trained runners, the tempo used for endurance tempo-3 is such that it can be maintained for approximately 1 h. The running intensity is 80–90% of HRR or 85–90% of HR_{max}. When maximum oxygen uptake is used as reference, the intensity corresponds to 80–90% of $\dot{V}O_{2\,max}$ or 85–90% of $_v\dot{V}O_{2\,max}$.

The scope of endurance tempo-3 can vary from 4 to 15 km, depending on the aim and degree of training. The substrate used in aerobic metabolism is almost entirely glycogen. Because the supply of glycogen in muscle is greatly lowered, any increase will be characteristic of adaptation resulting from endurance tempo-3.

Type	HR_{rest} (%)	HR_{max} (%)	$\dot{V}O$ (%)	$_v\dot{V}O_{2\,max}$ (%)
Endurance tempo-1	60–70	65–75	60–70	65–75
Endurance tempo-2	70–80	75–85	70–80	75–85
Endurance tempo-3	80–90	85–95	80–90	85–90

Table 4.3 Different types of endurance training and intensity

Better runners will be able to differentiate even further between a wider range of endurance tempos. When energy is mainly being generated aerobically, the tempo applied can range from 10 to 21 km/h. Obviously it will be easier for an individual running at a lower level of performance to differentiate even further. Generally, five subdivisions can be made for endurance tempos:

- recovery endurance training
- endurance tempo-1
- endurance tempo-2
- endurance tempo-3
- tempo endurance running.

This subdivision is discussed further later in this book.

Variable endurance training
In addition to the above-mentioned types of endurance running, one can also designate variable forms. These are characterized as being a combination of endurance tempo-1, -2, and -3. Because the tempo can be varied for endurance training, one is able to introduce a 'new' stimulus. In this manner, one can avoid any decline in training effect that might occur if endurance running was limited to a constant tempo. Variable types of endurance running can be categorized as follows:

- *Interval endurance running.* In this form of training the three endurance tempos are alternated randomly. One block in which a certain tempo is used will last from 2 to 5 min. The block tempo is chosen intuitively. When an athlete feels that he is running with ease, then relatively more blocks of tempo endurance tempo-3 can be run. On the other hand, if running becomes more laborious, more blocks of endurance tempo-1 are included.
- *Alternating-tempo endurance running.* Endurance tempo-1, -2, and -3 are used alternately in prescribed tempo blocks lasting a minimum of 5 min. An example of an actual choice for endurance running with alternating tempos could be 2–2–2–2–2 km endurance running at endurance tempos 1–2–3–1–3.
- *Climax endurance running.* The distances and corresponding running tempos are prescribed so that an athlete begins by using the slowest and completes the prac-

tice running at the fastest tempo. An example of climax endurance running might be: 4–4–2 km at endurance running tempos 1–2–3. As the intensity gradually increases, near the end of this type of training the athlete will be running at a high percentage of his maximum oxygen uptake. Being able to run for a long period at a high percentage of the maximum oxygen uptake is an important quality for a marathon runner (see Section 2.5.1).

Interval training

In the interval method periods of work and recovery are interchanged systematically. During periods of recovery, complete recovery is generally not achieved. The great advantage of the interval method is that one can increase the cumulative time over which a high tempo can be maintained in comparison to using a single workload with the same intensity until exhaustion occurs (Åstrand & Rodahl 1986). Furthermore, interval training has a unique effect on the cardiovascular system. The highest priority for the cardiovascular system is to maintain blood pressure. Blood pressure is determined by the V_{circ} and total peripheral resistance (TPR):

$$\text{Blood pressure} = V_{circ} \times TPR$$

V_{circ} is the product of the stroke volume (V_{stroke}) and heart rate (HR):

$$V_{circ} = V_{stroke} \times HR$$

During the first run in interval training, vasodilatation occurs in the muscles being worked, thus decreasing the TPR. In order to maintain the blood pressure, V_{circ} must rise. After the first repetition in an interval training session has ended, the heart rate falls rapidly within a short period of time. In order to avoid a rapid decline in V_{circ} and because a large quantity of venous blood is being returned, V_{stroke} must be increased temporarily. Due to this phenomenon, interval training becomes rather like strength training for cardiac muscle. The result is both an increase in volume and hypertrophy of the left ventricle. The period for which V_{stroke} is temporarily increased is only brief. Therefore, it is useless to repeat pauses lasting longer than 2 min.

Two subdivisions have been created for the interval method. The first division (extensive and intensive) is based on the intensity of the workload:

- Extensive interval training: lower workload intensity; shorter pauses; and serial pauses are generally not used.
- Intensive interval training: higher workload intensity; longer pauses; and serial pauses may be used, depending on whether fatigue develops quickly.

The second subdivision is based on the duration of the workload in order to differentiate between two types of interval training:

- short intervals
- medium-length intervals.

Long intervals, which are differentiated as a third type in much of the literature on training, have purposely been omitted here because the pause used in this type of interval training generally exceeds the 2 min considered optimum. In the terminology used here, types of training involving both long intervals and pauses exceeding 2 min are termed 'tempo training' (see other training methods, p. 231). In this book attention is given only to the first division.

Extensive interval training

The characteristic feature of extensive interval training is the application of many repetitions and few pauses. Because pauses are brief, the athlete is forced to run at a tempo that is 70–80% of the maximum that can be used to run the relevant distance. For example, if a distance of 400 m can be run in no longer than 60 s, then the intensity of the extensive interval training will be 75–85 s for 12 repetitions of 400 m with 1-min pauses.

Heart rate can be used to check whether the intensity is correct. After 3–4 repetitions, the heart rate may range from 10 to 15 beats/min less than the HR_{max}. One should only check the heart rate after 3–4 repetitions because it takes some time before the system for transporting oxygen is working optimally. It is suggested that the heart rate should be kept 20–25 beats/min less than the HR_{max} when running the first repetitions. After the transport of oxygen has adapted, the heart rate for which one is striving will rise to 10–15 beats/min less than the HR_{max}, although the intensity remains constant.

The length of a repetition ranges between 50 and 800 m. Recovery pauses should last no longer than 2 min. If the pause lasts longer, then the training effect will not be optimal. Interval training holds a special place of importance when the distance run is not less than 50 m. At first glance, it might appear that this type of training will involve in particular the creatine–phosphokinase reaction (see Section 2.2.3) and 'fast' glycolysis. However, there is a small supply of oxygen present in muscle that is bound to myoglobin. This oxygen reserve can be called upon when using short-term running workloads and is replenished after a brief pause for recovery. Interval training in which the duration of the workload is 10 s (about 50 m) and the pauses between repetitions are 5 s long can be continued for 30 min, while a continuous workload of identical intensity will cause the runner to stop because of exhaustion after about 4 min (Åstrand & Rodahl 1986). During interval training of this type, the concentration of lactate in the blood is remarkably low and the reduced supply of creatine phosphate is rapidly replenished by aerobic processes. These findings emphasize the effect of the small supply of oxygen on myoglobin. The duration of the pauses must not exceed 15 s. Thereafter, the concentration of lactate

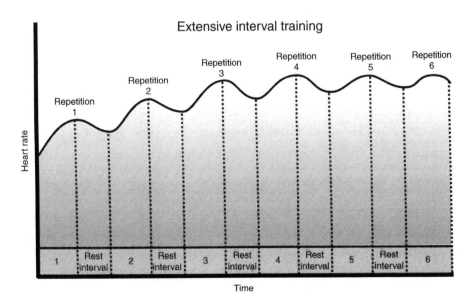

Figure 4.28 Heart rate and interval training
The heart rate targeted during extensive interval training can only be achieved after 3–4 repetitions. Only then will it prove useful to control intensity by measuring heart rate.

in the blood will rise, thus indicating an increased contribution from 'fast' glycolysis. The result will be a large reduction in the time for which an athlete can continue running. The total volume of extensive interval training varies from 2 to 8 km, depending on how well the athlete has trained.

Intensive interval training

In comparison to extensive interval training, here an athlete will run at a higher tempo, which will be 80–90% of the maximum speed that can be achieved for a certain distance. For example, intensive interval training consisting of three series of four repetitions across 300 m, with the fastest time clocked for 300 m being 36 s, can be run in 40–45 s across 300 m. In addition to the pauses between repetitions, in order to guarantee a high running tempo, serial pauses are also inserted. The repeated pause may not exceed 2 min, just as in extensive interval training. The duration of a single repetition ranges between 100 and 800 m, while the total volume of an intensive interval training session will not exceed 5 km.

Repetition training

This method is characterized by the use of repeated intensive workloads, between which are inserted periods for complete recovery. Usually this method is only used for well-trained runners. The intensity of the repetitions is very high, at 90–95% of the maximum tempo that can be run over a certain distance. For example, a repetition of 3×1000 m will be completed in a tempo between 2 min 40 s and 2 min 49 s, if the best recorded time over 1000 m is 2 min 32 s. When using this training method it is common to make an assignment based on the duration of the workload for a repetition:

- repetition training for short-distance running
- repetition training for medium-distance running
- repetition training for long-distance running.

Table 4.4 gives an overview of the length of the repetitions and the total volume for the three types of repetition training. Depending on the distance to be run during the competition, certain types of repetition training may be inserted more frequently into a training program.

Type of repetition	Length of repetition (m)	Total length (m)
With short distances	100–300	500–2000
With middle length distances	300–800	1000–3000
With long distances	800–3000	2000–6000

Table 4.4   Repetition training method

The contribution made by the creatine–phosphokinase reaction and 'fast' glycolysis to the total amount of energy generated during repetition training is much greater than in interval training. This is because the ATP/ADP ratio regulates itself after complete recovery. The ATP/ADP ratio must first decrease somewhat in order for the aerobic pathway to get started (see Ch. 2).

Competition or control training

The competition or control method uses a single competition-specific training load. The situation expected to be encountered during a competition is simulated or the athlete actually runs in a competition, starting with a certain assignment. The purpose is to ascertain, just before a series of important competitions, whether a runner is in good form and what are his strong and/or weak points. For example, an individual preparing to run a marathon can test himself during a half marathon by running the tempo intended for the actual marathon. In this manner, one can test whether the intended running tempo is indeed realistic. Furthermore, a certain tactic can be tested and practiced during a trial competition. Such competitions can be classified as build-up races and are indispensable for developing the high level of performance that must be produced during the main competition.

Other training methods

The methods that can be used during training form the last category, because they cannot be included in the methods already mentioned. The remaining methods are:

- tempo training
- Fartlek (i.e. 'playing' with tempo), where changes in tempo are usually dictated by the terrain on which an athlete will run (e.g. hills, loose sand)
- training on hills.

Tempo training

This means of training forms the link between interval and endurance training. Because the duration of the workload is longer, a short repeated pause, such as in the interval method, which lasts a maximum of 2 min is not sufficient. Although the 2- to 4-min pauses employed will not guarantee complete recovery, they make it possible for an athlete to run high-intensity repetitions. The aim is to stress the aerobic system completely. Therefore, the intensity is set at 95–100% $\dot{V}O_{2\,max}$ or 100% $_v\dot{V}O_{2\,max}$. Expressed in terms of heart rate, the running intensity is 98–100% of HR_{max} or 95–100% of HRR. The intensity can likewise be ascertained as 75–90% of the best performance over the relevant distance. For example, a tempo training of 5×1200 m with 4-min pauses will have an intensity ranging from 3 min 31 s (211 s) to 4 min 13 s (253 s) when the best recorded performance over 1200 m is 3 min 10 s (190 s).

The duration of the workload will not exceed 6 min, with a minimum duration of 2 min, because otherwise the aerobic system will start up at a lower percentage of the best performance. The scope of the workload will range from 3 to 8 km, depending on the duration of the workload.

Fartlek

This form of training resembles endurance running in that there are changes in tempo. The changes in tempo are dictated by the condition of the terrain. In this manner, one creates a hybrid form composed of a variety of ways in which to train for a sprint, running on hills, and tempo, as well as various types of endurance running. Therefore, this type of training is difficult to classify under the parameters used for workloads.

Training on hills

Training on hills is a specific form of strength training with a very small overload. When training on hills, there can only be a high degree of specificity if the total movement of the body closely resembles the movement being targeted. The gradient must not be too steep (a few percent to 10%) because otherwise the correct running technique cannot be maintained (see Section 5.1.4). When the overload is large due to a steep gradient, immediate damage will be done to the specific pattern of coordination for that movement. When running on steep hills the pattern must be adapted in such a manner that the ground contact time is longer (loss of reactivity) and other muscles (i.e. the hamstrings, gluteus maximus, and quadriceps femoris) must be used.

From the perspective of the physiology of exercise, it is advantageous to include hill training in a running program because more power is required from the muscles involved than when running on a flat surface. From this point of view, training on hills can be applied over distances of 300–2000 m. The aim of such training is to increase aerobic stamina. The intensity and density of this form of hill training are equivalent to those for tempo training. It should be noted that the pauses between repetitions will be longer because of organizational problems. The workload will range between 2000 and 8000 m.

One must be cautious when using the shorter (100–300 m) variation of hill training because of the above-mentioned low specificity coupled with a high overload when the angle of incline measures several percent. One might even consider replacing the extra resistance experienced when running up hill by running against the wind on a flat surface.

4.5.3 Overreaching and overtraining

When exercise and recovery are not in equilibrium, the intended adaptation will not be achieved, and thus there will be a temporary decline in performance. In the case of overreaching, such a decline in performance is compensated for by a recovery period of several weeks. Therefore, overreaching can be defined as short-term overtraining. If overreaching lasts too long, it may develop into the overtraining syndrome, which will require weeks to months of recovery.

It is difficult to differentiate between strenuous training, overreaching, and overtraining. In addition, when confronted with overreaching, a runner will usually experience a decline in his performance, which he will generally try to reverse by training harder. In this way, a runner may easily fall victim to an incorrect interpretation of the results that he has achieved during practice or competition.

Figure 4.29 The relationship between the weight of the workload and the increase in the level of performance
Training will only be optimal within a narrow range. Overreaching can be applied with the aim of increasing the level of performance beyond what can be achieved by training within the optimum range.

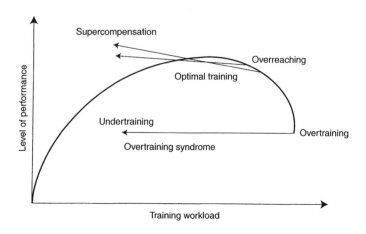

Moreover, trainers will apply overreaching with the purpose of bringing about greater adaptation than can be achieved by training within an optimum zone. A disturbed relationship between exercise and recovery may be the most important, but not the only, cause of overtraining. Additional factors that can increase the intended stress of the workload during training are, for example, emotional and social stress, climatological conditions, monotony during training, and an agenda filled to the brim with competitions.

The problem of overtraining occurs on a wide scale in runners. In interviews with long-distance runners, 60% admitted to having been confronted at some time by the phenomenon of overtraining (Hooper et al 1995). It is noteworthy that studies on overtraining have shown that a large increase in the scope of a regular training program can lead to overreaching and overtraining within the foreseeable future, while creating a program that is just as strenuous by increasing its intensity will actually result in improved performance (Lehmann et al 1991). One can presume that the explanation for this difference, which occurs more frequently in runners who have intensified their training programs, can be found in the fact that days of strenuous training are alternated with days of easier training. When the scope of is broadened, the separate training sessions begin to resemble one another, so that switching between rigorous and mild days of training will become more difficult. In other words, the training will become more monotonous.

4.5.4   Monotony during training

Extra attention should be paid to the problem of monotony, which can work to increase stress during training, because it is a factor that will play a key role in preventing overtraining. Moreover, it is easy to keep score of this factor in a training diary.

According to several of Foster's studies, one can quantify the daily training load by multiplying the sum of the duration of training by the degree of exertion experienced by the runner. The 'measure of exertion experienced' (MEE) will be a number between 0 and 10. A value of zero is equal to rest, while a value of 10 represents maximum effort. A weekly total can be determined by scoring the value of the workload each day. The weekly score appears to be a good measure for fatigue, although

RPE	Description
0	Resting state
1	Very calm
2	Calm
3	Reasonable
4	Lively
5	Heavy
6	
7	Very heavy
8	
9	Nearly maximum
10	Maximum

Complete list within 30 minutes of training

Figure 4.30   The table according to Foster The measure of exertion experienced (MEE) can be scored using these items.

233

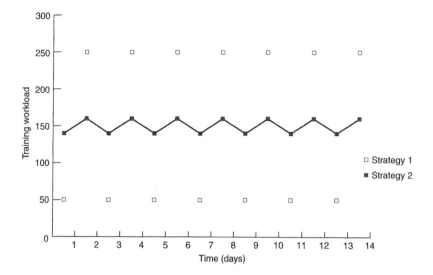

Figure 4.31a   Training strategy
Two training strategies using identical total workloads. Strategy 1: heavy and light workloads are continuously alternated during training. Strategy 2: the training workloads are almost equally strenuous.

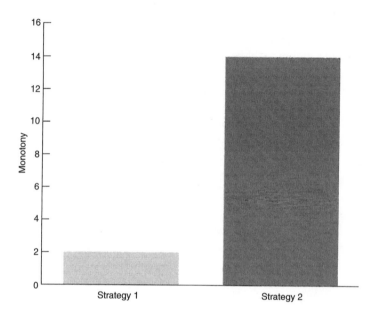

Figure 4.31b   Training strategy
The difference in monotony between strategies 1 and 2. Monotony can be defined as the weekly training workload divided by the standard deviation (SD). The training workload will be experienced as heavier the more monotonous a training strategy becomes.

it is of little value as an absolute measure. Rather, variability is much more important for calculating the stress caused by training. One can calculate the standard deviation (SD) for the weekly training load. The SD is a measure of deviation from the average: i.e. the smaller the SD, the less deviation from the average. By dividing the weekly score by the SD one obtains a new measure called the monotony score. The higher the monotony score, the more the training workloads will resemble each other. In addition to the daily average workload, SD, and monotony score, we can now easily calculate the weekly training workload by multiplying the daily average by 7.

The last measure that can be obtained from these factors used to monitor training is the level of stress caused by the workload. Stress can be defined as the training load multiplied by the monotony score. In one of Foster's studies, it was demonstrated that individual runners appear to tolerate a certain level of stress. If a runner

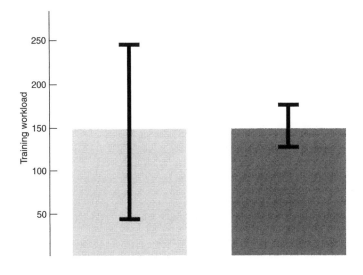

Figure 4.31c   Training strategy
The average workloads used daily in strategies 1 and 2 are identical. The standard deviation has a much wider range for strategy 1.

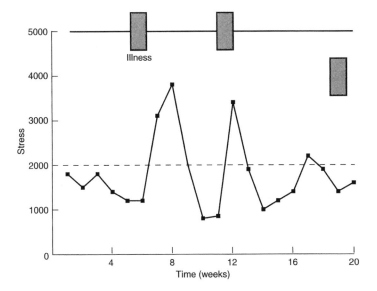

Figure 4.31d   Training strategy
The stress of training is registered each week for 20 weeks. Each runner has an individual level of stress that he finds tolerable. For the runner in this example, the threshold is at 2000. When this level is exceeded, this runner will be at greater risk of contracting an infectious disease, such as the flu, or developing a head cold. The runner in this example fell ill three times about 1 week after exceeding the 2000 line.

exceeds his stress level, the likelihood of adverse events (e.g. susceptibility to infections such as flu) is greatly increased.

It can be concluded from the relationship between the workload, variability, and stress of training that much variation is needed within a training program. Careful monitoring of the workload may offer the possibility to prevent overtraining.

5

Running techniques in practice

5.1 INTRODUCTION

Learning a motor skill is not an isolated process. The locomotor system is strongly interwoven with the body's sensory system and physical condition. This interrelationship is so complex that trying to make a distinction between variables for condition (strength, speed, stamina, etc.) and coordination would prove difficult, if not impossible and foolhardy. When training the locomotor system, one will observe a strong interaction between coordination and the sensory system and between coordination and physical condition. There must be a good interaction between these important requirements to be able to learn to move efficiently. Integrating the sensory system into the learning process makes good coordination possible which, in turn, is necessary in translating the training of one's physical condition into improved performance. On the other hand, an athlete must be in good condition in order to continue moving in a well-coordinated manner at the top level of his ability to perform. This interrelationship is not only found for complex patterns of movement such as running hurdles (sense of balance, awareness of the knee angle by way of proprioception, correct positioning of the trunk and swing leg when jumping hurdles, sufficient speed and strength for running in a three-stride rhythm, etc.). Even types of training, such as certain forms of strength training, in which coordination appears to be less important, the interrelationship between the sensory system, coordination, and physical condition is highly influential. In strength training, just as when using simple exercises, an important part of any improvement in performance can be attributed to an improvement in coordination. Therefore, during training it is important to maintain as well as possible this interrelationship between the three components (the sensory system, coordination, and physical condition).

5.1.1 Sensory system and coordination

Exercises in which little is demanded of an athlete's physical potential are particularly suitable, as well as necessary, for learning in detail how sensory information can be coupled with coordination. The motion of running is cyclic, which means that much of the information necessary for regulating the pattern of running originates in the motion of running itself (see Section 1.7). The effect that the reafferent sensory system has on the motor pattern is thus quite extensive. Being aware when such information is forthcoming is necessary if one wants to improve one's running technique according to a certain plan. Learning how to interpret sensory data about coordination (e.g. the position of the joints, pretension in the muscles) is also necessary when giving running instruction. Understanding the interrelationship between the locomotor and sensory systems is not only necessary in order to learn how to react to and correct errors in movement, but also to learn how to improve a pattern of movement so that errors will not occur. Being able to cope adequately with sensory information helps a runner learn to position his body more consistently and use push-off more advantageously.

This can be illustrated by the following example. The angle of the knee at the moment of initial contact (IC) determines how energy is loaded into and released from the elastic components. The magnitude and direction of the forces at work around the knee joint at the moment of IC change so rapidly that an athlete cannot direct them by reacting to information 'released' at the moment of IC. A pre-designed blueprint is needed with which one can perfectly anticipate what will happen at IC (Bobbert et al 1992). The information required to ensure that a perfect knee angle is 'designed' for the moment of IC can be derived from observing the external (type of ground surface, wind, etc.) and internal (how tension is built up in muscle, etc.) conditions. Only after integrating all this information correctly will it be possible to design a pattern of movement for the following strides, which will use elasticity optimally. With regard to timing and efficiency, for the hamstrings this will mean that the way in which the outward swing is organized just before IC, external forces are absorbed at IC, and the hamstrings transfer energy will be highly dependent on the way in which sensory information obtained from previous movements can be evaluated and incorporated in the ensuing pattern of movement (Cranenburgh 1997).

The hamstrings are a group of muscles for which it is not the amount of force they develop, but rather the way in which that force can be exactly adjusted during the process of running, which will determine the level of performance. In order to promote such fine-tuning between the sensory and locomotor systems, it is necessary to practice all sorts of running-related patterns of movement at a low intensity, without undergoing the related stress of a high tempo or a high level of force. If exercises are always carried out under physical stress, an athlete will never be able to refine his technique. The details of a running technique are so complex that an athlete will seldom, or never, be able to achieve absolute perfection, even when practicing calmly. Moreover, without constant practice, any refinement in technique will quickly be forgotten. Therefore, an exercise employing low-intensity movement is meaningful at all times and at all levels. The central concern is to sensitize the athlete to what his body is telling him.

The next step in this process is for the athlete to learn how to relate the sensory and motor systems when under conditional stress (maximum speed or extreme fatigue).

5.1.2 Condition and coordination

Good coordination is possible if it is facilitated by well-developed physical characteristics. For example, in order to execute a good running technique at high speed, one must be able to quickly build up a sufficiently high level of force, and contraction in the relevant muscle groups must occur fast enough. Conversely, it is also true that good coordination is an important vehicle for developing what is required of the body. The speed of muscle contraction, a high level of reactive force, etc., will only result when the patterns of movement in which these activities take place are correct and meaningful (see, e.g., how reflexes affect a pattern of movement; Section 1.7).

The strong interrelationship between coordination and physical condition often results in a simultaneous improvement in both aspects during training. For example, during speed running, the upper body should be held upright. To do this, the abdominal muscles must be strong. However, they must be strong for a specific function (i.e. working reactively as a corset). Holding the body correctly during speed running will cause the abdominal muscles to function with greater strength. At the same time, working the abdominal muscles reactively during strength training will ensure a better posture for running. Stronger abdominal muscles do not necessarily result when the physiological profile of the muscle increases, but will mainly result from improved muscle control and, therefore, improved coordination.

From this perspective, it is obvious that it is desirable to combine the aims of physical condition and coordination whenever possible. The habit of many trainers to interpret an athlete's training performance using only a stopwatch is a dubious practice. After all, an individual who runs a distance of 1500 m reactively will demonstrate a totally different type of performance (energy expenditure and coordination) than someone who runs an identical distance within the same time using a poorly reactive, energy-wasting technique. The effect of training for such effort will therefore also vary. In the first case, more will be demanded of properties such as elasticity, strength, and rapid build-up of force, while, in the second case, more will be demanded of the cardiorespiratory system and the quadriceps femoris, which is only partially active during reactive running.

In some cases, it is futile to combine condition with a correct pattern of running. For example, during strength training using heavy weights, it is almost impossible to achieve a pattern of movement that resembles good running. In such a case, from the perspective of training efficiency, it is better to put aside trying to combine improvements in coordination with condition for running. Rather, it is advisable in such situations to incorporate only one or two aspects of a running technique into the strength training employed. Moreover, limiting the combination of running technique and condition is quite important if strength training is to prove effective.

5.1.3 Principle of overload

Whether or not training is effective depends on the manner in which the body adapts to the training stimulus applied. If the body is not well equipped to carry out the task required, then the body will have to adapt to the demands made. However, once the body is able to implement what is being asked, it will cease to adapt further. A status quo will be reached in which no further change is achieved. If an athlete wishes to develop further his ability to perform, he must change the stimulus used during training and make it more difficult. A new stimulus will lead to improvement in performance until the body once again has adapted to the new demands. Therefore, the body will need to constantly experience a more strenuous training stimulus, which is called 'overload'. The principles of overload and adaptation not only hold true for the physiological aspects of exercise, but also for the way in which a runner's performance is coordinated, because condition and coordination are strongly interrelated. To improve patterns of coordination, the body also needs to experience an overload directed at the total pattern of coordination (i.e. running itself) or at one of its components.

If training only consists of running, it will be difficult to organize in such a way that adaptation in the area of coordination can be produced over a longer period of time. In practice, therefore, it is more effective to utilize other forms of movement during training in addition to running, i.e. placing more emphasis on various aspects of running. To adapt to a pattern of movement over a longer period of time, it is necessary to use many different (significant) stimuli during training.

5.1.4 Transfer of training

Not every sufficiently strong stimulus will automatically lead to an improvement in running performance. Overload will not automatically result in an improvement in the pattern intended. For example, a sprinter who only exercises with weights will not automatically become more coordinated and begin to run faster. Even after an individual has developed more strength throughout the sequence of extension by training, coordination must still be correctly trained in order to convert that strength into a practical running pattern. The conversion of training methods into practical movement is called the 'transfer of training', and this will only take place once the three demands for specificity have been met:

- equivalent internal structure of movement
- equivalent external structure of movement
- equivalent generation of energy (when applicable).

One pattern of movement can only be used to improve another pattern if the components of the two patterns are similar. Forms of exercise that closely resemble the motion of running itself will therefore transfer well to the running technique. A form of exercise such as pushing a bar-bell along the front of the body, which shares only a few similarities with the motion of running, will implement a transfer only to those few commonly shared aspects.

When practicing, therefore, one must attend to two opposing interests: the demand for overload and the demand for specificity. These opposing interests can be inserted into the central–peripheral model (see Section 4.2.2). Exercises that are peripheral with regard to the movement targeted supply a large overload but less specificity. Exercises that remain close to the target (central) have greater specificity but less overload.

From the perspective of coordination, for exercises that are far removed from the motion of running, the aim and implementation of training must first be described precisely before being implemented, with strict adherence to the assignment. If one fails to do this, the specificity, which is already slight, will quickly be lost and the exercise will become its own master, without contributing any improvement to the intended movement.

An example is 'pumping iron' during strength training. One such exercise is a vertical extension on two legs, which shows little resemblance to the motion of running. The transfer of coordination must be accomplished by adhering to the details exactly. The motion must be executed in such a way that the dorsal muscles help to keep the spinal column completely straight. If the spine is kept straight, it is possible to regulate well the movement in the pelvis (forward tilt). Consequently, the hamstrings will experience an eccentric moment which, through the motion of pushing the weight of the bar-bell, will cause the hamstrings to work well both isometrically and reactively. In this manner, improvement in coordination between the dorsal muscles and hamstrings is facilitated.

Less strict demands are made when carrying out exercises that are more closely related to the motion of running. Types of reactive jumping, on one or two legs, are not too far removed, with regard to ground contact time and body posture, from the body posture required during running. Ground contact times for speed running are about 0.07–0.11 s. All types of reactive jumping, for which ground contact times are similar and the hips and knees are kept more or less extended, will thus prove useful. Forms of exercise that are even more closely related to the motion of running entail even fewer restrictions on how they should be implemented. All the same, any description of how to perform such an exercise should be formulated specifically. An exact implementation of such an exercise will increase the transfer of the training to the movement targeted, and will therefore prove extremely effective.

5.1.5   Economy of training

A final factor in determining whether or not an exercise should be used is the principle of economy when coping with physical exercise. Exercises should be avoided when they carry a high risk of injury or result in such an assault on the body that a long period of recovery becomes necessary. For example, when strength training is carried out using relatively heavy weights, the investment that an athlete must make and the risks that he must take in order to work very specifically on a movement are so great that the cost–benefit equilibrium quickly becomes unbalanced. In such a case it is better for a trainer to refrain from trying to combine too wide a range of the properties required for the condition and coordination of the intended movement. Rather, it is advisable to direct the transfer at a single aspect of condition and coordination, while attempting to train other aspects by using different exercises.

The case becomes more complicated when coordination is linked to speed, as in supramaximal running. The chance of injury during such exercises, and the resulting need for a long period of recovery, is so great that failing to make a strong link between the manner of implementation and the movement targeted will not prove economical. In other words, it is only worth investing in supramaximal running if the transfer of training is worthwhile, i.e. if the specificity is quite high. Supramaximal running involves an athlete running downhill or being towed along by someone else. If the athlete then runs too fast, he will not be able to maintain the correct body posture for speed running. Such an implementation will clearly be too dangerous and is too far removed from the intended movement to justify the accompanying risks. If an individual runs slower (just a bit faster than maximum), the pattern of movement will demonstrate a good resemblance to that employed during speed running (according to the outermost shell of the locomotor system, see Fig. 3.1). One must ask, however, whether the internal pattern of movement also mirrors that used in speed running (according to the second shell of the locomotor system, see Fig. 3.1). In particular, do the hamstrings work like they do during speed running (to counteract knee extension during push-off), or is the rectus femoris working actively to generate (through both hip and knee extension) a greater vertical impulse during supramaximal running (Jacobs & Ingen Schenau 1992, Cranenburgh 1997)? If activity does in fact shift from the hamstrings to the rectus femoris, then the question arises of whether the relationship between risk and effect is still favorable enough for the exercise to be effective. If one wants to avoid such a shift in activity, then how closely should one adhere to the top speed during supramaximal training without help in order to avoid a change in the pattern of movement? Running within the supramaximal range makes such a great demand on specificity from the standpoint of costs and benefits that overload can be only minimal. Supramaximal training is a form of exercise which, in terms of the economy of training, is quite difficult to evaluate and which should be applied with extreme caution.

5.2 Basic components of running

Just as there are few differences between individuals in the anatomical blueprint of the body, there are hardly any interindividual differences in the manner in which patterns of movement are built up. A functional movement is always carried out by means of the same pattern of muscle activity in different individuals. Every pattern of functional movement is constructed on a fixed series of basic mechanisms. This is also true to a large extent for running (Doorenbosch et al 1997). Some mechanisms that are important in running are:

- the reactive muscle function of specialized muscle groups
- the fixed reflex-response patterns, which support movement
- the sensory function of, for example, the abdominal muscles and the sole of the foot
- the transfer of force from proximal to distal areas.

Because running is a very natural form of movement, such basic mechanisms also directly affect the way in which someone moves.

In practice, it appears extremely useful, as well as necessary, to train such basic mechanisms separately (as partial movements). When an athlete is able to cope well with the basic components of movement, it is often relatively easy to apply them during running to improve performance. It is also true that a runner will not be able to improve his running technique if he lacks sufficient control over the mechanisms upon which the targeted movement is based. For example, a runner wants to learn how to increase his stride, but he still has insufficient control over the mechanism for converting landing energy into a vertical impulse reactively. When he attempts to take longer strides during running, he cannot transfer the development of a longer stride into a faster running speed. However, if executed correctly, practicing types of reactive jumping will almost automatically lead talented runners to re-use landing energy during running. Lengthening the stride, which is rather easy to accomplish, will then result in an improvement in performance.

It is possible to practice the basic mechanisms of movement by using all sorts of training, i.e. when training for strength, jumping, or speed. In this chapter we discuss exercises for training athletes on the track and in the field. The elements of the basic drills used in strength training are presented in Chapter 6.

Because various mechanisms overlap and affect each other significantly, it is frequently difficult to differentiate between cause and effect when implementation is incorrect. The trainer must be quite adept analytically to unravel interrelationships and to begin re-training where mistakes have been made. Being able to understand, as well as to intuit, how the basic mechanisms of movement function is also of assistance. Thereby, one must recognize that many of the pertinent factors are still unknown. The information given in the following subsections is, therefore, based not only on published scientific data, but also on the practical experience that running instruction can offer regarding significant issues. The text is not intended to be complete, but rather we approach the practice of running from an adequate number of perspectives. The exercises presented for training are generally suitable for improving more than one basic aspect of running. It is useful to approach these exercises from different perspectives, and therefore some are repeated for more than one basic mechanism.

5.2.1   Function of the ankle and foot

The manner in which the foot functions during running has a large effect on the total pattern of movement. This is true not only during the swing (open chain) phase, but also during the support (closed chain) phase. By regulating the position and motion of the foot one can also control the total pattern of movement. It is therefore imperative to practice control of the feet during exercises. The function of the foot, and therefore also of the exercise program, can be divided into three categories:

- transferring sensory information from the joints and the sole of the foot to regulate locomotion
- storage and return of energy
- transfer of energy from the knee extension to the ground surface (via the gastrocnemius).

Sensory information

Information obtained from the sole and other structures in the foot is important for refining one's control over locomotion. For example, the progression of pressure through the sole of the foot signals how the transition from a closed to an open chain is timed. The ability to observe these signals correctly is often disturbed when strongly shock-absorbing shoes are worn. In addition, the regulating function of these signals often proves faulty because the runner has not been taught to incorporate and interpret them during technique training. Incorporating such signals in a good running pattern is not as easy as it might first appear. Pressure placed on the foot during the landing, which subsequently travels along the foot, does not result only from the speed of the body moving in horizontal and vertical directions. How joints are positioned and how they move in relation to the rest of the body (reafferent sensory system), and external influences (exteroceptive sensory system) also affect the way in which pressure travels through the foot during the support phase. A high degree of dorsiflexion halfway through the support phase will result in a different flow of pressure than when the transition to plantar flexion occurs early. Therefore, being aware of signals arising in the foot and incorporating them correctly in the total pattern of movement is essential in order to create a good running pattern. Experience has shown that controlling the position of the foot is an important mechanism in regulating locomotion in general (Pink et al 1994).

Good runners are almost always sensitive to the exact condition of the ground (hard, soft, or synthetic) and are able to adapt their running technique according to the nature of the surface. In contrast to landing on a softer base, the body will rebound faster on a hard surface, so that the running technique will require a somewhat shorter ground contact time and, therefore, different timing. During practice, emphasis should be placed on learning to interpret and use the signals sent from the foot.

The exercise program described in this book can be broadened in a number of ways. The exercises require little effort, but can still contribute significantly to making coordination more precise. Even top athletes should repeat these basic exercises frequently.

Figure 5.1a–i   Exercise 1: hopping on one leg, with and without ground taps

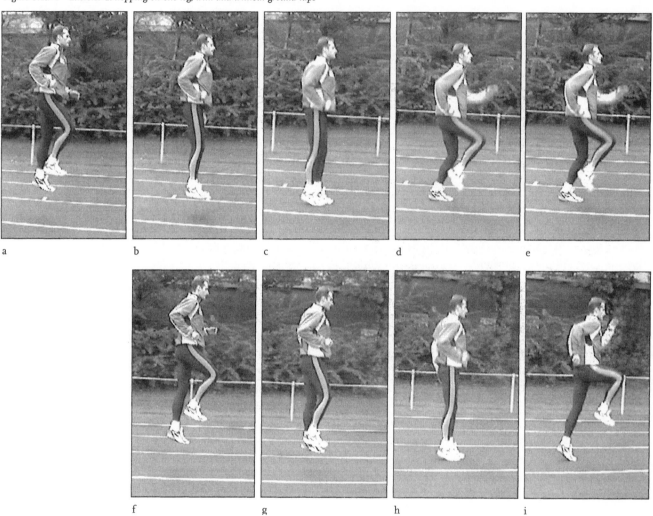

a   b   c   d   e

f   g   h   i

Exercise 1   Hopping on one leg, with and without ground taps

Here an athlete hops on one foot while slowly moving forward. While continuing to hop, the free foot repeatedly lightly taps the ground together with the hopping support foot. The free leg must touch the ground very lightly while the other (support) leg carries the weight of the body. The body is held as erect as possible with the knee of the stance leg only bent as little as possible. This so-called single-leg hop is done reactively, keeping the ground contact time as short as possible. Once an athlete has mastered the rhythm of the exercise, the knee of the free leg can be repeatedly lifted horizontally during the floating phase. By tightening the stance leg well, rebound will be higher. Like the two-leg hop, where each knee is lifted alternately, a single-leg hop is an important basic exercise used during running instruction. The athlete is asked to perform single-leg hops with a large range of movement in the free leg and brief ground contact, with the foot of the free leg tapping the ground as lightly as possible. After 5 m, the foot must no longer touch the ground while the leg continues to oscillate up and down in the same way. After 10 m, the foot must again repeat tapping the ground lightly. Hopping reactively will prove easier when the ground can be tapped. The signal received as the free foot taps the ground is apparently valuable in helping the stance leg to work reactively. The runner learns to be aware of signals coming from the free leg and to link them to reactivity in the stance leg.

Figure 5.2a–f   Exercise 2: hopping on one leg with small variations in height

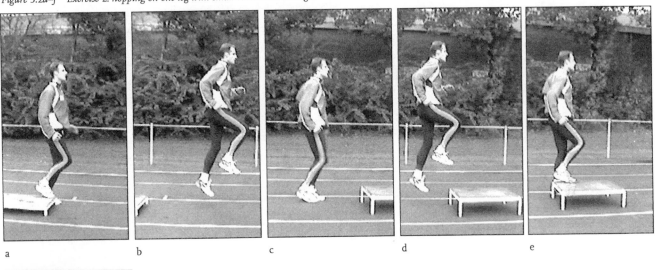

a   b   c   d   e

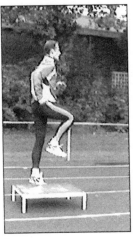

f

Exercise 2   Hopping on one leg with small variations in height

The athlete hops on one leg while moving forward along a number of obstacles, no higher than 20 cm, which have been placed, for example, 1 m apart. The free foot taps the elevation and the ground between elevations. These small differences in height cause the rhythm of the movement to change, so that push-off must be continuously readjusted. The signal sent from the tap is integrated into the constantly changing pattern of movement.

Figure 5.3a–e   Exercise 3: hopping on one leg using an elevation

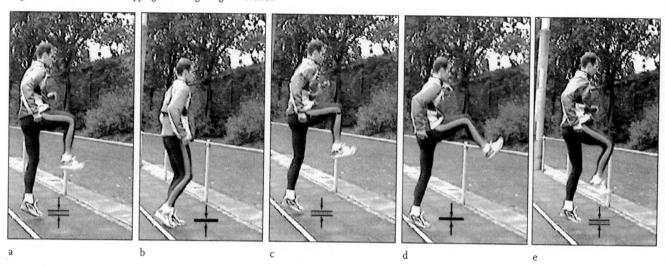

a   b   c   d   e

Exercise 3   Hopping on one leg using an elevation

After hopping twice, the free foot touches the ground and the edge of the elevation once (e.g. an 80-cm railing). This exercise begins at a slow tempo. Once the athlete has mastered the rhythm, the frequency is increased to what is maximally possible. Push-off from the stance leg and tapping with the free foot must be exactly coordinated to avoid disrupting the rhythm and causing the exercise to fail. To do this, the athlete must concentrate on the rhythm of the taps.

Figure 5.4   Exercise 4: skipping from a soft to a hard surface

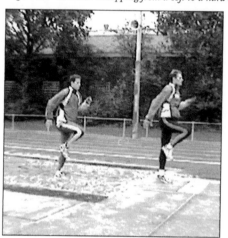

Exercise 4   Skipping from a soft to a hard surface

Signals sent from the foot change when the surface upon which the athlete is exercising changes. The pattern of movement must be attuned to these varying signals. For example, first a runner skips forward in sand before moving across a hard surface. Because the ground reaction force will change, he must adjust his pattern of movement. In addition to transitions between extremely different ground surfaces, there are also more subtle transitions. An athlete must learn to be alert to any such changes in order to fine-tune his movement pattern when small differences arise. Learning to be aware of such transitions and adjust one's pattern of movement can also be practiced using other forms of exercise (e.g. tripping, hopping, skipping with double ground contact).

Figure 5.5a–g   Exercise 5: skipping (single ground contact) with and without heel contact

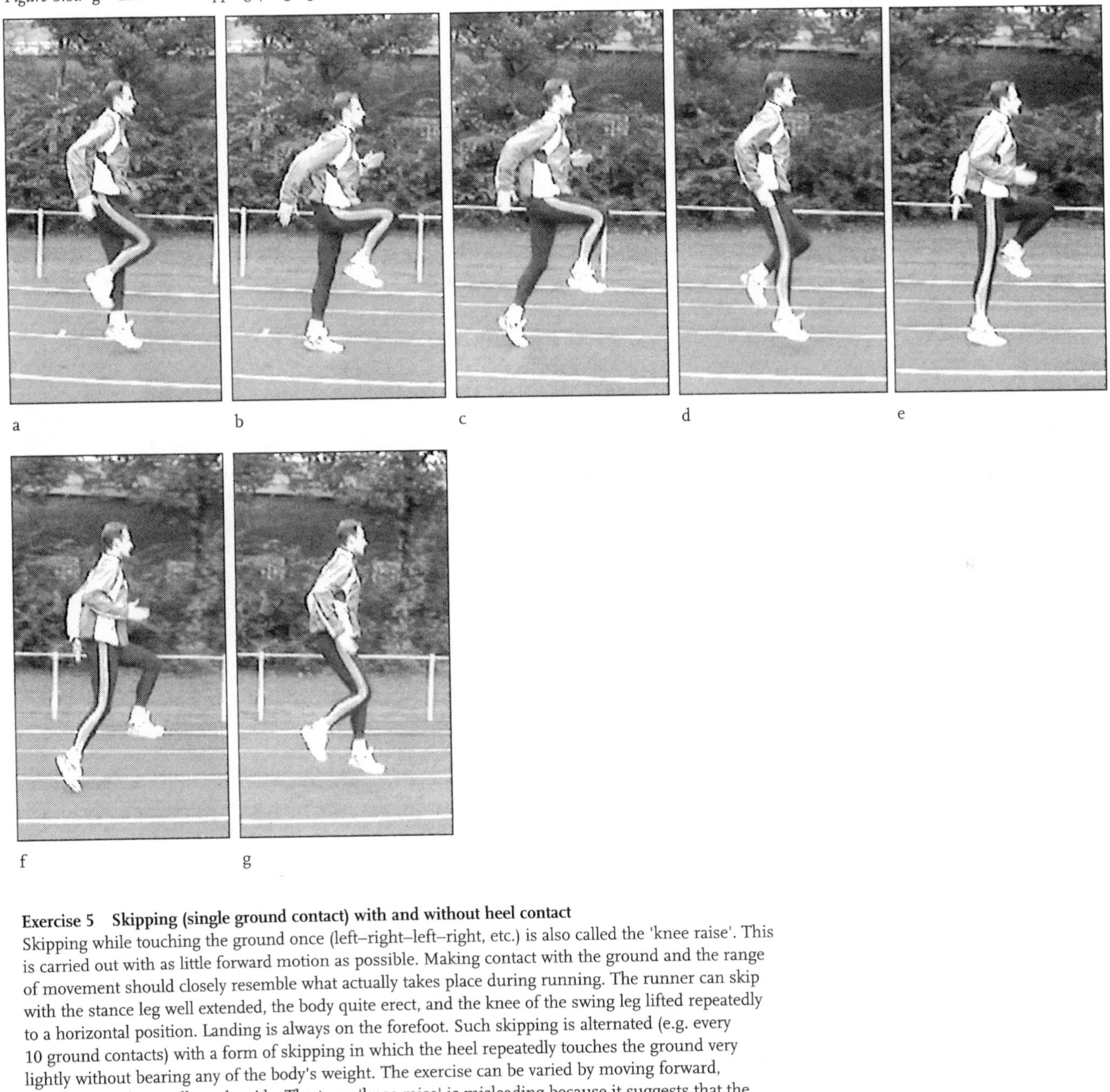

a   b   c   d   e

f   g

Exercise 5   Skipping (single ground contact) with and without heel contact

Skipping while touching the ground once (left–right–left–right, etc.) is also called the 'knee raise'. This is carried out with as little forward motion as possible. Making contact with the ground and the range of movement should closely resemble what actually takes place during running. The runner can skip with the stance leg well extended, the body quite erect, and the knee of the swing leg lifted repeatedly to a horizontal position. Landing is always on the forefoot. Such skipping is alternated (e.g. every 10 ground contacts) with a form of skipping in which the heel repeatedly touches the ground very lightly without bearing any of the body's weight. The exercise can be varied by moving forward, backward, or diagonally to the side. The term 'knee raise' is misleading because it suggests that the aim of the exercise is to train the muscles that lift the leg, particularly the iliopsoas. However, if one concentrates only on lifting the knee, the stance leg will not be extended and the ground contact time will be quite long. In this manner, the exercise will be of little use (even for the iliopsoas, which undergoes only slight exertion) and more rapidly lead to a failure rather than an improvement in technique.

Figure 5.6a–f   Exercise 6: hopping on one leg (variation)

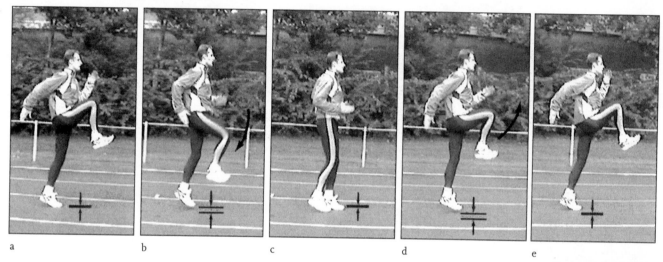

a   b   c   d   e

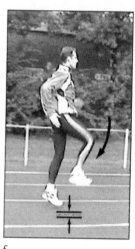

f

Exercise 6   Hopping on one leg (variation)

The swing leg taps the ground only after every other hop. During the first hop, the thigh of the swing leg has been lifted horizontally. The stance leg can now only hop within a small range of movement and with a very high frequency. Exercises 1 and 2 can also be practiced using this rhythm.

Storage and release of energy

In order to implement correctly all the functions of the ankle and foot, it is necessary to have good control over movement in the ankle. Because the external forces acting on the foot are very strong, it is important for a runner to tighten the muscles in the lower leg and foot just before foot placement. The tension that can be stored in the lower-leg muscles depends on the position of the upper tarsal joint. When plantar flexion is robust, there is always less tension than is possible in a neutral position. Therefore, just before foot placement the foot must be held in a neutral position so that, at the moment of IC, sufficient pretension is present around the ankle. Exercising control over tension around the ankle can be done by regulating the position of the upper tarsal joint.

This does not imply, however, that tension around the ankle can be regulated correctly by simply holding the foot in the correct position. Particularly after an injury (even for a brief period) to, for example, the Achilles tendon, many athletes appear to have more difficulty building up the necessary pretension. A reduction in the amount of pretension present will disrupt the running technique. Especially during speed running, any disruption in technique can have such a great effect that it can make or break a performance. Being out of condition is, therefore, not only a question (as trainers often think) of an individual's physical condition being under par. After a short-term injury to the Achilles tendon, coordination rather than strenuous condition training is a more suitable way to improve a runner's level of performance. During periods without injury, it is also useful to continue directing attention at controlling movement in the foot. When these muscles function well, they greatly benefit reactivity in the lower leg and foot. Certainly in less talented runners, there is always the danger that the stabilizing lower-leg muscles might become lazy.

Both the demands made on the lower-leg muscles (coordination combined with the sensory system, and a high degree of pretension during foot placement) are problematic from the perspective of training. Exercises that have a strong focus on coordination (e.g. balancing on teeter boards) generally require so little strength that their relevance for running is rather limited. Exercises that require more strength (e.g. types of jumping) can override, by means of the strong action of the soleus–gastrocnemius muscle group, the timely and correct tightening of the muscles that work to stabilize the ankle, and so corrections in the area of coordination fail to occur. The solution to this problem lies in the extensive and exact implementation of running instruction, for which the issues of pretension, immediate ground contact, and omission of compensatory movements when tension around the ankle is insufficient stand central.

Figure 5.7a–f   Exercise 1: skipping with double ground contact

a   b   c   d   e

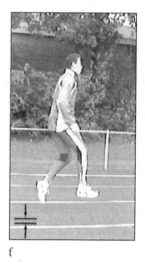

f

Exercise 1   Skipping with double ground contact

While skipping (moving forward minimally) an athlete makes left–left–right–right–left–left, etc., ground contact instead of using a left–right–left–right pattern. The periods of ground contact and the intervals between contacts are equally long, with the rhythm kept as even as possible. The body is held erect and the leg swung up horizontally with the knee bent. During the support phase, the heel does not touch the ground. The exercise should be carried out with minimum movement in the ankles. The ankle should not move (no plantar flexion in an open chain) in either the support phase or the swing phase. Once skipping is implemented correctly, one can increase the rhythm. The athlete must maintain his balance and not lean beyond his point of support.

Figure 5.8a–j   Exercise 2: skipping with double ground contact

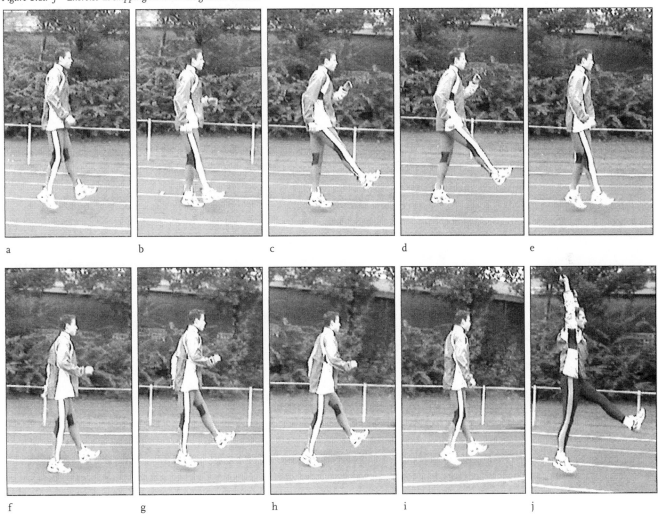

a   b   c   d   e

f   g   h   i   j

Exercise 2 Skipping with double ground contact

The legs remain constantly extended and the swing leg is repeatedly lifted to the front until the foot is about 10 cm above the ground. In addition, a weight (e.g. a 10-kg bar-bell) is held as high as possible above the head. The athlete skips on the forefoot. The ankle is in a neutral position, which should change little during the swing phase.

Figure 5.9a–f   Exercise 3: skipping with single ground contact

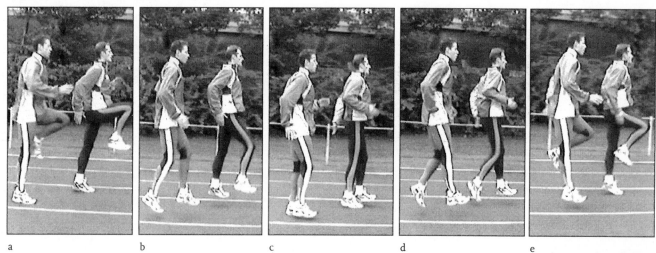

a   b   c   d   e

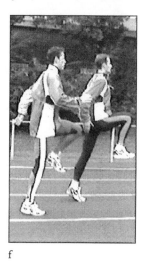

f

Exercise 3 Skipping with single ground contact

One leg with the knee bent repeatedly swings horizontally, while the other knee remains extended. There is maximum tension in the ankles, which remain in the most neutral position possible during the swing phase. Because the muscles in the extended leg are well tightened, they can work reactively. Once the athlete has mastered the exercise sufficiently, he can also skip forward. Keeping the ground contact time short is essential.

Figure 5.10a–e   Exercise 4: skipping with increasing forward speed

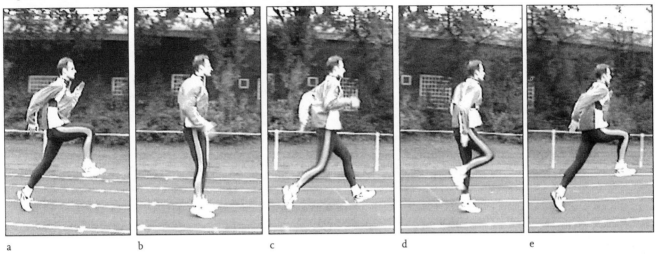

a   b   c   d   e

Exercise 4   Skipping with increasing forward speed
While making single skips, the forward speed is gradually increased, with attention being placed only on keeping the position of the ankles neutral. This exercise is particularly useful for runners who tend to relax the foot too much during the open chain, thus allowing it to droop (plantar flexion).

Exercise 5   Alternating speed
Running while changing speed: slightly accelerating then decelerating. The knees are repeatedly raised. When slowing down, one tends to allow a lot of dorsiflexion during the support phase. However, the ankles must be held rigid and the heels may not touch the ground as speed reduces.

Exercise 6   Hopping on one and two legs
The exercises previously described for one- and two-leg hops can also be used with emphasis placed on holding the ankle rigid. During the floating phase, neither foot should be allowed to droop (neutral position).

Figure 5.11a–d   Exercise 7: hop–stretch–jump

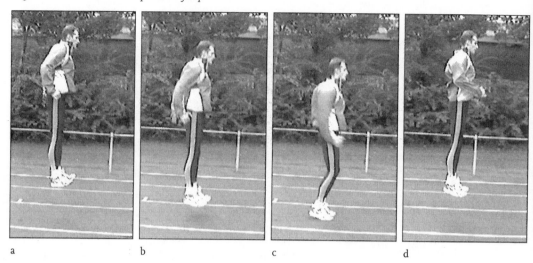

a   b   c   d

Exercise 7 Hop–stretch–jump

Two-leg hopping while holding the body extended. There is dorsiflexion in the foot (the so-called hop–stretch–jump) during the floating phase and the ground contact time is kept short. This exercise can be done while moving horizontally (e.g. forward, or forward and backward). Using a skipping rope can prove useful, especially for middle- and long-distance runners.

Figure 5.12a–e   Exercise 8: skipping with the ankles held rigid

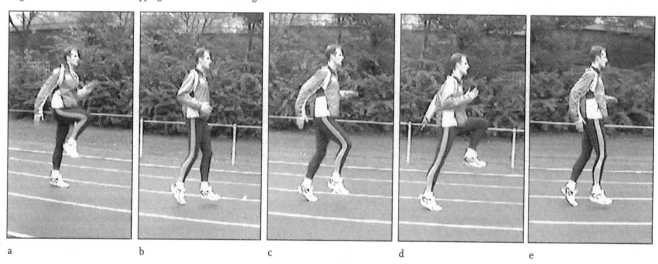

a   b   c   d   e

Exercise 8   Skipping with the ankles held rigid

The knees are raised only slightly so that foot strike will not be too hard. It should be made as difficult as possible every second, third, or fourth stride, by bending the knee and lifting it horizontally as rapidly as possible. A large degree of dorsiflexion threatens to develop when foot strike is hard. This can be avoided by maintaining good tension in the foot.

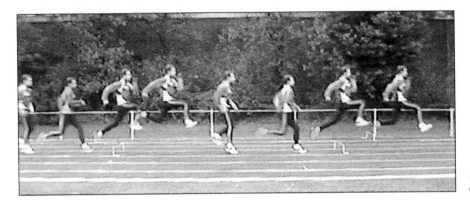

Figure 5.13   Exercise 9: running jump on one leg

Exercise 9   Running jump on one leg
Here 15-cm-high barriers are placed 3–5 m apart (depending on the ability of the runner). The runner jumps, pushing off horizontally on one leg across the barriers (not too high) and repeatedly touches the ground twice between barriers (e.g. repeating right–left). The assignment is to touch the ground twice between barriers rapidly in succession. If the ankle (right) drops too much during the landing, then the two ground contacts will not occur rapidly in succession. The drop in the body's center of mass can quickly be absorbed, so that the second contact will follow rapidly when there is optimum pretension in the ankle and it is in a neutral position.

Transfer of energy

An extraordinary amount of force is placed upon the Achilles tendon during the support phase (Jacobs et al 1993). This force develops as the gastrocnemius transfers energy during knee extension. To some extent, the transfer mechanism can be made to function well by regulating movement in the upper tarsal joint. If, during the support phase, too much dorsiflexion is allowed, the calf muscle will not be tightened correctly and the transfer of energy is limited or occurs too late. A runner can avoid too much dorsiflexion by exerting more pressure on the forefoot during the support phase. The instruction, which has become almost a classic for endurance tempos, to complete the movement of the foot from heel to toe is incorrect. When a runner complies with this instruction, he causes so much dorsiflexion to develop that it counteracts the mechanism used by the gastrocnemius to transfer force. In fact, when a runner has reached a certain level of competence, one can barely discern completion of foot movement when he is running at an average tempo. While it is true that the heel touches first, when the landing pressure has been completely built up a lot of pressure will already be felt in the forefoot.

When receiving running instructions, one can practice controlling the position of the ankle together with the knee extension in order to improve the transfer of energy from the knee to the foot. It is useful to practice this basic mechanism until a high level of control and precision have been achieved. The mechanism for energy transfer between the knee and the ankle has a large effect on the progression of the entire cycle of movement. The mechanism comes into action just prior to the transition from a closed to an open chain (the most decisive moment during running), and therefore regulates this transition to a certain extent.

Figure 5.14   Exercise 1: running hurdles

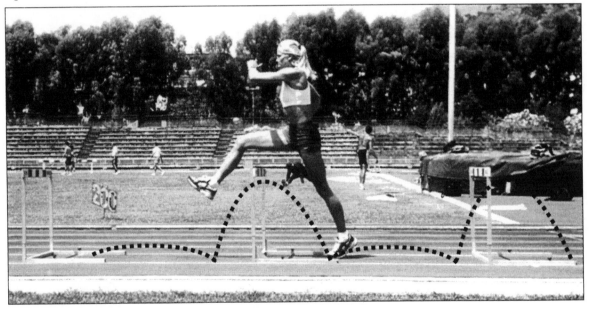

Exercise 1   Running hurdles

Barriers (hurdles) are placed 1.5 m apart. The athlete runs the hurdles, repeatedly touching the ground twice between hurdles on the same foot (left–left crossing the hurdle, right–right crossing, left–left, etc.). The swing leg must point directly forward when crossing the hurdle, while the knee of the trailing leg is held to the side. The stance leg must push off forcefully during the second ground contact between hurdles. The foot must remain well tensed during push-off so that energy from the knee extension can be transferred to the ground correctly. The knee of the support leg should not be bent too far during the support phase. Once the exercise has been mastered, the speed of implementation can be increased or the hurdles made higher or placed further apart. The exercise can also be intensified by holding the arms stationary (e.g. hands behind the head) or by carrying a weight. Running hurdles is a form of exercise that requires much tension around the hip and in the stance leg. The exercise is frequently used following a period of injury to rebuild good morphology.

Figure 5.15a–f   Exercise 2: hopping on one leg while moving forward

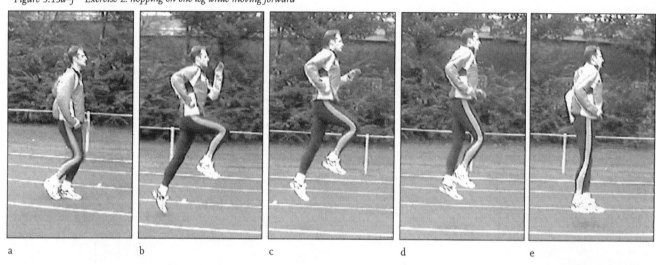

a   b   c   d   e

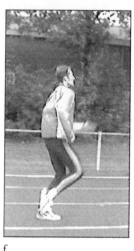

f

Exercise 2   Hopping on one leg while moving forward

The impulse of the motion is not only upwards but also directed vertically and horizontally. When hopping on one leg, the stance leg is always slightly bent. By hopping forward, the bending–stretching motion of the knee becomes more rapid. Both the transfer of force by the gastrocnemius and movement of the foot must be coordinated with this motion. When the forward speed is increased, it becomes difficult to maintain the correct pattern of movement. When the forward velocity is too fast, the pattern cannot be maintained correctly, so that increasing the speed will not prove beneficial.

Exercise 3 Skipping up steps with tension in the ankle

Skipping up steps while making one ground contact. The ankles must remain rigid and there must not be much plantar flexion in the foot during the open chain. Once the exercise has been mastered, one can practice skipping up stairs, but now landing on every second step. One must make certain that the ground contact time remains short and that the knee of the stance leg is bent only very slightly when touching the stair. At the end of push-off, the knee should be well extended. Because skipping is done up the steps, the knee must extend more actively because of the greater vertical displacement. This emphasis on knee extension will result in an increased transfer of energy from the knee to the ankle (especially when missing out one step). Therefore more pretension will be needed in the ankle.

Figure 5.16a–e Exercise 4: reactive skipping on one leg

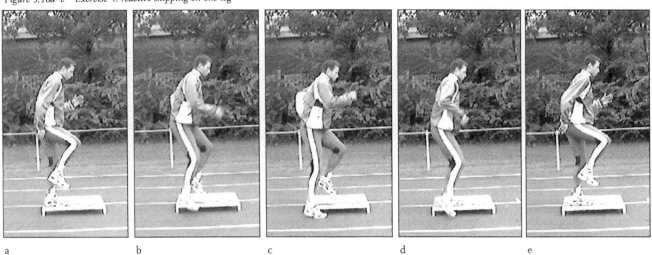

a b c d e

Exercise 4 Reactive skipping on one leg

Start by standing on the left leg (knee and hip slightly bent) on a 5–15 cm elevation. The right leg is placed next to the elevation with the foot above the ground. The left leg is bent rapidly, while the right leg is extended. Because of the drop, the right foot will land hard. The heel will barely touch the ground, if at all. Tension in the right foot must be maximum. The support phase on the right leg is kept as brief as possible and, using a powerful push-off, the athlete again shifts his stance to the left back on the elevation. Once this shift has been mastered, the exercise can be carried out in succession at a high tempo. The better the implementation, the faster the exercise can be done and the more exhausting it will be. It is thought that this type of skipping can provide one (right) leg with a training overload by stimulating the other leg with an underload.

Figure 5.17a–c   Exercise 5: skipping while touching the ground twice

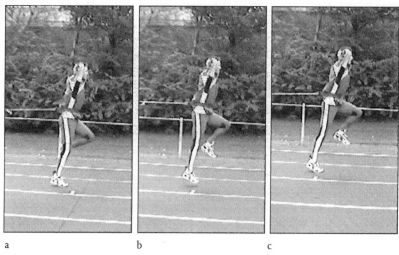

a   b   c

Exercise 5   Skipping while touching the ground twice
A drag weight is attached around the waist. The upper body must remain upright. Repeatedly, thrust
is generated by forcefully pushing off from the second ground contact. Because of this second ground
contact, there will be slight or no prestretch, so that the ankle must be purposely tightened while
extending the knee and transferring energy from the knee to ankle.

Figure 5.18a–e   Exercise 6: simple skipping

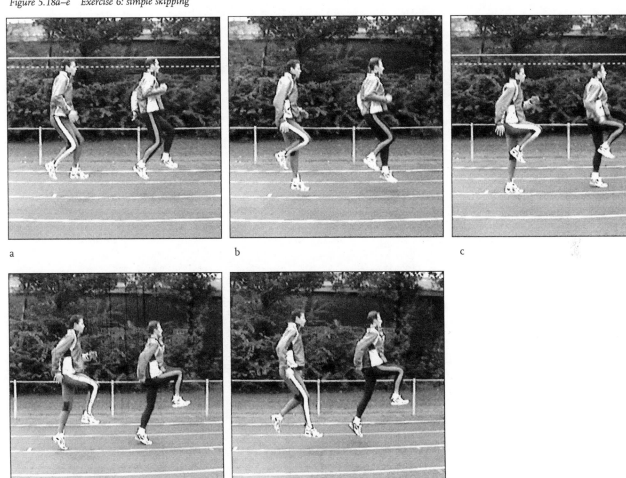

a   b   c

d   e

Exercise 6   Simple skipping

The athlete is asked to skip simply at a low frequency, keeping the ground contact time short and the floating phase long. This will only be possible if the knee of the stance leg is bent only slightly during foot strike (otherwise ground contact will be long) and if the vertical component of push-off is large. Therefore, all the muscles that function during the transfer of force from the hip to the ground must work on time and have good pretension. This is also the case for the muscles that provide pretension in the foot.

Figure 5.19a–i   Exercise 7: forward leap

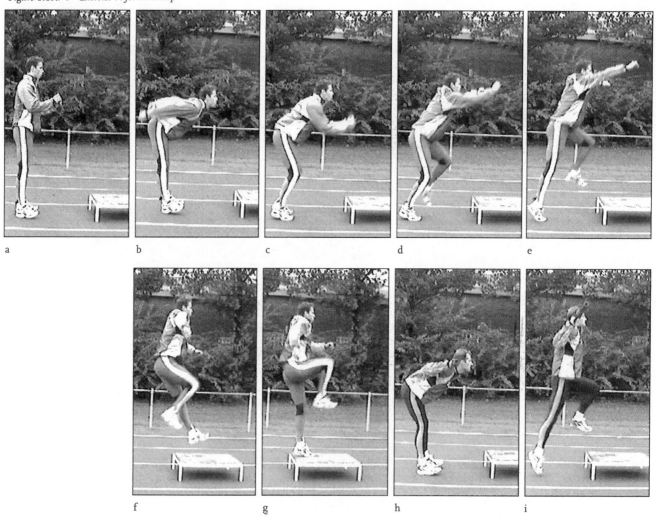

a   b   c   d   e

f   g   h   i

Exercise 7   Forward leap

Start by standing with the feet together, knees slightly bent, upper body leaning forward, and back well extended. From this position, the body extends explosively outward. Halfway through the extension, the right leg is lifted, while the left leg pushes off with force. The runner then leaps up toward the front, landing upright with the right foot on an elevation and the left leg in front bent at the knee and hip. The more tension that is present in the right foot at the moment of extension, the more forceful push-off will be and the faster the foot can begin swinging forward after the foot has left the ground. Once the exercise has been mastered, it can be intensified by holding a bar-bell (from 10 kg to a maximum of 60 kg) at neck level.

5.2.2   Technique and reactivity

Reactive conversion of landing energy

To a large extent, reactivity is a skill associated with coordination. Regulating the extension and discharge of elastic muscle components demands that timing be anticipated exactly. To function reactively, muscle fibers must work near isometry, and the elastic tissues must stretch until they reach a length at which they can store a lot of energy (see Section 1.4.3). This means that tension in the muscles must be built up and coordinated very accurately. In addition, there is only a very small interval in which to release energy. Because muscle reactivity plays a very significant role in the management of energy during running, exercising coordination for reactivity will prove particularly useful. It is not always necessary to associate practice directly with the motion of running. Vertical jumping on both legs, a pattern of movement that differs considerably from running, can also contribute to an improvement in reactivity. When practicing reactivity, one must pay attention to three requirements:

- The posture of the body must remain relatively straight. Small deviations from the correct posture can quickly result in a decline in reactivity. For example, the range within which the pelvis may move is of the order of centimeters.
- The ground contact time (when using a rebounding motion) must be very short. The energy stored into the body during running is also released very quickly. By keeping ground contact times brief while jumping in different ways, one will learn how quickly energy is stored and released during running. Moreover, it is possible to lengthen the interval between the storing and release of energy. Being able to coordinate slower reactive activity, however, deviates so much from what occurs during running that the transfer of training from slower types of exercise is quite limited. It is only advisable to use both slow and faster forms of exercise when training the hamstrings. The function of the hamstrings is so important that using exercises that have even a low transfer of training will also prove helpful.
- Within the period in which energy is being stored and then released for use, there should be little other movement in the joints upon which forces are working. Avoiding any further movement aims to keep the muscle function close to isometry. There is a strong relationship between isometry and reactivity. Moving as little as possible during the reactive phase helps guarantee isometry.

In practice, reactive types of jumping are very strenuous or even dangerous. The relationship between risk and effect might, therefore, be so unfavorable (large effect, but at a great risk) that one must be advised to avoid reactive jumping during training. However, if one follows the three above-mentioned requirements and does not forget that training should be aimed at technique, not at an energy process, then some types of jumping will not necessarily be more dangerous or exhausting than other forms of training. The relationship between risk and effect is actually quite beneficial here. However, when the varieties of jumping are hybrids of reactive and explosive muscle activity, or when an eccentric moment is present in the muscle fibers (e.g. when jumping from a level that is too high, or when bending the knees too much during landing), then the risk of injury will be high while the effect of the training will be minimal. Understanding exactly how such exercises should be implemented is therefore indispensable. High-jumpers are true specialists in reactive jumping, but even when training top performers, hardly anyone today would consider using larger workloads (e.g. jumping from extreme heights). Rather one would strive to improve performance by learning exactly how to implement different types of exercise.

Because reactive jumping is a form of coordination training in particular, it must not be used as an exercise when an athlete is suffering from neuromuscular fatigue. The number of repetitions should be restricted, and these types of exercise should always be planned at the beginning of a training session.

Vertical jumping

During vertical reactive jumping, an athlete will drop from a certain height and convert the landing energy as he rebounds into a vertical push-off. The most important characteristic of this type of jump is that the amount of energy stored during the landing is greater than that stored during running. Each time the height of the drop is changed, another adjustment is asked of the contractile segments. As the height of the drop increases, more pretension must be present. Moreover, when the drop is quite high, the elastic fibers threaten to extend further. Therefore, the length that muscle fibers must reach in order to function isometrically depends not only on the positions of the joints but also on how far the series-linked elastic components (SEC) segments have been stretched. No linear relationship has been found between joint position and the length to which muscle fibers must extend. Consequently, it is not easy to determine the correct length for contractile segments. In addition, it is also difficult to establish, through coordination, the correct amount of pretension needed and the required length of the contractile segments. Practicing by means of vertical jumping requires a wide variation in the height of the drop in order to learn how to make such adjustments. When training for reactive coordination, not only the upper range of heights that an athlete can reach (and still meet the three requirements for reactivity) but also, and in particular, the minimum drop are important.

In addition to variations in the height of the drop, the reactive pattern can be affected by changing the way in which the jump is implemented. Any variation (e.g. by mixing vertical and horizontal displacement) will lead to a change in the timing of when a muscle must work. Being able to regulate many such variations will help a runner to cope more precisely with landing energy. It is essential that the type of jump selected for an individual athlete is fitted to his personal potential. Because endurance runners will jump using smaller strength peaks, they must jump from lower heights compared to sprinters. In addition, other factors, such as body structure, weight, and natural talent, play a role. Customizing an exercise program to fit an individual's needs is an important basic requirement if reactive jumping is to be trained efficiently.

When practicing vertical reactive jumps, a number of exercises are suitable. These have already been described when discussing instruction on how to position the ankle (i.e. hop–stretch–jump using two legs and hopping on one or both legs). These exercises can be done in several ways. However, one must pay attention not only to tension and foot movement, but also to the manner in which the entire extension sequence functions. Tension and how the muscles around the hip and trunk work reactively is particularly important.

For all types of jumps, positioning the direction of the hips from front to back is important. If the hips are held backward (or the trunk leans slightly forward), reactivity will decrease. Holding the hips well to the front is also important and will require a sufficient amount of pretension in reactively working muscles, namely the abdominals.

When hopping on one or both legs, one can talk of a swing–support pattern of leg movement. Because this pattern contains the crossed-extensor reflex, there must be precise coordination between the correct extension and tightening of the push-off leg and the rapid bending of the knee and hip of the free leg. When carrying out rebounding jumps on one or both legs, a significant part of the reactive push-off will originate from movement of the pelvis in the frontal plane. The free half of the pelvis drops during the landing only to rebound upwards thereafter. For this to occur, tension is needed in the muscles on the side of the hip (the small gluteal muscles and the upper part of the gluteus maximus by way of the iliotibial tract). Especially when bouncing on one leg, athletes frequently tend to release tension from these muscles by twisting the upper part of the body toward the side of the stance leg. The runner must hold his trunk well upright and remain aware of whether tension in the relevant muscles is high.

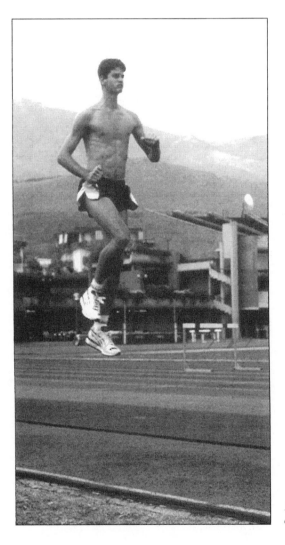

Figure 5.20 A very high, rebounding jump, exactly executed

Figure 5.21a–f   Rebounding jump on one leg

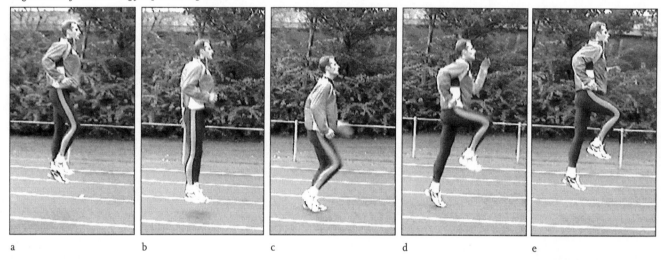

a   b   c   d   e

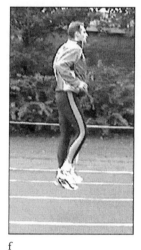

f

Exercise 1   Rebounding jump on one leg

These exercises are generally carried out in succession. The height of one jump is identical to the height of the drop from which the next jump will be made. In addition to the height of the drop, the forward velocity at the moment of push-off will influence how the action progresses reactively. It is useful to use as many variations as possible for this exercise so that the runner can learn how to adjust his movements more precisely for reactivity. Some examples:

- hopping on one leg in succession: low–high–low–high–low–high, etc.
- hopping on one leg: low–low–high–low–low–high, etc.
- hopping on two legs: low and far upward without displacement–high without displacement–low and far, etc.
- hop–stretch–jump: backwards and low to the front and low–high without displacement, etc.
- alternating hop–stretch–jump: low and high rebounding jump on one leg.

Exercise 2   Hopping on one leg varying the height of the drop

Elevations (10 cm high, 50 × 50 cm) are placed in a row 1 m apart. The runner makes a series of rebounding jumps on one leg, as high as possible, landing alternately on and between elevations. The height of the previous jump is no longer equal to the drop height of the next jump. Therefore, the athlete must anticipate the landing and build up pretension in his body differently. Obviously, this exercise can be executed in a variety of ways. For example, the elevations can be placed 2 m apart so that there is space on the ground to hop twice and once on the elevation. Hopping on elevations is a good way to learn how to position the hips. The runner will tend more than usual to hold his hips too far to the rear or to lean his upper body toward the side of the stance leg.

Figure 5.22a–f   Exercise 3: zigzag hopping on two legs

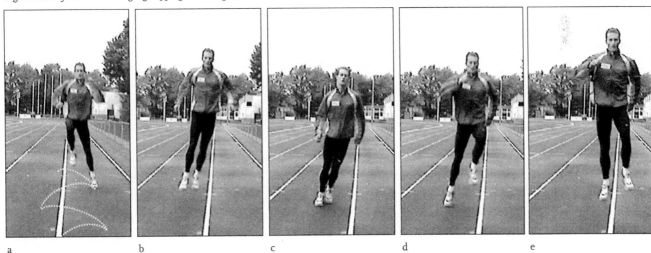

a   b   c   d   e

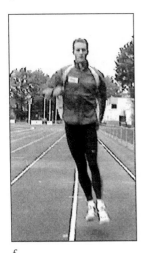

f

Exercise 3   Zigzag hopping on two legs

Start to hop forward on both legs. Gradually the body begins to move sideways, alternating from left to right. Displacement must be to the left when the left leg is pushing off for the next jump. The contact time for push-off is kept as brief as possible.

Figure 5.23a–f   Exercise 4: hop–stretch–jump over hurdles

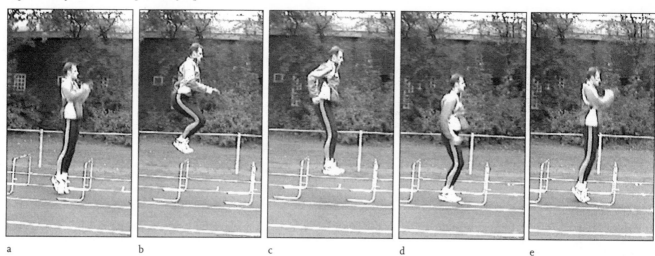

a b c d e

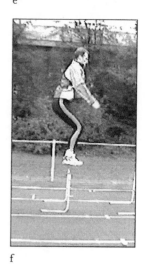

f

Exercise 4   Hop–stretch–jump over hurdles

This is an important standard exercise for teaching reactive jumping. The hurdles are placed about 1.2 m apart and are low enough that the knee need hardly bend to cross. The runner tries to hop over the hurdles, moving the body as little as possible and keeping the ground contact time short. There is only one ground contact between hurdles. It is not advisable to place more than eight hurdles in a row. Because the hop–stretch–jump exercise is carried out across hurdles, implementation must be very precise. There is little room for varying the height of the jump or for horizontal displacement. Such restrictions will provide a good instrument for refining the reactive technique further.

Figure 5.24a–f   Exercise 5: hop–stretch–jump from an elevation across a hurdle

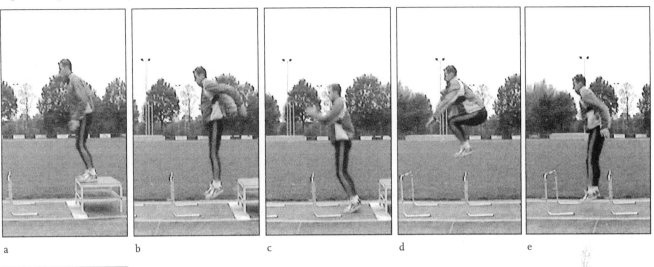

a   b   c   d   e

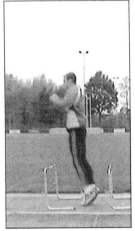

f

Exercise 5   Hop–stretch–jump from an elevation across a hurdle

The height of the drop in this exercise can be greater than when jumping in succession. However, because there is a greater chance that the exercise will be done incorrectly, it is only suitable for the very best athletes and should never be used as a basic drill. Moreover, the number of repetitions must remain very limited. A skillful athlete can use this exercise to 'dot the i' during training. The maximum height from which one can jump is determined individually, but will seldom be higher than 50 cm.

Exercise 6   Hop–stretch–jump (variation)

Although the basic form of reactive jumping over hurdles is always a useful practice, even for the best athletes, instruction can be broadened further using other variations in the set-up. Some examples are:

• Hurdles are placed 3 m apart. Hop–stretch–jump over the hurdle, followed immediately after landing by a flat hop–stretch–jump with horizontal displacement up to the next hurdle, followed by a high hop–stretch–jump over the hurdle with slight horizontal displacement, etc.
• Hurdles are placed 2.5 m apart with a 10-cm elevation placed in front of each hurdle. Hop–stretch–jump over the hurdle, followed after landing by a hop–stretch–jump on the ground, a hop–stretch–jump on the elevation and over the next hurdle, etc.
• Hop–stretch–jump over four hurdles, followed by a long rebounding jump into sand.

Horizontal jumping

For horizontal reactive jumps carried out on one leg, one can speak of a swing–stance pattern of leg movement. Although the jumps used in training are more often horizontal reactive than vertical reactive, the former type is technically more difficult. Therefore it is advisable to first learn to regulate reactivity before practicing horizontal jumps.

For horizontal jumps, one must also comply with the three requirements for reactivity. In particular, the need to keep ground contact time brief is problematic. Because the landing and push-off are done using the same leg, it is extremely difficult to absorb and immediately release landing energy without giving rise to an eccentric moment in the contractile muscle segments. In particular, during the classic running jump, an eccentric moment will develop rapidly in the muscle fibers, making reactive push-off impossible. During horizontal jumps, one must pay careful attention to whether the three criteria for reactive jumping have been met.

Just as for speed running, the way in which the knees are positioned at IC will give a good indication of the quality of the jump. If the knees are close together at IC, it is possible to convert landing energy reactively. However, if a runner is still holding the knee of the swing leg behind the knee of the stance leg at foot placement, it will be impossible to carry out the jump reactively. In that case, it is better to omit this type of jump and look for an alternative and easier form.

In addition to the fact that one must jump reactively, the pattern of movement for a jump must not counteract the pattern observed for running. Rapidly bringing the swing leg forward linearly is essential during running. However, for the classic running jump, the floating phase lasts so long that an athlete will tend to trail his back leg before initiating forward swing. Anyone who performs a running jump this way would be best advised to avoid using it during training and to choose a different type of horizontal jump in which the swing phase can be initiated rapidly. The same problem occurs, albeit to a lesser degree, in horizontal hopping. The same rule applies for a running jump using both legs and for hopping as applies to reactive jumps off an elevation: the exercise is only suitable for the very best runners, and even for them it is only used to 'dot the i'.

Figure 5.25a–f   Exercise 1: running jump on one leg

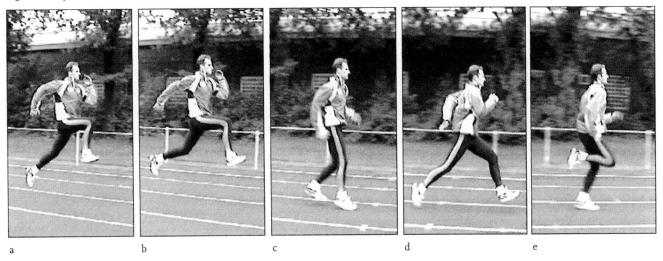

a   b   c   d   e

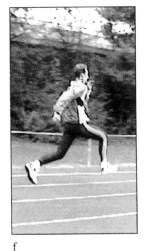

f

Exercise 1   Running jump on one leg

The safest and most technically relevant horizontal jump is the running jump on one leg. The athlete runs a few strides (3 or 5) to gather speed. Thereafter, he pushes off for a running jump (left). During the floating phase that follows, the swing leg (right) is kept bent at 90° at the knee and hip. The upper body is vertical. The swing leg is more or less 'presented' for the next landing. The landing is hard on the right foot and the ground contact time is as short as possible. The left foot rapidly touches the ground after the right foot, by which the next running jump is initiated. Here the right leg assumes the bent 'presenting' position as rapidly as possible. By increasing the height of the running jump, the drop for the landing on the 'presented' leg will increase. The load can be varied by increasing the height of the jump or by jumping more horizontally. Both high and horizontal running jumps on one leg are useful for training. Attention must always be paid to how the swing leg is presented and how quickly that leg can be repositioned after push-off. Generally, the exercise can only be implemented well over a distance of 30 m.

Reactivity and transition from closed to open chain

In practice, it appears that runners, especially those with well-coordinated hamstrings, are able to jump well reactively if the legs are retracted rapidly after leaving the ground. The hips and knees then bend forcefully at the same time, after the feet have left the ground. Apparently it is difficult to push off just before retracting the legs by means of concentric explosive muscle action. Therefore the only possibility remaining during push-off is reactive muscle work. It is possible that the relationship between how the muscles work reactively during push-off and how the legs retract rapidly thereafter is involuntary. Such a pattern of movement is given 'preferential' treatment and can be carried out more rapidly and with more force than can other patterns that do not depend on reflexes.

Reactive jumping followed by retraction of the legs is a useful practice for runners. After all, the same thing happens during running. Such types of reactive jumps only function well, however, if the foot is placed directly beneath the hip before the reactive push-off. If the foot is placed in front of the projection of the hip on the ground (during a breaking step), the total pattern will be so disrupted that retracting the legs after push-off will prove useless. This means that when jumping on both legs the forward velocity must be nearly zero.

One can place different emphases on these exercises when practicing. The aim might be to learn only how to push off reactively (i.e. a push-off in which the reactive phase is not followed by an explosive phase) or to practice making a rapid transition from a closed to an open chain. Because the movements are so closely interconnected, these various aspects allow for several different ways of using the exercise. It is true for these types of jump also that the height from which the jump is made must be changed if the exercise is to be sufficiently well rounded.

Exercise 1   Running start and single-leg jump
Jumping on one leg after a running start, such as described above, is quite suitable for coupling reactivity with a transition from a closed to an open chain. Having good pretension during the floating phase is essential for a reactive push-off.

Figure 5.26a–g   Exercise 2: hop–stretch–jump across high hurdles

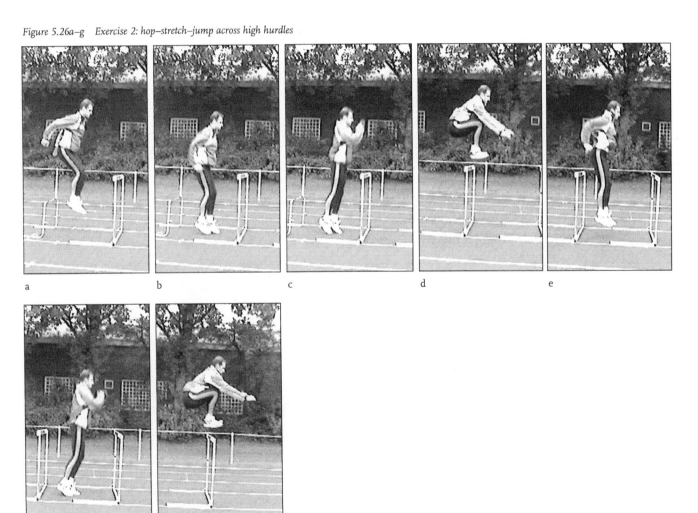

a   b   c   d   e

f   g

Exercise 2   Hop–stretch–jump across high hurdles
Because the hurdles are high, the legs must quickly be retracted directly after push-off. The exercise is carried out using a series of 5–8 hurdles in a row. The advantage of jumping in series is that reactivity often improves when the movement is repeated. When using a series of 8 jumps, the best jumps usually occur between the 3rd and 7th hurdles. Emphasis is placed on retracting the legs as quickly as possible, although one must also take care that the body is sufficiently extended at the moment of landing. The body squats as it crosses the hurdles. If the body is not extended enough just before landing, reactivity will decrease and the push-off will take too long.

Figure 5.27a–c   Exercise 3: reactive jumping while landing on an elevation

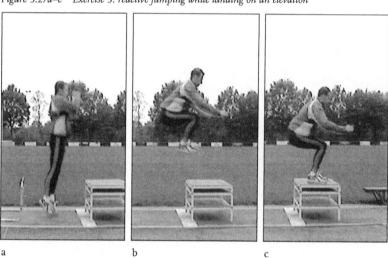

a   b   c

Exercise 3   Reactive jumping while landing on an elevation

When jumping over hurdles, some athletes make the mistake of keeping their hips too extended although their knees are bent. This can be compared to the mistake made during running when first the knee and then the hip bends after push-off. By landing in a squat on an elevation, the athlete is compelled to bend at the hips immediately after push-off. Push-off for the jump towards the elevation is preceded by one or more jumps. For example:

- reactive hop–stretch–jump across hurdles
- hop–stretch–jump backwards and forwards
- stretching vertical jump with the feet spread apart and knees bent.

Figure 5.28a–g   Exercise 4: rebounding jump with the feet spread apart

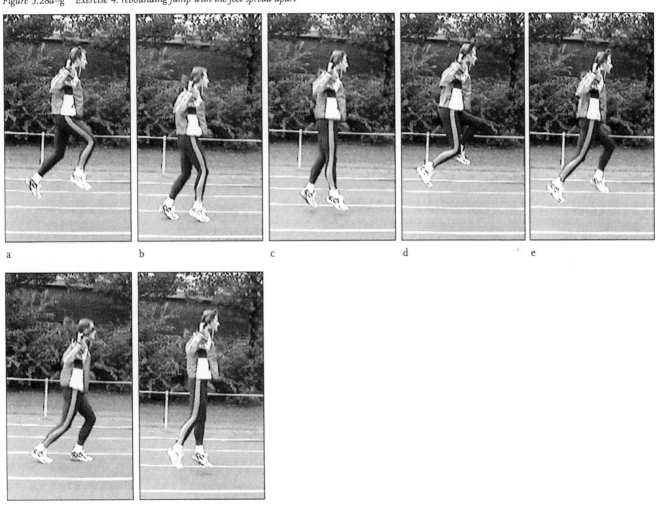

a   b   c   d   e

f   g

Exercise 4   Rebounding jump with the feet spread apart

Stand with one foot placed 30 cm in front of the other foot. Bounce forward while repeatedly switching the forward position of the foot. The exercise can eventually be carried out holding a bar-bell at neck level. While bouncing, the knees are raised higher and higher. Both hips and knees therefore bend increasingly during the floating phase. The contact time of push-off remains short. Finally, the legs are retracted as powerfully as possible in combination with a reactive push-off.

Figure 5.29a–f   Exercise 5: skipping in combination with heel strike

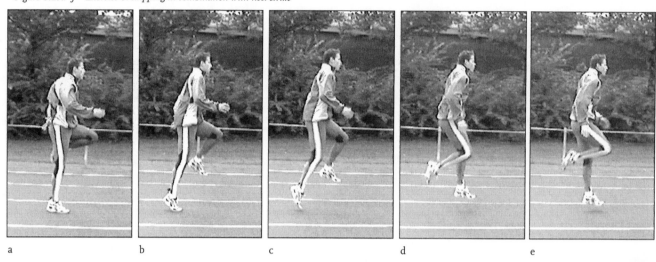

a   b   c   d   e

f

Exercise 5   Skipping in combination with heel strike

Skipping with single ground contact. The hip of the swing leg bends up to 90° while the knee is bent as far as possible, allowing the foot to touch the buttocks. The contact time is kept short. During the support phase, the knee is almost extended. The forward velocity during the exercise is very low, and the frequency of movement decreases slowly. Even at a lower frequency the ground contact should be short and the leg continue to be retracted, thus requiring the push-off to be more forceful. The exercise can be followed by slowly accelerating forward until a running speed has actually been reached.

Figure 5.30a–e   Exercise 6: reactive skipping on one leg with resistance

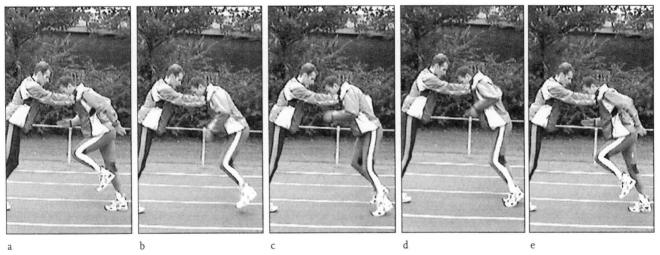

a   b   c   d   e

Exercise 6   Reactive skipping on one leg with resistance

Start by standing on the left leg, which is extended with the body leaning forward. An assistant helps by pushing against the shoulders. The right leg is in a starting position, bent to 90° at the hip and knee. Thereafter, the left leg is quickly bent (to about 45° at the hip), while the right leg is rapidly extended and as tense as possible when placed on the ground for the stance phase. The stance phase is very short, after which the right leg again bends as the legs exchange positions and return to their starting positions. The exercise is carried out in a series. The stance phase of the left leg may last longer than that for the right leg. During the exercise, the athlete must push as hard as possible against the helper's hands while supporting himself on his right leg. Due to the high pressure, he will tend to keep the hip of the stance leg bent. Hip extension is improved and strengthened. The helper walks backward, foot by foot, during the exercise, which is performed rapidly in succession. During this exercise, one (right) leg is overloaded by providing the other leg with an underload (see also reactive skipping on one leg without resistance).

Body posture and reactivity

As far as the lower extremities are concerned, muscles cannot work rapidly and reactively in just any position. When the knee and hip are extended and the ankle is in a neutral position, reactivity is optimal and will occur particularly rapidly. The reactive potential declines rapidly if the body deviates even slightly from this posture. When the knee and hip are bent at 45°, it is almost impossible for the muscles to work rapidly and reactively. The way in which the hips are held, therefore, plays a crucial role in muscle reactivity during running and jumping. If the hips are held somewhat backward, which many runners do under pressure, reactivity is not used optimally. This will have a greater influence on performance, especially at high speeds when it is quite difficult to maintain an optimum body posture. Because elastic energy is 'free' energy, investing in learning how to maintain an optimum body posture under pressure will prove worthwhile. Even learning how to adjust the position of the hips better within a margin of a few centimeters (i.e. the hips further forward) will be highly beneficial. Holding the pelvis correctly will cause the abdominal muscles to work faster and with more force during running. Good coordination and morphology for the abdominal muscles are therefore basic requirements for having a good posture for the sprint.

Figure 5.31a,b   Exercise 1: high-frequency skipping

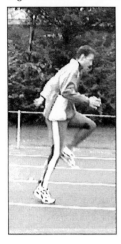 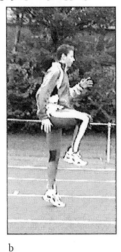

a   b

Exercise 1   High-frequency skipping

Start by standing with the upper body leaning forward by about 45°. The back must remain extended. In this position, the runner skips while making a single ground contact. The frequency of movement is very high. In contrast to standing erect, by holding the trunk forward the frequency will be higher and the forward velocity low. Thereafter the trunk slowly assumes a vertical posture and the position of the hips shifts further to the front. The further the trunk is raised, the more difficult it will be to maintain a high frequency. The runner will increasingly realize that more reactivity and pretension are needed to move rapidly. The exercise only ends when the trunk is erect. As a variation, the forward velocity can be increased as the trunk is being raised upright. The exercise ends here in good reactive running, with a high forward velocity and the trunk held precisely upright.

Exercise 2   Hopping on both legs

The starting position is identical to that described in Exercise 1. Instead of skipping, the athlete now hops on both legs. While the trunk is still leaning forward, the athlete hops rapidly, but not too high, in succession. As the body slowly becomes erect, tension in the body is purposely increased and vertical displacement becomes greater. The trunk finally reaches a perfectly vertical posture so that the height of the hops will be maximum. As a variation, the exercise can be done on one leg. Care must be taken that the trunk does not tilt sideways toward the push-off leg. In that case, tension in the gluteal muscles would decrease, so that they could no longer work well reactively.

Figure 5.32a–f   Exercise 3: squatting leap on two legs

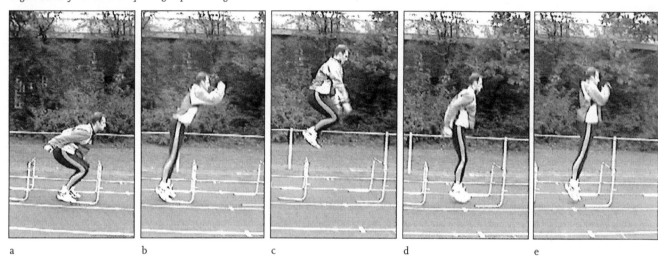

a   b   c   d   e

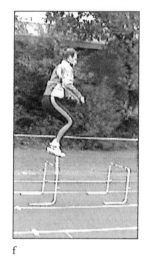

f

Exercise 3   Squatting leap on two legs

A vertical leap on two legs across a series of low hurdles (about 1.2 m apart). The runner leaps across the first hurdle (about 70 cm high) from a half-squatting position. At the start, the angle of the knees is 90°, the trunk leans slightly forward, and the back is well extended. The leap is done explosively as the body is extended. After landing beyond the first hurdle, keeping the ground contact time short, a reactive leap is made over a second 50-cm high hurdle. The third leap is once again made from a squatting position, while the fourth leap is again reactive, etc. This series of leaps is made difficult by the fact that it must be repeated from a different position. Attention must be paid in particular to keeping the body well extended while leaping reactively.

Figure 5.33a–f   Exercise 4: skipping while making a single ground contact

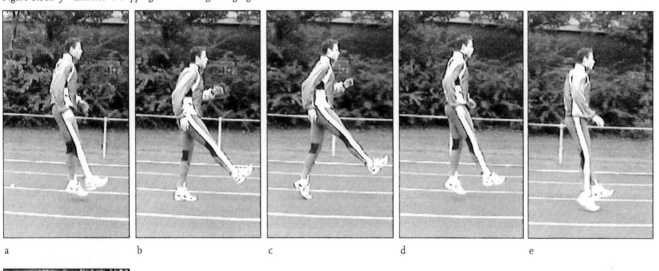

a   b   c   d   e

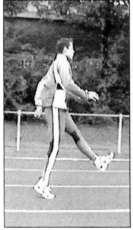

f

Exercise 4   Skipping while making a single ground contact
The knees remain extended throughout the entire exercise. The body is extended and kept highly tensed on purpose. Ground contact should be quite brief. Subsequently, the frequency with which the exercise is carried out decreases slowly, without lengthening the ground contact time. Implementation is only reactive when the body is sufficiently tense and has a correct posture. As a variation, the frequency can be suddenly rather than gradually changed.

Figure 5.34a,b   Exercise 5: running while keeping the legs straight

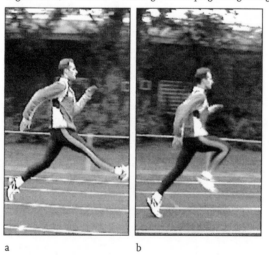

a   b

Exercise 5   Running while keeping the legs straight

Running with the legs extended (knees kept constantly straight) and the upper body erect. The shoulders may even be held somewhat behind the hips. The ground contact time must be kept as brief as possible. After 20 m, a sudden transition is made to ordinary walking. The trunk remains vertical, the ground contact time brief, and the tension used for reactive push-off maintained. In this way, the runner can learn to build up tension in his body when running, and thus regulate the reactivity of push-off.

5.2.3   Coordinating the hamstrings

The hamstrings play a very important role during running and represent the spider in the web of locomotion. They have important reactive properties and have the potential to transfer energy between the hip and knee so that the force of push-off can be directed. Particularly when running under pressure, such as at high speeds or with increasing fatigue, the way in which the hamstrings work has a determining influence on performance. Because the function of the hamstrings is both complicated and important, runners should find it beneficial to practice coordinating these muscles frequently and in various ways.

Most athletes have little understanding of how the hamstrings function. In contrast to the quadriceps, for example, the hamstrings muscles are not visible to the naked eye. They work within the deep recesses toward the back of the body. Moreover, in comparison to other muscles, it is more difficult to be aware of how tension in the hamstrings feels during a contraction. Furthermore, the hamstrings are biarticular. The most important task for monoarticular muscles is to initiate movement (by doing positive work), while biarticular muscles are responsible for absorbing external forces and regulating movement. Because the hamstrings possess all these properties, a runner will frequently be less aware when these muscles have begun to function poorly and so will develop a less effective pattern of running. In comparison to other muscle groups, this makes it more difficult to improve coordination when the hamstrings are not functioning optimally.

Frequently, injury to the hamstrings is thought to result from a lack of strength. Injury is also frequently blamed on the quadriceps, which might be too strongly developed in relation to the hamstrings, thus causing a lack of balance. However, the cause of nearly all injuries to the hamstrings is loss of coordination. Such injuries result because the muscle contracts at the wrong time or with an incorrect amount of force. The muscle actually injures itself. Therefore, coordination training is an important way to prevent this from happening. Coordination training will also play an important role during the period of recovery following injury. Injury to the hamstrings frequently requires a long period of recovery. During much of this time, however, the athlete's coordination will be seriously disrupted. Training various relevant movements can greatly help reduce the period needed for the body to recover.

Because it is useful to train the hamstrings in various ways, one should also consider using exercises, in the area of coordination, for which transfer to the motion of running is limited. Every improvement in the way in which the hamstrings function will be of value. An important part of a training involves the use of bar-bells (see Ch. 6), while another part of a training involves different types of jumping and running. One can differentiate two groups of exercises:

- Exercises in which one learns to cope with reactivity. Hamstrings work reactively in many forms of movement. During certain types of jumping, for which the ground contact time is longer, there are large external forces on the hamstrings. Using other forms of exercise will make it difficult to build up the degree of pretension needed. Especially for sprinters, extensive training using many different types of impact can prove useful. In the long term, these exercises will have a strongly positive effect on speed running, in addition to helping prevent injury.
- Exercises in which the hamstrings are trained in many different positions and movements (involving knee and hip angles). The degree of impact of these exercises will be lower than that of reactive types of exercise, but being able to adjust the timing when the muscle must work will prove more difficult here. Exercises

in this category need not resemble too closely the characteristics of running in order to contribute significantly.

Once a runner has achieved a thorough command of both types of exercise and can practice skillfully, the hamstrings will be able to tighten and relax more rapidly and 'freely' during running. The hamstrings will also function better in terms of the build-up and release of extension, and therefore the running technique will be more effective. When the hamstrings function optimally, an athlete can continue increasing his level of performance over a very long period of time.

Hamstrings are very specialized muscles. Within the framework of training, this means that only a specialized activity may be used to train them. This will have a number of consequences with respect to the exercise program:

- Because their structure is pennate, the hamstrings are only able to exert a lot of force over a limited range. During training it is important to stay within this optimum range. Contracting too far, such as in the leg curl and when training in an open chain, will prove detrimental to the hamstrings because the equilibrium between active and passive tissues and the regulation of elasticity is disrupted. It is better to train these muscles within a closed chain. Changes in the angle of the knee can be more or less compensated for by changes in the angle of the hip, so that the total length of the muscle will remain approximately constant.
- The hamstrings do not themselves generate positive work, but rather direct forces generated by other muscles. Thus when training hamstring coordination, the hamstrings should never be exercised in isolation but always together with the other muscle groups. Coordination between those other muscle groups and the hamstrings must be functionally correct during training. For example, the dorsal muscles must never be allowed to relax or permit flexion in the spinal column when a force is operating upon the hamstrings. To a large extent, the dorsal muscles regulate prestretch in the hamstrings.
- The hamstrings have been designed to function reactively. Therefore, they are quite capable of dealing with the force of impact.

Hamstring exercises 1

The first group of exercises is based on the following principle. Pressure can be placed on the hamstrings by bending forward from an upright posture with the knees almost straight. In this posture the dorsal muscles are well tensed and so the spinal column remains straight. Therefore, the body will only tilt forward when the hip joint changes position. Tilting the pelvis forward will cause prestretch in the hamstrings, which can eventually be compensated for by bending the knees slightly. Because the knees will be either straight or slightly bent, the projection on the ground of the partial center of gravity for the mass above the hip joint will travel along the front of the knee. Therefore, the moment that develops must be compensated for by, for example, the force exerted by the hamstrings. (When the knees are flexed quite far, this projection on the ground travels along the back of the knee so that the quadriceps femoris will need to generate a counter-force.) The forward motion of the trunk provides prestretch in the (pretensed) hamstrings, which will discharge reactively during the next extension.

The more powerful the motion of the trunk as it moves forward and returns upright, the greater the (landing) load will be on the hamstrings. While a beginner will exercise in a controlled and not too powerful manner, an advanced runner can exercise so forcefully that a type of jumping will develop in which the hamstrings will be severely stressed reactively.

The speed at which the reactive trajectory is traveled using such forms of exercise is obviously slower than in running. However, because the hamstrings play an important role during running, exercising in this way will still prove useful.

Figure 5.35a–n   Exercise 1: bending leap from an upright position

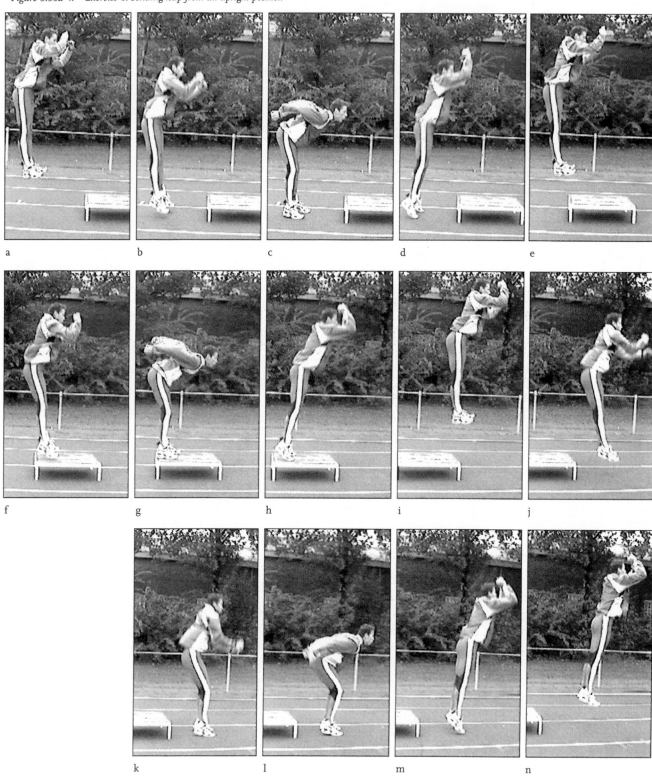

a   b   c   d   e

f   g   h   i   j

k   l   m   n

Exercise 1   Bending leap from an upright position

Start by standing upright with the dorsal muscles tensed. The trunk is tilted forward under control. Here the body must not tilt further forward than is permitted by pelvic movement alone. The body is then extended forcefully. To do this, the spinal column must be kept stable and extended. If enough force is used for the extension, the feet will leave the ground (see Figure 5.35d–g). Once this basic technique has been mastered, the leap can be done with greater force and a low elevation can be used for the landing. When an athlete recovering from an injury to the hamstrings wants to begin coordination training for this muscle group, it will prove useful to do mild exercises over a longer period of time using these movements (also with a 10-kg bar-bell held at neck level). The exercise can be made more strenuous by implementing it with more force or by keeping the arms stationary (e.g. with the hands behind the head). In this way, arm movement cannot dissipate the energy generated as the body drops forward, and thus a heavier load can be placed on the hamstrings.

Exercise 2   Bending leap from an elevation

Start by standing upright on a low (10 cm) elevation. Then leap off the elevation on both legs. Just before the landing, the body begins to bend. Because of the speed of the fall, the trunk will tend to be flung forward forcefully after the landing. The hamstrings and the gluteus maximus will absorb the landing energy elastically, and subsequently reconvert it into a vertical push-off (see Figure 5.35h–n). The higher the elevation from which one leaps, the more landing energy there will be for the hamstrings to store. The landing energy must never exceed what the hamstrings are able to absorb. The dorsal muscles must continue to hold the spinal column extended. If the back bends or the landing cannot be converted rapidly into a push-off, the drop has been too high and the exercise too strenuous. If such mistakes are made when carrying out the exercise, it will prove useless to practice so intensively and an easier form of practice should be found.

Exercise 3   Bending leaps in succession from an elevation

Instead of jumping once from an elevation, the height of the drop can be achieved from a number of jumps done in succession. The height that can be reached by jumping is also the drop height from which the subsequent jump will be made. In order to execute a series of leaps in which the trunk is flung forward, it is particularly important to time correctly the forward motion of the trunk just before landing (see Figure 5.35a–n). This will be an especially intensive exercise if the athlete is able to perform it masterfully. When implemented as rapidly as possible and from the greatest possible height, 12–15 leaps done in succession will be exhausting for a top athlete.

Exercise 4   Types of jumping (variations)

Jumping can be carried out in a number of ways.

- Instead of repeatedly jumping vertically, one can also jump horizontally (e.g. a series of jumps in which vertical and horizontal jumps are alternated).
- Instead of exercising on a flat surface, one can jump on a slight upward or downward incline. In addition, one can alternate landing on a small elevation and the ground. Using such variations, one can repeatedly place different loads on the hamstrings and learn how to incorporate such alternating loads elastically.

Figure 5.36a–d   Exercise 5: backward weight throw standing on two legs

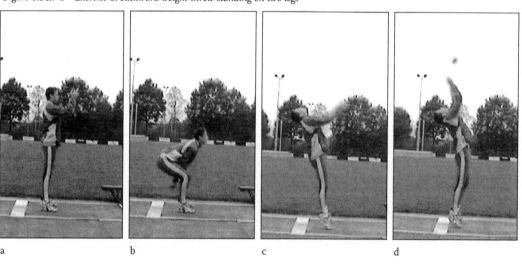

a   b   c   d

Exercise 5   Backward weight throw standing on two legs

One form of exercise widely used in athletics is the backward weight throw while standing on two legs. The runner begins by standing erect with the legs spread slightly apart, while holding a weight in the hands in front of the chest. After bending forward to move the weight in the direction of the feet, the runner swings the weight with both hands upward, throwing it as high and far behind the head as possible. In this manner, extension of the body is maximum. One can direct the load particularly to the hamstrings, just as in previous exercises, by bending the knees only slightly when leaning forward and by keeping the back very extended as the trunk bends forward. The hamstrings will be exerted even more during the backward throw. One must be cautious during implementation that sufficient pretension is built up in the muscles as the body bends forward. Moreover, it is important that the back remains extended during the entire throw. This exercise places a large load on the dorsal muscles. If the back cannot be kept extended, it is better to use lighter weights.

Figure 5.37a–e   Exercise 6: weight throw standing on one leg

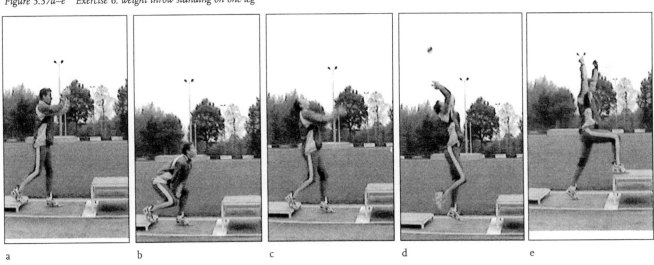

a   b   c   d   e

Exercise 6   Weight throw standing on one leg
Throw a weighed ball while standing on one leg. The stress placed on the hamstrings will be greater than when standing on both legs. Moreover, during a single-leg throw, a swing/stance leg mechanism, which is similar to running, comes into action. Start by standing on one leg, with the upper body leaning forward and the knee not bent too far. The other leg is extended to the rear with the foot just resting on a low (10 cm) elevation. The throwing motion proceeds like that for a two-leg throw. The back leg swings forward during the throw and ends with the hip and knee bent with the foot resting on a 40-cm elevation. The swing leg must move forcefully and be supported in a manner similar to running, with the hamstrings prestretched and the stance leg extended (see Sections 1.7.5 and 3.2). The balls that are being thrown are naturally lighter in weight than those used when exercising on both legs.

Figure 5.38a–f   Exercise 7: bending leaps with one foot in front of the other

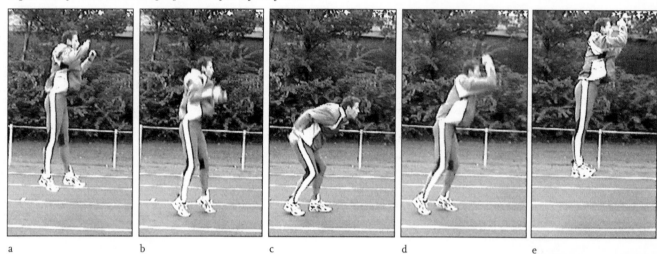

a   b   c   d   e

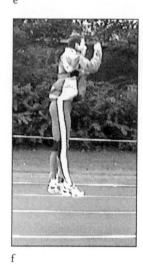

f

Exercise 7   Bending leaps with one foot in front of the other
The jumping exercise described above (Exercise 1, pp. 286–287) can be carried out with one foot in front of the other instead of spread apart sideways. One foot is about 30 cm in front of the other. When the upper body is flung forward during the leap, a heavier load is placed on the hamstrings of the front leg. When performing a series of leaps, one can either continue keeping the same leg in front, or alternate between the left and right legs. One can vary the direction of displacement: leaping only vertically, beginning vertically then gradually changing to more horizontal leaps of increasing length, or leaping horizontally as far as possible, while maintaining a correct technique. The more horizontal the jump, the earlier the hamstrings (the force of push-off directed to the rear) will start to work during push-off.

Figure 5.39a–g   Exercise 8: more strenuous leaps

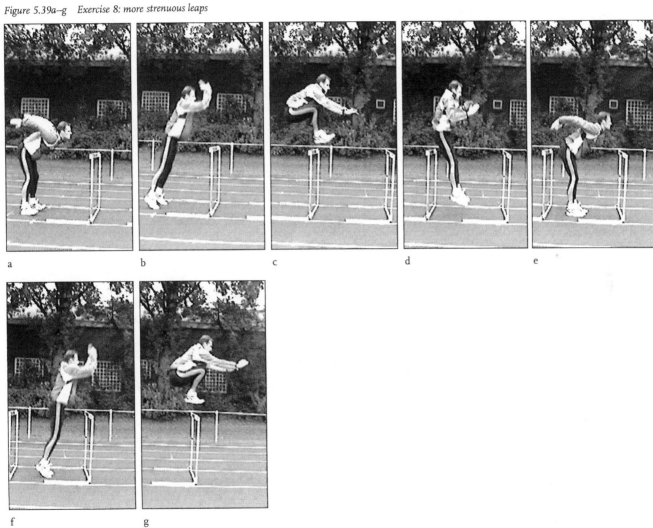

Exercise 8   More strenuous leaps
Exercises can be intensified in a number of ways (coordination). After push-off, the legs can be retracted explosively (e.g. when leaping across a hurdle). However, bending downward during the next landing will be extremely difficult and only possible for the best athletes. Landing after the following leap with the feet spread slightly apart (about 1 m), like when performing a long lunging stride, will make the exercise more difficult.

Hamstring exercises 2

In the second group of exercises, the hamstrings are less severely stressed but the coordinating movement is more difficult. Emphasis is placed on directing the force of thrust toward the rear and on absorbing external forces in unusual knee and hip angles. In addition to the exercises described below, there are many other ways in which one can learn to coordinate the hamstrings better (e.g. running jump on one leg with the trunk held vertically).

Exercise 1   Running with straight legs

The trunk should be held upright, or tilted slightly backward. The knees remain in the same position (straight or very slightly bent) throughout the entire exercise. The runner must try to reach the highest speed possible in this position. This can only be kept up for about 40 m if implemented with maximum intensity. By keeping the knees more or less extended, the working of the quadriceps and gastrocnemius (transfer of force from the knee to the ankle) is almost completely inhibited. By holding the trunk erect or slightly backward, it will be difficult to direct thrust. Both factors contribute to the fact that the hamstrings must function well if the target speed is to be attained.

Exercise 2   Running while alternately extending the legs

One can run while alternately (e.g. every 10 m) extending and bending the knee and hip very rapidly after toe-off. The function of the hamstrings must remain intact during very sudden changes in dissimilar patterns of movement. When carried out intensely, the exercise can only be continued over a distance of 60 m. Moreover, the posture of the trunk requires that there be a lot of tension in the muscles around the waist.

Exercise 3   Accelerating from a stationary position

Start by accelerating from a stationary position while holding the trunk erect. In this position, only the hamstrings will be able to direct thrust toward the rear. The runner must concentrate while performing this exercise because the trunk will always tend to lean forward during acceleration. The contact time must be kept short and there should be a lot of tension in the trunk. The lower the velocity, the more difficult it will be to accelerate when the upper body is erect. The exercise can best be carried out over a short distance (e.g. 20 m). It can also be practiced over a longer distance while wearing a light weight around the waist. The trunk must be held upright, ground contact times should be short, and there must be tension in the trunk.

Exercise 4   Skipping while making two ground contacts

Begin skipping, making two contacts with the ground (left–left, right–right, etc.) while wearing a drag weight around the waist. The trunk is held erect and the ground contact time is short. Because of the double ground contact, push-off cannot be made after a hard landing and will therefore not be reactive. The pretension needed in the hamstrings to direct thrust backward cannot develop from prestretch and must therefore be generated especially for this purpose. By increasing the resistance, the hamstrings can be tightened further. However, resistance must not be so high that a short contact time becomes impossible.

Exercise 5   Skipping while making one ground contact

Bend one leg quite far at the knee and hip, while keeping the other leg extended at the knee and slightly bent at the hip. The forward velocity is low, and the ground contact time short. After 5 m, the forward velocity is suddenly increased as much as possible. By keeping one leg straight, the trunk will remain vertical. Because the ground contact time is brief, the action of the hamstrings (in both the extended and bent leg) must be timed well.

Exercise 6   Types of exercise with the feet spread apart

Spread the feet far apart with the back leg extended and the front leg bent to about 90° at the knee. By leaning the trunk (back extended) forward from this starting position, the load on the hamstrings in the front leg will be increased. Exercises in which the feet are spread far apart will, therefore, be more strenuous for the hamstrings the further the trunk leans forward.

- While keeping the feet spread apart, jump without much vertical displacement as the legs change position very rapidly. During the landing, there must be little or no spring in the knee and hip of the front leg, while the knee of the back leg must remain as extended as possible. The athlete continues to jump around without pausing, while maintaining brief ground contact. By avoiding long ground contact and spring, the muscles in the thigh will be required to work well together.
- This type of jumping must now be done so that the knee of the back leg is extended during the support phase and the trunk permanently held forward with the back extended. The load placed on the hamstrings will be increased, making it more difficult to avoid spring. This exercise can also be performed while holding a bar-bell (no heavier than about 40 kg) at neck level (see Figure 5.40).
- Instead of jumping around without much vertical displacement, now jump as high as possible. The landing that follows will require a lot of power, but should be executed without spring, holding the back extended and trunk slightly bent forward (see Figure 5.41).
- Push-off is made with the feet spread apart. During the floating phase, the feet tap together before landing again with the feet slightly apart, keeping the same foot forward. The exercise can be intensified by leaning the trunk forward and keeping the knee of the back leg as extended as possible during the support phase.
- With the feet slightly apart, try to jump vertically, as high as possible. The body lands with the feet spread apart and, keeping the contact time short, jump around once as fast as possible (see Figure 5.42).

The exercises described above will have the greatest effect on how the hamstrings are coordinated when implementing with precision the various details (ground contact time, position of the back, angle of the knee during landing, etc.).

Figure 5.40a–d   Leaping with the body held low

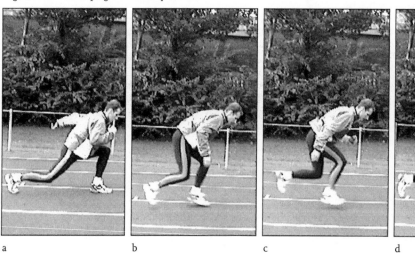

a   b   c   d

Figure 5.41a–e   Leaping with the body extended upward

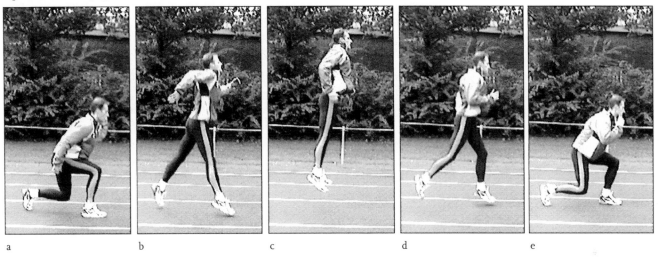

a   b   c   d   e

Figure 5.42a–f   Leaping while bending and extending the body

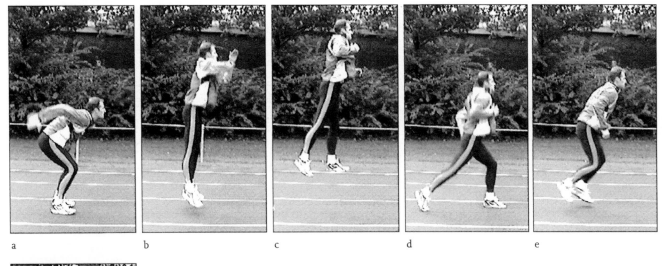

a   b   c   d   e

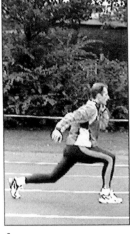

f

5.2.4 Frequency and reflexes

Pathways along which reflexes travel can be called the highways of the central nervous system (CNS). Motor patterns that can use these reflex highways will travel faster and be implemented with more force than will other motor patterns for which reflex responses are not available. During running, the work produced by various muscles alternates quickly. Therefore, a rapid exchange between tightening and relaxation in muscle is an important requirement for achieving a good level of performance. The way in which reflex patterns work to make tension and relaxation possible should be incorporated as fully as possible in a variety of types of training. One requirement is that during the exercise, when one leg moves, at the same time there must always be a corresponding but counteractive movement in the other leg.

During an exercise emphasis can be placed on the speed at which a muscle tightens and then relaxes (frequency training) and on combining reflex response with a high peak force. Because both categories of exercise are regulated by the CNS highway, fatigue will occur at a neuromuscular level (i.e. at the level of stimulus transfer). When the exercise has been implemented optimally, a typical image is observed. Directly after exercising, the athlete will appear to be extremely exhausted, more so than when having undertaken any other form of exercise. However, recovery will occur quite rapidly and the athlete will soon be able to exercise again. Moreover, athletes who are most proficient at practicing such exercises (i.e. those with the most power and speed) will be unable to continue exercising as long as athletes who have yet to gain more control. Apparently practiced athletes can exhaust their nervous systems more rapidly than less practiced athletes.

In this exercise program, emphasis is placed on the stumble and inverse-extension reflexes, which are incorporated in a pattern of movement with regard to running. In frequency exercises, the rhythm of motion is faster than during running. Exercises in which greater force is combined with reflex action are frequently used during strength training (see Ch. 6). A number of exercises can be practiced on an athletic track.

One must be able to exercise the same control over the basic mechanisms of movement which resemble running. For example, being able to regulate movement around the ankle is an important requirement if reflexes are to function optimally. Therefore, one must make certain that the exercises are implemented correctly (e.g. sufficient tension must be present around the ankle during the exercise). If an athlete performs the basic mechanisms carelessly, it will be impossible to optimize the movements.

Figure 5.43a–d   Exercise 1: skipping while making one ground contact combined with heel strike

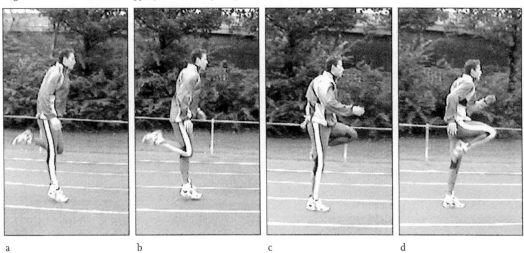

a   b   c   d

Exercise 1   Skipping while making one ground contact combined with heel strike
A frequently used exercise during training is the heel-strike move. Skip while making one ground
contact, where the hip remains extended and the free leg only bends at the knee after the foot has
left the ground. The knee bends so that the heel touches the buttocks (a, b). Although this exercise
is widely practiced, it has little value because the movements are in no way linked to one of the reflex
patterns (stumble reflex and inverse-extension reflex). A more useful exercise would combine extreme
flexion in the knee and flexion in the hip (c, d). The leg is lifted horizontally, with the foot touching
the buttocks (skipping–heel strike). When both forms of exercise are performed using the highest
frequency and the greatest degree of movement, it will become clear that the skipping–heel strike,
but not heel strike, is supported by reflexes. The heel strike can be continued for a long period of time,
while the skipping–heel strike rapidly leads to neuromuscular fatigue.

Figure 5.44a–f Exercise 2: skipping while making two ground contacts

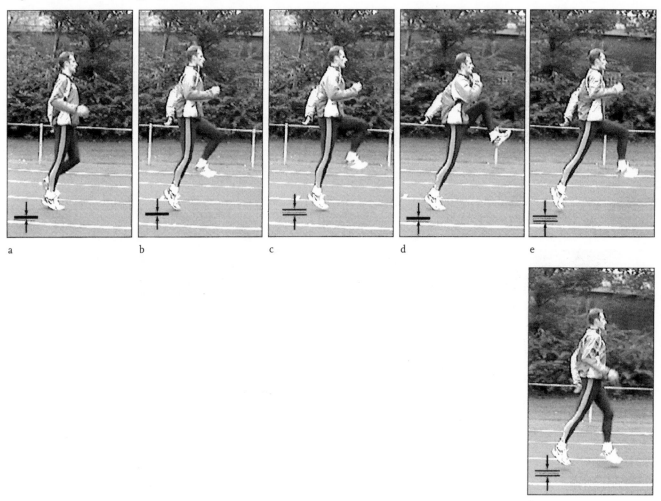

a   b   c   d   e

f

Exercise 2   Skipping while making two ground contacts
Both a very high frequency and a large degree of movement are used to perform this exercise. The swing leg is lifted horizontally as rapidly and as early in the cycle of movement as possible, thus 'pushing' the total movement onwards.

Figure 5.45a,b Exercise 3: skipping while making one ground contact

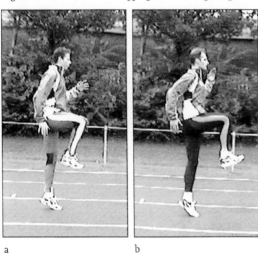

a   b

Exercise 3   Skipping while making one ground contact
First, skip a number of times before suddenly standing still. Now balance on the forefoot of the stance
leg, which is kept extended. The free leg is bent at the hip and knee, with the foot raised. The upper
body is erect, with one arm in front and one arm behind the free leg. When the exercise is performed
well the body will already be positioned correctly by the time the foot of the stance leg touches ground.
After foot strike, there must be no further movement. After standing still for about 1 s, again begin to
skip as fast as possible, with the knee of the swing leg repeatedly lifted horizontally. One should make
certain that the trunk does not lean toward the side of the stance leg. The rhythm of the exercise can be
varied (e.g. standing still after every second, third, or fourth skip; alternating standing still after every
fourth and third skip; etc.).

Figure 5.46a–f   Exercise 4: skipping over low gates

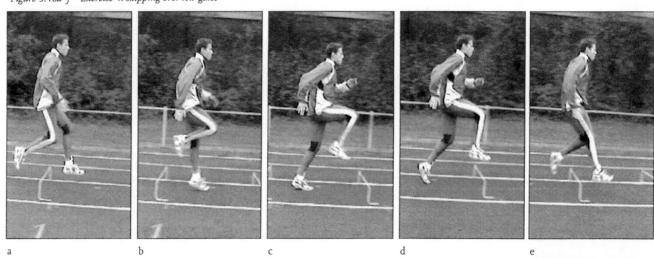

a   b   c   d   e

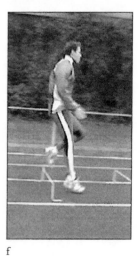

f

Exercise 4 Skipping over low gates
Ten gates (15 cm high) are placed in a row, 1 m apart. Skip on one leg, repeatedly touching the ground once between gates. The more rapid the forward velocity, the higher the frequency must be. The assignment is to run across the gates, keeping the frequency as high as possible, while maintaining a sufficiently large degree of movement. The distance between the gates and the number of ground contacts between them can be varied so that there are numerous possibilities available for instruction.

Exercise 5   Tapping

Sprinters frequently use an exercise (so-called tapping) which aims to achieve the highest possible frequency of movement (i.e. skipping while touching ground once with the knees raised only minimally). The idea behind this exercise is that this extremely high frequency will be good practice for training the general coordination of the body. The disadvantage, however, is that any support gained from reflex responses will be more or less overlooked. Repeated high-frequency tapping alternating with skipping, whereby the knees are lifted horizontally, will provide a better form of exercise. The frequency will decline during the transition, but more will be demanded of the runner on a central level because movement will involve reflexes. This variation of the exercise can also be practiced in several ways (e.g. high-frequency tapping while the trunk bends slightly forward, exchanged for skipping while the trunk moves to an upright position).

Exercise 6   Running jump on one leg

The running jump on one leg has already been described (see p. 255) where the frequency is raised as high as possible. The rhythm (right–left–floating phase–right–left–floating phase) is carried out rapidly. The sudden change from right to left is the factor that will restrict the frequency. During the floating phase, the center of mass of the body will rise slightly, so that the running jump remains short.

5.2.5   How the pelvis and trunk move

Even though it takes place within a narrow range, movement in the trunk and pelvis will nevertheless play an important and frequently underestimated role during running. Practicing how to move the pelvis and create torsion in the trunk will prove worthwhile. One must also understand how the abdominal muscles function here. During speed running, the abdominal muscles are worked strenuously while the trunk is held upright. Abdominal muscles that function well are able to cope with such large external forces. In addition to working with large external forces, one must learn how to control and maintain tension in the muscles that cause the pelvis and trunk to move in situations where coordination is difficult. In addition to the abdominal muscles, one should also train the dorsal muscles and short muscles surrounding the pelvis.

Figure 5.47a–i   Exercise 1: running sideways

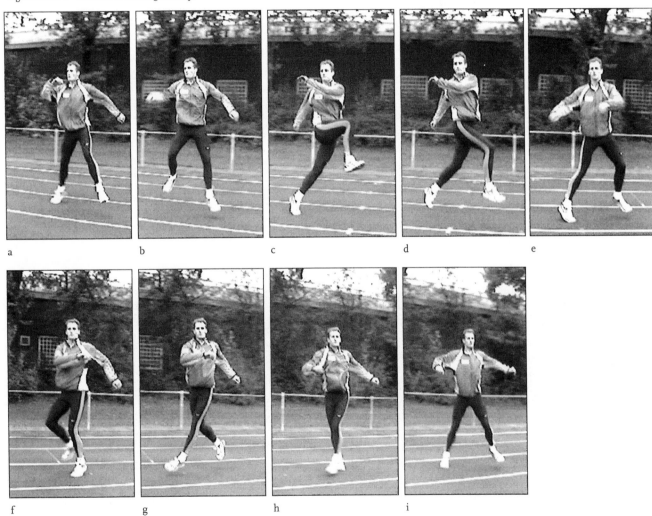

a   b   c   d   e

f   g   h   i

Exercise 1   Running sideways
Run sideways toward the right, as the left leg alternately crosses in front and then behind the right
leg. In this manner, the hips will repeatedly rotate to the left and right. The trunk does not rotate,
but rather remains stationary. In order to help keep the trunk stationary, the arms can be raised to
shoulder level and extended sideways. The exercise can be done in a number of ways. The knee of
the back (left) leg can be kept low during the entire practice so that either the cadence or torsion will
be increased as much as possible. The knee of the back leg can also be lifted high as it crosses in front
of the other leg and then swung rapidly with force in the direction in which the athlete is running.
Moreover, the arms and trunk make a powerful countermove. A lot of tension is required in the
abdominal muscles, regardless of how the exercise is implemented.

Exercise 2 Skipping with single ground contact
Here the frequency is not too high and the knees are lifted to an angle of 45° with the hips. During skipping, tilt the pelvis slowly forward and backward. It is important to regulate this movement correctly. Once the exercise has been mastered, then, after tilting the pelvis forward and backward several times, it can be held as far to the back as maximally possible while increasing the skipping frequency as much as possible.

Figure 5.48a–c   Exercise 3: skipping with single or double ground contact

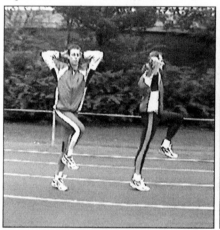 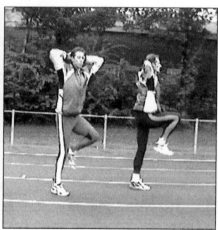 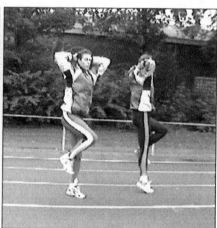

a   b   c

Exercise 3 Skipping with single or double ground contact
Hold the trunk vertical and clasp the hands behind the head with the elbows pointing sideways. While skipping, rotate the trunk slowly, with the left then the right elbow pointing forward. The knees continue moving in the line of progression. The abdominal muscles must have a great deal of pretension due to the torsion created by this motion. As a variation, the exercise can be carried out as follows: the left elbow is slowly moved forward, after which the right elbow is suddenly brought forward with a jerk as rapidly as possible, etc.

Exercise 4   Bouncing on two legs

Clasp the hands behind the head and point the elbows to the side as far as possible. During each hop, torsion will develop in the trunk: when the right leg swings upwards, then the left elbow is brought forward, and vice versa. Attention should be paid to holding the elbows exactly horizontal on one line and to turning the entire trunk. The degree of movement for torsion cannot be too large.

Figure 5.49a–e   Exercise 5: hopping (variation)

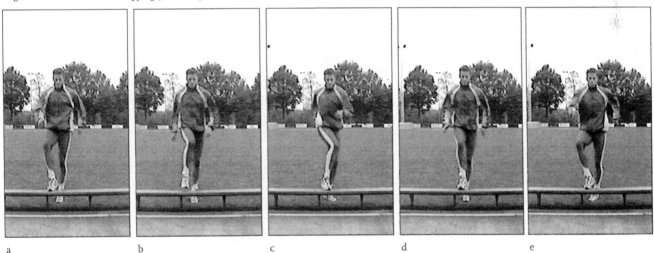

a   b   c   d   e

Exercise 5   Hopping (variation)

Start by standing upright on one leg, with the free leg bent at the knee and hip and the foot placed on a 30-cm high elevation. The weight of the body rests only on the stance leg. The arms are extended down at the sides of the body, with the muscles tightened well. Thereafter, the knee of the front leg is rotated inward and then outward, keeping to the rhythm of the hop. The arms move in the opposite direction. Once the rhythm and motion have been mastered, the frequency and force of the motion can be increased. Here the trunk must remain upright. When the exercise is performed with as much force as possible, the abdominal muscles will require a lot of tension, making the exercise quite strenuous for the medial and lateral rotators in the hip.

Figure 5.50a–h   Exercise 6: running hurdles with double ground contact

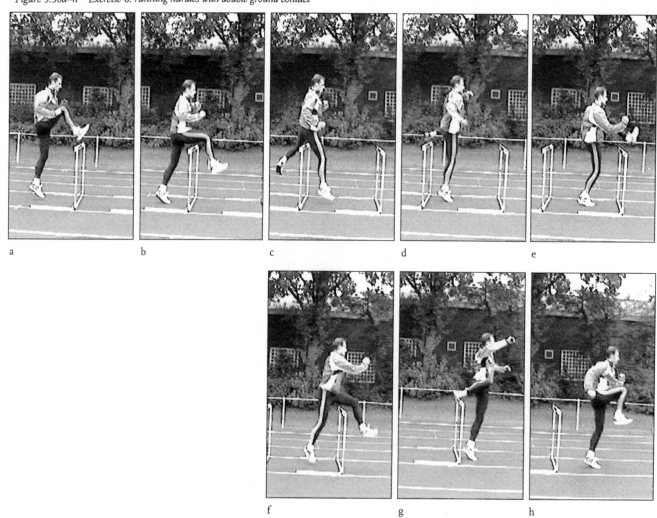

Exercise 6   Running hurdles with double ground contact
Run across the hurdles touching the ground twice between hurdles (see training the ankle, Section 5.2.1). When the hurdles (about 1.2 m apart) are high enough, much will be demanded of the muscles responsible for moving the pelvis (the dorsal and abdominal muscles and the short muscles around the hip). Hurdles can be run in a number of ways (e.g. forward as well as backward, with the arms free or kept fixed, touching the ground three or four times instead of twice, with or without ballast, etc.).

5.3   CONSTANT-SPEED RUNNING

When practicing the basic mechanisms of running, one can link a large specificity with a (very) large overload. The quality of the blocks from which the motion of running is built up can be greatly improved in this manner. When training the total pattern of movement (i.e. running itself), if specificity is very high it will be impossible to use a large overload because it would greatly disrupt coordination and the basic mechanisms would cease to function as expected. For example, when using some sort of resistance (e.g. running with a cord fastened around the hips and attached to a drag weight), it must not be made so heavy that it becomes impossible to reuse the energy generated during the landing. If that is in fact the case, running will no longer be reactive, but rather the athlete will have to propel his body forward during each push-off, causing his running technique to deteriorate. During supramaximal running (where the athlete finds himself being dragged along by the rope, see Section 5.1.5), the pattern of running will likewise change unfavorably if the drag weight (i.e. the overload) is too heavy. At the moment of IC, there will be a change in the way that the hamstrings and the rectus femoris direct force. The horizontal component of push-off will decline, while its vertical component will increase. The hamstrings will work less, while the rectus femoris will be required to work more. Moreover, the athlete will tend to place his foot in front of the projection of his hip on the ground, so that the leveraged deceleration will support the vertical push-off and a longer stride, therefore making a lower frequency possible. Although to the naked eye this might not appear to differ from speed running, an unfavorable running technique can still be provoked during supramaximal running. For this reason, one must use a very small overload. The margin is so slight that one can ask whether, during supramaximal training, it is wise to use a tool such as a drag cord, or whether it would be better to limit oneself to running with tail wind or downhill on an incline not exceeding a few tenths of a percent.

Practicing the complete motion of running must therefore only be done when the overload is very restricted, so that all the basic movements can be regulated well. Most trainers have learned through practice generally to stick to this rule. However, inexperienced trainers can be quite impressed by the way in which athletes become exhausted when using a large overload, and fail to understand that this type of training will not improve the level of performance, and might actually have the opposite effect.

The aim of using the complete pattern of movement as a way to practice is to teach a runner how to incorporate and use more precisely all the relevant basic mechanisms of motion in order to develop as efficient a running technique as possible. Two strategies can be used: (1) linking a movement to an assignment; and (2) using repetitions.

Using the first strategy, an athlete is asked to run in a specific manner. Depending on his level of competence, the assignment is designed to make either global and rough or meticulous and strict demands upon him. For example, a suitable assignment for an athlete who has had little training might be to raise the trunk slowly to a more or less upright position as speed increases. Alternatively, a well-trained runner might be asked to start by falling forward and after exactly 30 m bring his hips forward in a single move to a position exactly appropriate for speed running. The better the runner, the more precise the assignment must be to lead to an improvement in his technique. Here the runner must have a good power of imagination as well as an exact sense of his body as it moves. The most difficult assignments are those in which the motion of the pelvis plays the central role (e.g. raising the pelvis on the side of the swing leg, or strengthening medial rotation by means of torsion in the spinal column during the support phase). Only 'masterful' runners will be able to change the motion of the pelvis on purpose while running.

In addition to requiring that an assignment be carried out precisely, implementing a technique in a specific manner can be achieved by changing the conditions in which one must run. For example, the stride can be regulated by asking an athlete to run over low barriers. In addition, a technique can be modified by using some form of resistance or drag weight, by running slightly up or down an incline, by running on various ground surfaces, etc. In contrast to following verbal instructions, one is now forced to pay greater attention to ensuring that the overload used is not too large and that it does not have a detrimental effect on how one should run correctly.

Repetition learning plays an important role when trying to discover the most efficient way to run, in addition to influencing the technique by giving instructions and practicing exercises. For athletes who are reasonably talented but have had little running instruction, it appears that a technique will become fairly efficient in the long run using only explicit instruction. Apparently the body itself is quite capable (up to a certain degree) of discovering which movements are efficient. Repetition is therefore a good means of instruction and should be included in a training program. Technique training is thus as an interaction between instructions provided and assigned by an external source (i.e. the trainer) and an automatic process of development (i.e. within the body itself). The result is that exercising and incorporating changes into a technique will only show an improvement in performance after a longer period of time.

This process can best be illustrated using an example. A very talented sprinter has been suffering from an injury to his Achilles tendon for a long time. Although he is not able to run fast, he can still train all the important basic mechanisms and run on grass at submaximum tempos. After his injury has healed, he can again train optimally for high-speed running and will quickly be using a good technique. The runner has little voluntary control over the angle of his knee at the moment of IC during speed running, even though this is considered to be a performance-determining factor. After a period of time (say 2 months), the angle of the knee at IC will have changed somewhat (becoming slightly smaller), and the sprinter's level of performance will have improved. Apparently, the body has needed time to coordinate movement around the knee with the running technique now being used. The efficiency that has developed is derived from calculations made in a much more complex field of mechanics than a trainer or general sports scientist is able to utilize (Bobbert et al 1992). In particular, the ideal angle of the knee at IC can only be found by automating the movement. While one runner will run more efficiently when the knee is nearly extended, another runner will prefer to bend his knee further (i.e. a 'sitting' running technique). Seen from this perspective, particularly instructing an athlete to run as 'high' as possible (i.e. with the knee nearly extended at IC) is dubious to say the least.

The art of training the total motion of running therefore lies, on one hand, in allowing the body room to find those aspects of a technique that can best be perfected automatically and, on the other hand, in purposely regulating those aspects that will clearly prove detrimental to performance. In the past, it has been shown more than once that incorrect ideas have managed to creep into technique training when the function of the locomotor apparatus has not been clearly understood. A number of such incorrect ideas were upheld as standard for years. In addition to the fact that athletes were particularly expected to 'run high', according to most trainers, the upper body should not be permitted to lean backward, for example, during the last leg of a sprint. Reactive running and avoidance of long-axis rotation, however, are actually facilitated by such a body posture, and perhaps should not be discouraged when an athlete has reached the limit of his ability to perform. The running culture frequently eclipses what Nature would normally dictate. A good trainer should be able to find an ideal synthesis between the two factors.

When instructing a technique for the entire motion of running, various aspects can be emphasized. Later the exercise program is divided according to such particular points of interest.

5.3.1 Avoiding long-axis rotation

Axial rotation may develop because force is still being applied during the latter part of the support phase. At the beginning of the next support, one must compensate for any rotation that has occurred, which will thus result in a decline in speed. In addition, torsion in the spinal column can develop during push-off (see Section 3.2). Torsion can be favorable and contribute significantly to thrust. It is important, however, that a runner learns to create good torsion while simultaneously avoiding long-axis rotation. To do this, the runner must understand how torsion feels and what the implications of axial rotation are. In addition, he must be able to sense that, when thrust occurs at the beginning of support, it will cause less axial rotation and result in a more consistent pattern of running.

A good way to experience this is by keeping the arms immobile while running. Arm movement can both increase torsion and absorb any disturbance in equilibrium resulting from axial rotations. When a compensatory movement can no longer be made, the negative effect of long-axis rotation will definitely be experienced as an imbalance, and the runner must find a way to run whereby any disruption to his equilibrium can be avoided. Subsequently, arm movement can be re-inserted into the motion of running, albeit within a smaller range of motion. Now the runner will only exert force when his elbows are located next to his body. It is specifically then that arm movement can contribute optimally to torsion. Through these exercises, the length of the support phase can be decreased. However, the runner will be required to learn how to hold the upper part of his body erect. If the trunk is permitted to hang toward the front, any advancement made after exercising will have a very restricted effect, certainly when the runner himself does not naturally work reactively. In athletes who have already developed a good running technique, and therefore almost never demonstrate axial rotation, the same exercise program can be applied to improve the way in which the abdominal muscles and hip rotators function. The exercises are then practiced at a higher running speed to make them more difficult.

Figure 5.51   Exercise 1: running with the arms held stationary

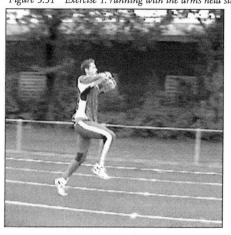

Exercise 1   Running with the arms held stationary

The running speed is constant across a distance of about 40 m, with the arms kept stationary in one of many ways: with the hands clasped behind the head, with the arms crossed in front of the chest, extended sideways, with both hands holding a pole or piece of rope, etc. Ground contact must be kept brief and the trunk should remain quite vertical. Once this has been mastered during slow running, and the abdominal and dorsal muscles are able to control movement around the long axis (torsion), the velocity may be increased. The athlete will try to find the highest speed at which to run while still keeping the ground contact time as short as possible. When the running speed is too fast, the contact time will increase. Stronger rotation in the lower body can no longer be compensated for by a counter-movement in the trunk, so that compensation will have to be regulated during the support phase. The transition between speeds (i.e. a speed that makes brief ground contact possible and one that results in a longer contact time) will be rather abrupt. In this way, the runner can learn to intuit when long-axis rotation will develop.

Exercise 2   Running a distance of 20 m with the arms held stationary

The arms can be kept from moving in various ways. After 20 m, the arms can be allowed to move again. However, the pattern of leg movement and the posture of the trunk may not change. Now the runner can move without causing long-axis rotation to develop, and arm movement will only increase torsion. Once the intended pattern of running has been achieved, learning to maintain the correct technique may be made more strenuous. For example, the runner can accelerate while moving the arms until reaching the maximum possible speed. The length of the stride can be adapted (e.g. by running after 40 m over low (15 cm high) obstacles placed a certain distance apart and between which one or two ground contacts must be made).

Figure 5.52a–c   Exercise 3: skipping–heel strike with very well-controlled arm movement

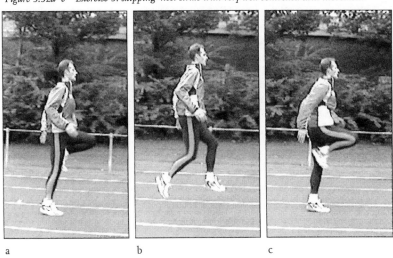

a   b   c

Exercise 3   Skipping–heel strike with very well-controlled arm movement
See also information on training frequency (p. 224). The arms move within a very small range,
with emphasis being placed on moving them backward with force when they are alongside the body.
Starting from this pattern of movement, the forward velocity can be increased, although this pattern
must not be changed substantially. At first the running technique will feel somewhat uncomfortable
and may appear to waste energy. After a number of repetitions, one can look for a transition that will
feel better. However, the basic properties (short ground contact, erect upper body, brief arm action)
must remain intact.

Figure 5.53   Exercise 4: running in curves

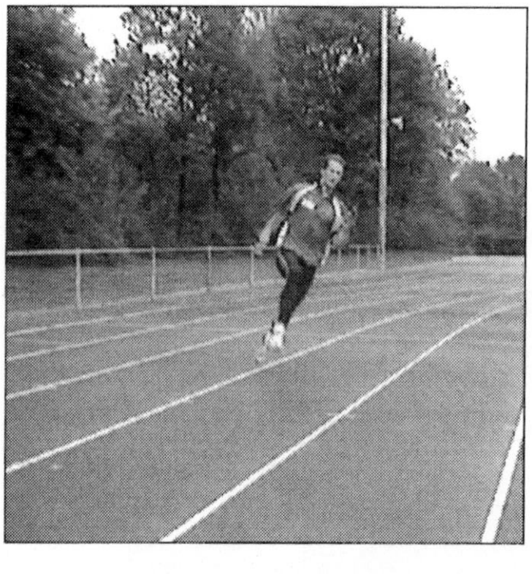

Exercise 4   Running in curves

The athlete runs rather rapidly around a curve of an ample radius. When running in a curve, long-axis rotation will be quite disruptive. Running on a curve is made particularly difficult by long-axis rotation, which develops when force is exerted for too long by the leg on the inner side of the curve. A running pattern can be easily developed in which the inside leg makes very brief contact with the ground while the outer leg forcefully exerts thrust reactively. After running a 30-m curve, the athlete should run another 30 m on the straight, while trying to maintain the technique used for the curve (running reactively, avoiding long-axis rotation) as well as possible.

Exercise 5   Variations in running

Many variations can be created based on the previous exercises. For example, running 30 m followed by 10 strides curving toward the left (where the left leg touches the ground briefly and long-axis rotation to the right is avoided), then 10 strides curving toward the right (now brief ground contact on the right side) and finally running 30 m straight ahead while both legs make brief ground contact and the arms swing slightly toward the back.

Figure 5.54   Exercise 6: running while jumping rope

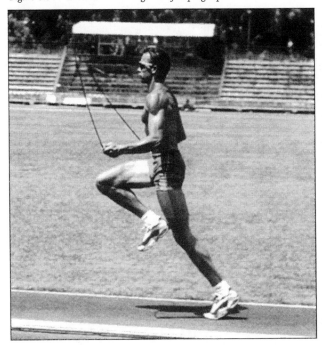

Exercise 6   Running while skipping with a rope
Run while holding one end of a skipping rope in each hand. The rope swings beneath the body during
the floating phase, turning one cycle each step. Because the arms cannot oscillate, and in order to
avoid the danger of tripping over the rope, push-off must be short and reactive. Therefore, there
will be no rotation around the long axis. The forward velocity can be increased while skipping. By
using a skipping rope, the total pattern of running will automatically be aimed in the right direction
(i.e. reactivity and no rotation). The learning process is intuitive and thus suitable for young athletes
as well as for runners who might find it difficult to translate abstract instructions into correct
movements. The disadvantage of this exercise is that it will take some time to master the technique.
However, this form of exercise will be useful even for the most highly skilled athletes. It is possible
to create different combinations for the forward velocity and the frequency with which the rope is
turned (e.g. a high running speed using low-frequency rope turning will result in a long stride and
reactive push-off).

5.3.2 Emphasis on reactivity

Because the various movements from which the motion of running is built are strongly interrelated, one can affect the reactivity of push-off by emphasizing one particular aspect. The running pattern described for the exercises makes it difficult to replace reactivity by any other (e.g. explosive–concentric) muscle action. The exercise 'compels' an athlete to run reactively. Exercises that are aimed at avoiding rotation around the longitudinal axis can also contribute, for example, to reactive running. The shorter push-off time that results when one tries to avoid axial rotation gets the athlete on the right track toward using his muscles reactively and, in turn, is required before one can run reactively. One can approach the issue of reactivity from perspectives other than avoiding axial rotation. Of course, one can best begin by choosing an approach that addresses the particular mistake being made.

Reactive running and knee action

The way in which muscles work reactively is dependent on the amount of energy being loaded into the muscle. For running, this means that reactivity will depend on the way the foot is placed on the ground surface, and therefore on the velocity of the leading leg in the direction of backward flexion at the moment of foot placement. Backward flexion is directly related to forward flexion in the trailing leg. Both legs work together during the swing phase, like a pair of scissors. In practice, it appears that concentrating on forward flexion in the trailing leg is the best approach to understanding this scissor-like motion. Forward flexion must be initiated early and with force. Moreover, the movement must be linear (i.e. the hip and knee must bend simultaneously). If the knee bends first before being brought forward, time will be wasted and backward flexion in the leading leg will take place too slowly. When the movement has been executed correctly, one will observe a sudden, decisive moment in which the trailing leg is lifted off the ground and forward flexion becomes a powerful, supporting effort, rather than a relaxed swing.

Figure 5.55a–d   Exercise 1: skipping with a single ground contact

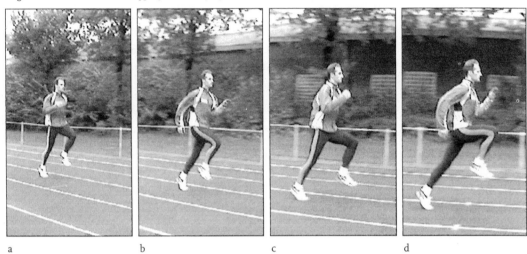

a   b   c   d

Exercise 1   Skipping with a single ground contact
Begin by skipping, touching the ground once, with a frequency that is not too high. The knees will remain low because there is little flexion in the hip. Next, skip forcefully in a predetermined rhythm with the knee lifted horizontally (e.g. every second, third, or fourth skip is powerful; three low skips are followed by two high skips; etc.). When skipping is done with force, the hip and knee must bend simultaneously and the foot should not be allowed to droop (no plantar flexion). The forward velocity is slowly increased starting from this pattern of motion. As the speed increases, the low skips can be done within an increasingly larger range of movement. In the end, both legs will continue to demonstrate the same pattern of movement, in which the swing leg is moved forward linearly with force after the transition from a closed to an open chain. After the gradual transition, the athlete will continue running at speed for about 20 m.

Exercise 2   Increasing the running frequency
Run at a submaximum speed, and subsequently increase the frequency but not the forward velocity. Here the swing leg moves as linearly possible. Next, the forward velocity will increase without causing any change in the pattern or rhythm of the movement. Even at high speed, one must try to increase the frequency a fraction more than required for that running speed.

Exercise 3   Running slightly downhill or with a strong back wind
Run at high speed while trying to increase the cadence somewhat by bringing the knees forward as quickly as possible during each stride. Forward thrust will be less of a problem when running downhill or with a back wind than during vertical push-off. The runner will tend to place his foot somewhat further ahead of the body during foot strike (in order to push off more vertically), consequently leaving the swing leg to trail somewhat further behind. Making a conscious effort always to bring the swing leg forward is therefore a major intervention in this pattern of movement.

Reactive running and ankle rigidity

Before the moment of toe-off, there is plantar flexion in the foot. If it is initiated from a strong position of dorsiflexion (halfway through the support phase), it will take the foot too long to leave the ground. Lifting the foot rapidly from the surface, and also running reactively, can therefore be improved by learning to regulate the amount of dorsiflexion in the support phase. Being aware of how the ankle moves during reactive running amounts to trying to hold the ankles in a more or less rigid position. By doing this, there will be more tension in the muscles and less dorsiflexion permitted halfway through the support phase. Plantar flexion in the foot will be completed earlier, the moment of toe-off will be reached sooner, and moving the knee forward will take place more rapidly.

For all exercises aimed at increasing tension in the ankle, it is important to hold the upper body erect. The way in which the body moves must give the impression that the stance leg is like a spring, so to speak, which has been wedged between the upright trunk and well-tensed ankle, and which is repeatedly squeezed together before springing open.

Exercise 1   Running uphill, into the wind, or with a drag weight
The resistance with which the runner must work may be reasonably heavy. However, the ground contact time should remain very short. If this causes the forward velocity to be a bit lower, there will be no problem. The ground contact time can only be kept short using such resistance if there is sufficient tension in the ankles. If not, then the resistance will immediately cause a great deal of dorsiflexion to develop and the ground contact time will increase.

Exercise 2   Faster tripling
Start the exercise by tripling, keeping the ankles rigid and bending the legs only slightly during the swing phase. The knees will therefore remain low. Starting from this tripling, the forward velocity is increased while keeping the knees low for as long as possible. Ground contact is brief. Because the knees remain low, a lot of tension will be needed in the ankle during a short push-off in order to accelerate effectively. When it becomes impossible to accelerate further with the knees low, they can be raised higher and the velocity increased. Tension must be maintained in the ankle.

Exercise 3   Running across a distance of 100 m
Here hold the trunk well upright while not running too fast. The ground contact time must be kept brief throughout the entire exercise. The floating phase will take a long time, and consequently the stride will be long. Because the ground contact time must remain short, the landing energy must be rapidly converted into a vertical push-off by tightening the total chain of muscles (and also the ankles) correctly.

Exercise 4   Running at constant speed with very short ground contact times
Every 10 m, alternate running at a high frequency with the legs extended and running at a low frequency with the knees bent. For the latter combination, much more tension will suddenly be needed in the ankle joint and must be built up very rapidly.

Reactive running and increased frequency

Some athletes who naturally run quite reactively demonstrate, as a result of faulty practice, poor coordination between the movements taking place in the stance and swing legs. Because of their natural talent, energy will be rapidly discharged soon after foot placement. The action of the swing leg, however, is timed in a way that does not agree with such natural reactivity. As a result, the motion of the swing leg will neither support nor regulate reactivity, but rather will be counterproductive. A vertical component that is much too large develops at the beginning of the support phase and passes as a shock through the body before then ebbing away. After the energy has been discharged rather ineffectively, the stance foot remains temporarily on the ground before the swing phase begins. The runner's movements are jerky and a comfortable stride cannot be found, certainly at submaximum speeds. By varying the frequency while keeping the speed constant, and vice versa, one can improve the rapport between reactivity in the stance leg and the effect that the swing leg has on that reactivity. By varying the relationship between the variables speed and frequency, a runner can begin to realize when the knee of the swing leg should lie next to the knee of the stance leg in order to regulate the pattern (dominant for him) of reactivity correctly. Such running exercises naturally have the greatest effect when used together with other exercises.

Figure 5.56 Exercise 1: running over low barriers

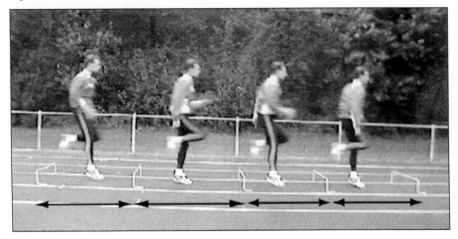

Exercise 1   Running over low barriers
Barriers are placed between 1.8 and 2 m apart. Start by running 20 m before crossing the barriers, touching the ground once between them. Ground contact time must remain short. Changes in the length of the stride required here must be achieved by repeatedly varying the frequency. The distance between barriers can be varied in a number of ways (e.g. a series of barriers placed close together followed by a series placed farther apart). One should take care that any adaptation in the running pattern is caused only by changing the frequency.

Exercise 2   Running 3 × 80 m

Run 80 m three times at a submaximum speed using a good reactive technique. (1) During the first run, the frequency should remain constant while the stride, and therefore the forward velocity, must be varied every 10 m. (2) During the second run, the speed should remain constant, while both the frequency and the stride should be varied every 10 m. (3) During the third run, the speed and frequency remain constant while the range over which the swing leg moves is varied every 10 m. By performing the required variations using a good technique, the runner will learn to coordinate accurately the actions of his support and swing legs.

Exercise 3   Running with a low forward velocity and low frequency

The knees are only lifted halfway. After running three strides, three more high-frequency strides are run actively, lifting the knee high and increasing the forward velocity. Thereafter, three more low-frequency strides follow, with the knees being held low and the velocity not increasing. Then three more active strides follow, with the frequency and velocity increasing, etc. The exercise must be carried out in such a way that one can observe a large difference between the active and passive strides and such that the transitions and acceleration occur abruptly. In the end, the athlete will be running at high speed. Coordination between the stance and swing legs can be improved by making the transitions abrupt.

Exercise 4   Running with a drag weight around the waist

Ground contact times remain short and the frequency varies at constant speeds. Due to the effect of the drag weight, timing the coordination of the push-off with the action of the swing leg will have to be adjusted precisely. When the timing is poor, increasing the frequency will prove difficult and any mistakes will be emphasized.

Reactive running under great pressure

It can be very educational for a runner, in particular a sprinter, to practice reactivity during running by pushing his body to the limit of its ability. Under great pressure imposed by extra resistance (e.g. weighted vest or drag weight), which must be overcome during each stride or by increasing the length of the stride (e.g. across low hurdles), a runner can be taught the way in which reactive and non-reactive running differs so greatly. On one hand, the overload should not be so extreme that reactive running is made impossible. On the other hand, the overload must not be so slight that it will be easy to correct mistakes in the running pattern. The assignment is to run while maintaining very short ground contact. When a certain stride length causes the ground contact time to increase, a runner will find himself unable to revert to a short ground contact time and running will cease being reactive. In this manner, a runner will come to understand which body posture allows running to be reactive and which will have a detrimental effect. Moreover, such exercises are particularly suitable for better runners, but may prove too strenuous for beginners or recreational runners.

Figure 5.57   Exercise 1: running over barriers

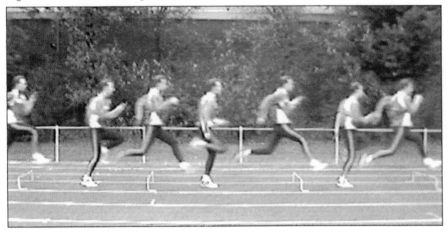

Exercise 1   Running over barriers
First, run 20 m before crossing 15-cm high barriers as rapidly as possible, keeping the ground contact time between barriers very short. The barriers are placed at increasing lengths from each other until reaching a distance at which it is still just possible to keep the ground contact time short. For good runners this distance might be as long as about 2.5 m. At this critical distance, when the ground contact time is too long, the runner will not be able to take his next step reactively. In this way, he can become aware of the exact difference between reactive and (non-reactive) explosive muscle action during push-off. Moreover, this exercise is very suitable for learning how reactive running is affected by a certain body posture. Namely, when a runner begins to stretch forward in order to bridge a large distance, he will bring his shoulders in front of his hips so that the body cannot be extended during the landing, thus making it impossible to push off reactively.

Exercise 2   Running with ballast

The ballast can be, for example, a 10-kg weighted vest. The running speed is not very fast, the ground contact time is short, and the stride is long. These requirements can only be met when there is sufficient tension in the body and when it is positioned exactly with regard to using the muscles reactively. The ballast reduces the margin within which errors can be made. Mistakes (e.g. a step that makes a long ground contact) cannot readily be corrected, and so the runner must learn to optimize his reactive movements.

Exercise 3   Running while wearing a heavy drag weight

By increasing the resistance caused by the drag weight, reactive running can be made more difficult. By training near the boundary where reactive running is still just possible, the runner can better learn to feel the differences between reactive and non-reactive running, just like in the previous exercise.

5.4   HOW TO START AND ACCELERATE

Learning how to start and accelerate holds a special position when instructing an individual how to run, as this part of the running technique is only of interest for sprinters. For other types of runners who only have to accelerate submaximally, no benefit will be gained from training in how to take off from the starting block. During practice, a trainer will search for a way to combine using the most power possible for the most favorable direction of thrust. Furthermore, as a byproduct, rotation will only be permitted to develop if it can be compensated for without slowing the body down. Because the forward velocity will change continuously during acceleration, a runner will constantly be forced to adjust how he must compromise between the magnitude and direction of thrust and compensation for rotations (i.e. also for an optimal body posture).

During speed running, maintaining an optimum body posture will be mainly determined by the demands made by reactivity and the need to avoid rotations around the longitudinal and lateral axes. On the one hand, there is only a small margin in which a running technique can deviate and still remain functional to do this. On the other hand, during the start and acceleration, there is a broader range in which to work. Because it will be possible to compensate for rotations, there will be more ways in which to develop and direct the force of thrust optimally. The way in which the body is built and the athletic potential of the runner are important factors influencing optimization and, in contrast to speed running, will more greatly affect the technique for starting and acceleration. Practicing how to start and accelerate will require a runner to look for a suitable technique geared to his individual needs. When observing a 100-m race, one will find that differences in technique during and just after the start are more pronounced than at the finish, assuming that all the runners are equally adept.

Large interindividual variations make it difficult to determine whether an athlete has actually chosen that one particular technique, from the many existing possibilities, which will prove optimal for himself. Many athletes try to imitate how other (successful) athletes start off at the block, even when they do not have the same physical requirements. For example, just before a start, for which an enormous amount of force is required, a runner may decide to expend a great deal of his strength on one thrust, even though he has neither the necessary level of strength nor suitable lever arms to do this. When instructing a technique, one must remember that there are many possible ways to achieve the goal. In particular, with regard to practicing the complete motion of running, estimating whether an individual and his technique are mutually suitable will prove decisive. Further consideration is given below to several aspects of the start and acceleration.

5.4.1   Basic components of the start and acceleration
On the whole, the basic mechanisms upon which the start and acceleration rely are identical to those for speed running.

Positions for the ankle and foot
The positions of the joints in the ankle and foot will change more during start and acceleration than while running at speed. This is because there will be more time at the end of push-off to return to a position that fits the transfer of force. Halfway through the support phase, therefore, much dorsiflexion will be permitted if, and only if, good plantar flexion can develop again thereafter. The exercises used to

teach a runner how to position the ankle when running at speed will also be of value during the start and acceleration.

Explosive push-off technique

During the start and acceleration, the explosive concentric action of muscles plays an important role, whereas reactivity only comes into the picture after an increase in velocity. The technique for explosive muscle work is quite simple compared to reactive muscle function. The positive work that is generated concentrically mainly develops in groups of large monoarticular muscles (i.e. the gluteus maximus, the vastus segments of the quadriceps femoris, and the iliopsoas). In practice, timing when these muscles should act almost never poses problem. During the start and acceleration phases, a great deal of activity is demanded of the rectus femoris, which has an important task in coordinating extension of the knee and hip. Forms of exercise that help coordinate knee and hip extension will contribute to an improved start. In particular, during the first strides after leaving the starting block, being able to adjust the coordination between the knee and the hip can prove beneficial.

Figure 5.58a–e   Exercise 1: vertical jump with the foot on an elevation

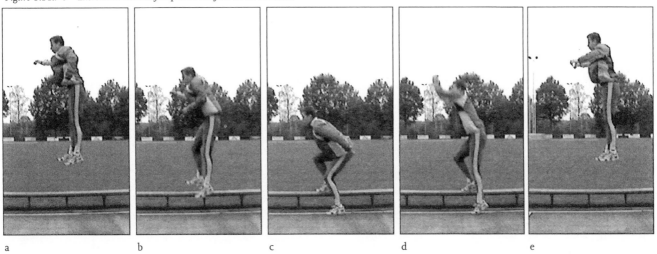

a   b   c   d   e

Exercise 1   Vertical jump with the foot on an elevation

Start by standing upright with one foot on a 20–30 cm high elevation. Allow the body to sag somewhat before making a vertical jump. After the landing, the body is once again in the starting position. The jumps can be carried out in succession. The back must always be extended during push-off. By varying the posture of the trunk before push-off one can emphasize either the function of the hamstrings or the quadriceps. When the trunk is held forward before push-off, hip extension will demand more force than the knee extension, so that the hamstrings will need to exert much more force. When the trunk is held nearly upright, knee extension will require more force than the hip extension, so that more force will have to be generated by the quadriceps (the rectus femoris). Jumping in succession can be done in a number of ways. For example: five jumps with the trunk upright and five with the trunk bent forward; jumping back and forth with the trunk upright or bent forward; or beginning with the trunk upright and then bending it gradually forward with each successive jump. To a certain degree, the last variation imitates what takes place during the start: first the quadriceps femoris exerts a great deal of power and thereafter the hamstrings take on the load. Otherwise, similarities with the start go no further than the way in which load is transferred between these muscles. From the perspective of coordination, the differences are too great to guarantee transfer to the start and acceleration.

323

Figure 5.59a–e   Exercise 2: squatting jump across hurdles

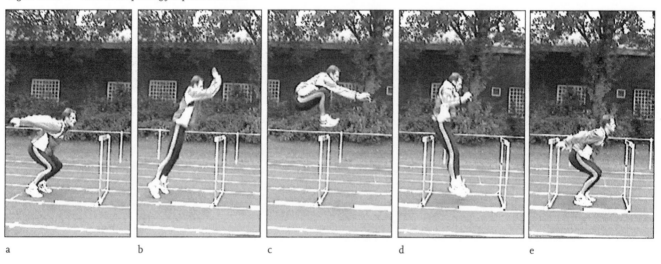

a   b   c   d   e

Exercise 2   Squatting jump across hurdles
Jump across a series of hurdles (1.2 m apart) from a squatting position. Using this exercise, the runner can also shift the load from front to back in the upper thigh by holding the trunk further forward in the starting position.

Figure 5.60a–f   Exercise 3: squatting jumps (variation)

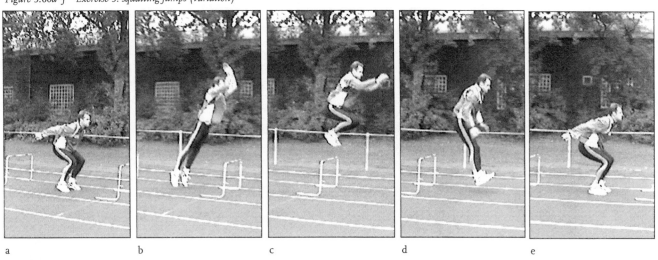

a   b   c   d   e

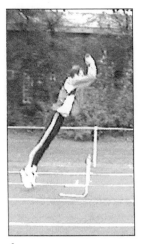

f

Exercise 3   Squatting jumps (variation)

Jump from a squatting position across a low hurdle, covering a long distance horizontally with each jump. The jumps are done in succession without pausing. Horizontal and vertical displacements are combined. The posture of the trunk, where push-off is initiated, can also be designated. By performing this exercise in various ways, one can instruct combined hip and knee extension.

Reflex techniques and explosive action

One of the most serious errors to occur at the start is not extending the stance leg through completely. The reason for this is nearly always found in a failure to swing the leg high enough. Because the runner is leaning too far forward, he tends to put his leading leg down on the ground too quickly. Therefore, the supportive response of, in particular, the inverse-extension reflex is not used optimally and the stance leg does not extend completely. By means of specific exercises, a runner can learn to direct push-off (knee and hip extension) by moving the swing leg. Movements taking place during the start can be compared to a horizontal jump on one leg, and thus learning to extend the stance leg correctly can be trained in this way.

Figure 5.61a,b   Exercise 1: vertical jump with one foot on an elevation

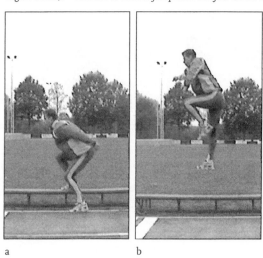

a   b

Exercise 1   Vertical jump with one foot on an elevation
Start by standing upright with one foot on a 20–30 cm high elevation. Allow the body to sag somewhat before pushing off for a vertical jump. During push-off, the leg that does not push off from the elevation rapidly swings high with the knee bent. After landing, the body is once again standing in the starting position. Jumps can be carried out in succession. In the starting position, the trunk can either be held upright or allowed to lean forward. Push-off from the elevation must be well coordinated with the action of the knee. The swing leg may be raised above a horizontal level. It is useful to vary the height of the elevation, which will require a different fine adjustment for push-off and the motion of the swing leg.

Exercise 2   Horizontal running jump beginning from a stationary position
The number of running jumps should be limited to five or six, because thereafter the forward velocity will be so rapid that reactivity will play a dominant role during push-off. However, a running jump is quite difficult to execute reactively and will provide insufficient transfer to both the start phase and the running speed.

Exercise 3   Climbing stairs
Climb the stairs trying to step over as many stairs as possible per step. It is only possible to run upstairs if the swing leg is raised high during each step while the stance leg is repeatedly extended correctly.

Pelvic, trunk, and arm movements

The trunk and pelvis move within a wider range during the start and acceleration phases than when running at speed. Trainers are in error when they try to restrict such movements and instead instruct an athlete to use only his legs at the start. A runner is generally aware of any movement taking place around the longitudinal axis. Almost every runner everts his foot when placing it on the surface, and much medial rotation develops in the hip of the stance leg during push-off. However, many runners are unable to feel how the body moves within the frontal plane, and further instruction will be needed. This training can also be done using vertical jumping on one leg, which must be implemented with precision.

Figure 5.62a–f   Exercise 1: vertical jump on one leg with a foot on an elevation

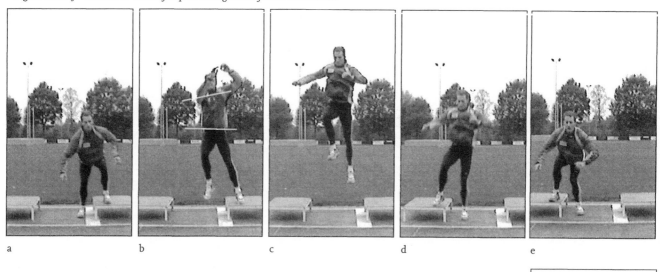

a   b   c   d   e

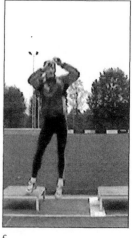

f

Exercise 1   Vertical jump on one leg with a foot on an elevation
Start by standing between two 30-cm high elevations with one foot on an elevation. After a preparatory movement downward, jump vertically from a squatting position. At the end of push-off, the shoulder is raised on the side of the elevation. At the same time, the hip of the swing leg is lifted. As the foot leaves the elevation, the hip and shoulder on the side of the push-off leg are further apart than on the side of the swing leg. The foot of the swing leg lands on the other elevation, while the other foot lands on the ground. Thereafter, a vertical push-off follows while the shoulder on the side of the push-off leg is moved upward.

Figure 5.63a–e   Exercise 2: 'skating' jumps in succession

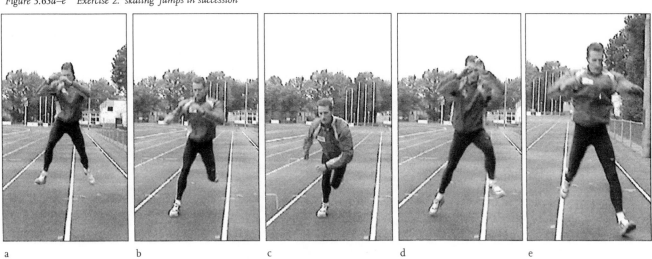

a   b   c   d   e

Exercise 2   'Skating' jumps in succession
A number of skating jumps are made in which the body is extended as completely possible. Thereafter, the runner begins accelerating over a distance of 20 m, thus trying to integrate movements occurring in the frontal plane, which are very prominent during skating jumps, into the start.

5.4.2 Total pattern of running: the start and acceleration

Many interindividual differences can be observed in the way in which a good start and acceleration can be carried out. This means that when instructing a runner in how to start, one can almost never predesign the final form that will be optimal for that individual, but rather the form will develop gradually during the training, which is itself learning process. In order to allow a technique to unfold in this way, all basic errors must first be eradicated. Once an athlete has stopped making fundamental errors and has learned to regulate the mechanisms relevant to movement, one can begin searching for an implementation that will fit the individual.

5.4.3 Errors during the start and acceleration

Some of the following problems can occur at the starting block or during acceleration.

- At the moment of foot placement, the hips are positioned far behind the foot of the stance leg. As a result, knee extension must be delayed and the hamstrings are forced to work much more actively. This type of start is often seen in runners who naturally carry their bodies correctly when running at speed. However, placing great emphasis on the hamstrings at the start will generate less power, and thus acceleration, than when placing emphasis on the quadriceps (which includes the rectus femoris) at the start.
- By applying an overload in the form of a drag weight hanging from a cord fastened around the shoulders instead of around the hips, a runner will quickly learn that holding the hips toward the rear is not a suitable posture when one must exert a great deal of force. The hips must be held further forward and the hamstrings should be less active than the quadriceps.
- Runners will frequently try to exert too much force. They are searching for a lot of force while forgetting that the movement must be executed rapidly. With this incorrect idea in mind, the swing leg will be brought forward while there is still insufficient flexion in the knee. Therefore, the knee will not end high enough and the stance leg will not be extended adequately.
- By running over low hurdles just a few centimeters high after the start, a runner will learn instinctively to bend his knees somewhat further. When he also realizes, particularly early in the start phase, that extending the leg completely can prove very effective, a runner will learn to rotate his body less and try to find a better compromise between moving rapidly and applying too much force.
- For runners with very long levers (i.e. long legs), the margins for compensating for forward and long-axis rotations are not very large. In contrast to runners with short legs, their body postures should be better attuned to speed. When the upper body is allowed to lean forward a bit too long or when it is erected too early, an immediate decrease in acceleration will result. A runner must learn to develop a good sense of balance at the starting block. A good way to practice controlling one's balance is by correcting the position of the knee of the swing leg at the end of push-off. Lifting the knee higher will cause the body to become more erect, while letting the knee hang will cause the body to lean further forward. Teaching a runner how to achieve balance cannot be done quickly. Some good sprinters are less concerned about using a poor technique at the start block because improving the speed of running will prove much more beneficial.
- The position of the hips during the start must not only be correct as seen from the front and back, but must also be correct vertically. If the hips are held too low during the start, the angle of the knee will be so acute at the moment of IC that

the runner will not be able to extend it quickly enough. Although the force being exerted is very powerful, it will nevertheless always come too late. Being able to hold the body erect in an optimal position will depend on the entire posture of the body and on the athletic potential of the runner. Sizeable differences can be observed between individuals.

- Runners who have good control over their feet when running at speed will sometimes seem to use their feet less well during the start phase. Strong dorsiflexion, combined with pronation in the foot and a leg that is turned outward, is difficult to convert into the plantar flexion necessary at the end of the support phase. This error can usually be corrected by paying sufficient attention to tension in the feet during the start.

6
Strength training for runners

6.1 INTRODUCTION

For athletes, certainly for middle- and long-distance runners, strength training is an area that often appears to have little association with the nature and instinct of running. The organization of strength training will offer runners few obvious points of departure. Many trainers view strength training as something that should be used with particular caution. Consequently, many middle- and long-distance runners will try to avoid strength training completely, or will set up a training program based on what they happen to find familiar. For sprinters, the situation is different. One need only observe the musculature of top sprinters to understand that strength is important. Furthermore, one often overlooks the fact that even an athlete running at a lower level of competence will generally appear to be just as muscular as a champion. However, sprinters often are blinded by the importance of musculature and strength, and consider only an increase in muscle mass (hypertrophy) to be a true sign that strength training is working successfully.

For years, therefore, it was assumed that an increase in strength achieved after a strength-training program was exclusively the result of hypertrophy. The increase in strength after several months of power training can reach spectacular values, even as much as 100%. However, one must question whether an increase in strength is always accompanied by an increase in muscle mass. In a number of situations, increased strength cannot be explained by the presence of more muscle mass. For example, female athletes are able to increase their strength substantially and progressively, just like their male colleagues, without showing any further increase in bulk. Another situation relates to the increase in strength during the first phase of a strength-training program that takes place without an increase in the number of sarcomeres linked in parallel. Furthermore, one can give numerous examples in which individuals have appeared to possess superhuman strength during life-threatening situations. In the theory of training, this strength reservoir is called the 'autonomous protective backup'.

Finally, while evaluating a 6-month strength-training program for athletes who were accustomed to practicing strength training, it was found that the higher level of strength of an individual could not be attributed only to hypertrophy (Costill & Wilmore 1994). As soon as 3 months after beginning the program, no further changes in hypertrophy were observed, but the athletes continued to become stronger. This research supports the conclusion that there must be other processes, in addition to hypertrophy, that are also responsible for increasing strength (Häkkinen et al 1985). The only possible explanation is that these processes are related to an improvement in coordination, which is a function of the neural system. In many cases, an increase in strength can be explained by neural adaptation. In the following sections, therefore, attention is given not only to hypertrophy, but also to neural adaptations after following a strength-training program.

6.1.1 Definition of concepts

In order to make strength training an instrument that can be incorporated in the total structure of training, it is first necessary to define some concepts. What is strength, how can different types of strength be characterized, and how is strength related to functional movement? What is the relationship between strength and coordination, or between power and other conditional requirements? How does strength training cause adaptation?

Force, muscle strength, and strength training

In physics, force is defined as the cause of a change in motion (Ingen Schenau & Toussaint 1994). Force exerted upon a body (e.g., on a bone or leg) is a measure of magnitude and direction. The common way to represent force is by using a vector which can be specified by using the variables magnitude and direction.

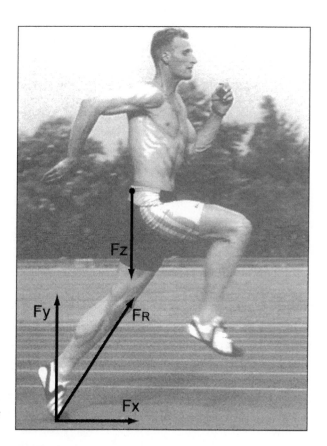

Figure 6.1   How some forces play upon a runner
The forces illustrated are gravitational (Fz) and foot reaction (FR), resolved horizontally (Fx) and vertically (Fy).

During running, there is an interplay between muscle strength and the forces caused by friction and gravity, which are responsible for accelerating and slowing down the mass of the body. During training, one is almost always concerned with the ways in which one can adequately influence muscle strength. As early as the 1960s (Scholich 1965, Nett 1968, Schröder 1969), three manifestations of muscle strength were defined, which today still greatly influence which methodology is used for strength training in the field of athletics. When the criterion for categorizing the manifestations of muscle strength is the nature of the muscle contraction, then, after roughly subdividing force into either static or dynamic, one can differentiate between maximum strength, fast-power, and strength endurance. Thereby, one should note that dynamic force can be subdivided further into concentric and eccentric muscle contractions.

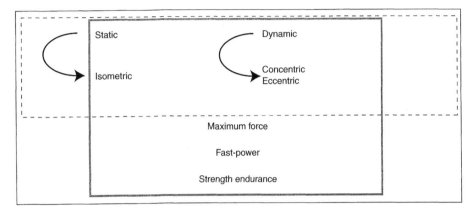

Figure 6.2 Classification of different types of force
A traditional classification of the manifestation of the basic motor property 'force' dates back to the 1960s and is still used to determine the methodology for strength training. According to the criterion 'muscle contraction', one can determine three manifestations (maximum strength, fast-power, and strength endurance) for static and dynamic muscle contraction.

Definition of maximum strength: the ability to realize the highest possible value for strength with the help of maximum random muscle contractions against an insurmountable resistance (Kibele 1995).

Definition of fast-power: the ability to realize the greatest force possible per unit of time (Hollmann & Hettinger 1980).

Definition of strength endurance: the conditional requirements for power that, on the one hand, are determined by maximum strength and fast-power and, on the other hand, by endurance (Harre & Leopold 1986).

Based on this division of the manifestations of force, one can subdivide strength training further into a number of traditional categories. This division is aimed in particular at the relationship between force and velocity with regard to muscle fibers. Exercises that can be executed as forcefully as possible without causing a shortening muscle contraction fall in the category of maximum strength. Exercises that can be implemented dynamically using a heavy weight so that maximum power output is possible fall in the category of maximum power training. Exercises that are implemented rapidly using relatively lightweight bar-bells fall in the category of fast-power or explosive power. There are, in addition, other categories that are not based on the force–velocity relationship for muscle fibers, such as strength endurance and hypertrophy training.

Some important comments can be made on this subdivision into different types of strength training and on the assumed relationship between the various types. In Chapter 1 (see Section 1.8), many anatomical data were presented that lie somewhere between the realm of isolated and, according to the rules of the force–velocity diagram, contracting muscle fibers and the realm of functional movement. Functional movement is only slightly related to the force–velocity diagram for muscle fibers, and therefore this diagram is of little use in strength training. Nevertheless, it is necessary to group the different forms of strength training.

Because it is not useful to take the force–velocity diagram as the orientation point for muscles, it is necessary to reformulate the reasons for integrating a certain type of strength training in a training program The different categories of power training are discussed further in Section 6.1.2.

Strength and coordination

In the previous chapters, it has been shown that the different facets of athletic power (stamina, explosive force, reactivity, coordination, strength, etc.) have a strong influence on each other. Thus it is only useful up to a certain point to make a firm differentiation between these various facets. Moreover, the quality of a training will actually depend on the way in which these different facets can be made to interact during practice. If one loses sight of this interaction and only approaches each of the aspects individually during training, there is a very great danger that the training will have little effect. This is especially true for strength training, because it generally is practiced in an environment far removed from the actual activity of running. Moreover, strength exercises and the actual practice of running are experienced quite differently by a runner. Because the character of strength training is totally different from running, the transfer of training is often not designed into the methodology, but rather is expected to take place automatically. Therefore, in practice, strength training often becomes an isolated ritual that is frequently used too often by sprinters and not often enough by distance runners.

The relationship between coordination and power is quite strong, so strong in fact that it could be suggested that power training is actually to a large extent coordination training. This close relationship is illustrated by the way in which power develops through training. When an individual begins power training, his performance improves in three stages. In the first stage his level of performance increases

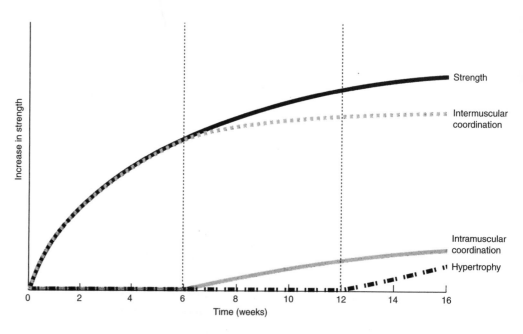

Figure 6.3 The three phases in the development of strength over time
The development of strength through training can be divided into three phases. First, the increase in strength can be attributed to an improvement in intermuscular coordination. Second, there is an improvement in intramuscular coordination. Third, an increase in strength results from hypertrophy.

as he improves his movement and learns to carry out the movement targeted more effectively. While muscle strength may remain unchanged, the muscles are now better able to work together, i.e. intermuscular coordination has improved. In the second stage, individual muscles become stronger, even though their physiological cross-section may not have increased in size, i.e. intramuscular coordination has improved. How this mechanism works is still generally unknown. The reason might be an improved stimulus transfer or 'rearrangement' of active and passive tissues in the muscle. During the third stage, there is only an increase in performance after about 12 weeks. It is only at this point that both an increase in strength and an increase in the physiological cross-section of the muscle will be found. Thus not only the cooperation between muscles, but also the ability of one muscle to exert more force (phases 1 and 2), are functions mainly of coordination.

Much is still unknown about the entire mechanism by which strength is increased through training. It is clear, however, that the phenomenon of strength must not be sought just among the properties of active muscle structures, but it is also influenced to some extent by the properties of the nervous system (both the central nervous system and at a lower level, where the nerve to muscle stimulus transfer takes place).

Because the concepts of coordination and strength are inseparable, the efficiency of training also depends on the specificity of the exercise (see Section 5.1). The pattern of movement in the strength exercise must resemble the intended movement (running), with regard to its internal and external structure and, if applicable, with regard to the area of energy supply. If there is no similarity, then the strength exercise will only be slightly effective, i.e. the exercise will contribute little to improving performance.

There is an old adage in the world of athletics that you become a champion beneath a bar-bell. This illustrates the greater possibilities that bar-bell training provides in the area of coordination compared with non-specific training using various types of strength equipment. When training with bar-bells, it is possible to simulate closely the movements in the working muscle and moving body when running. Reactivity during running is very important for certain muscle groups. By training with bar-bells, these muscles can be loaded by way of prestretch, and therefore become able to work reactively. When using power equipment, one's movement is dictated by how the apparatus has been constructed and whether the muscles can be worked reactively. This is particularly true for movements in which tension must be loaded and released in the muscle very rapidly. Moreover, when using power equipment, injury can easily occur if the body is forced to move too rapidly; synergists and antagonists cannot carry out their supplementary work as needed and the joints are thus not well protected. The use of power equipment is only suitable when training those muscles that are easy to coordinate and that work concentrically during running, i.e. the gluteus maximus, the iliopsoas and, for sprinters (at the start), the vastus segments of the quadriceps. With the exception of these few groups of muscles, the use of bar-bells is always preferred over other training equipment. Important aspects of coordination, such as the build-up of strength, anticipation of external forces, and reactive muscle action can be trained well using bar-bells. In fact, bar-bells offer the best way of training all types of movement in all sports in which speed, and thus reactivity, plays a role.

The most important argument usually made against the preferential use of bar-bells is that other equipment is safer to use. Two objections can be raised here. First, it is not useful to train most muscle groups with heavy weights when one cannot regulate the force that is required with regard to coordination. In this case, the transfer of training to an improved running performance will always fail. Correctly coordinated strength training using a relatively lightweight bar-bell is therefore useful for an individual with less strength and will be just as safe as when using equipment and a heavy weight but without regard for coordination. Furthermore, the argument for safety will only partly be true. There might be less danger of injury resulting from workouts using strength equipment (certainly for less skilled sportsmen with a poor bar-bell technique), but the danger of injury will be 'exported' outside the workout room. In other words, injury will occur more rapidly during running than when using bar-bells during strength training. This is especially true for groups of muscles, such as the hamstrings, that work together in a complex, coordinated manner.

Any type of strength training suitable for runners will therefore require, from the perspective of coordination, exercises that have an explicit transfer to the movement targeted. When training with bar-bells, it is possible for muscles to work and cooperate together within patterns of movement that resemble the running movement intended. Just as when learning how to run, it is more effective not to train the entire movement in one training session, but rather to improve partial segments of the motion. For these reasons, it is advisable to use a wide variety of exercises so that various aspects of running can be given an effective overload.

During strength training it is useful to differentiate between 'dumb' and 'smart' muscles. The greater the complexity of coordinating a group of muscles during running, the greater the variety needed in the exercise program. For example, the gluteus maximus is a 'dumb' muscle that hardly requires any variation in exercise program, while the iliopsoas needs to be trained in different ways because its action must be precisely coordinated with the action of, for example, the abdominal muscles. In particular, for the muscle groups for which coordination is most complex (e.g. the 'smart' biarticular hamstrings) it is advisable to provide a widely diverse exercise program for strength training. In addition, it holds that the exercises must be set up according to the specialized structure of the muscles concerned.

6.1.2   Description and definition of different forms of strength training

Hypertrophy training

Only after a 12-week period of strength training will one clearly find hypertrophy in the muscle groups that have been worked in athletes whose previous practice has included very little strength training. However, the power training must be set up in a specific way. The most important requirement for hypertrophy is the major breakdown of muscle protein in stressed muscle fibers. The amount of contractile proteins in a muscle fiber is the result of the continuous breakdown and synthesis of muscle proteins. During strength training the breakdown of muscle protein dominates, while during recovery the muscle protein will be resynthesized. The speed at which muscle protein breaks down is most rapid when using workloads that demand maximum force output. When a lower percentage of the maximum force is applied, the speed at which muscle proteins break down decreases. When less of the available energy in muscle cells is needed to fuel cross-bridge interactions, there will be more energy available for anabolic processes, such as the resynthesis of muscle protein (Zatsiorsky 1995).

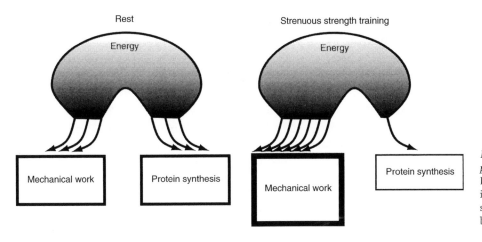

Rest

Strenuous strength training

Figure 6.4 Available energy for anabolic processes in a resting state and during exercise In a resting state, more energy is available in the muscle cell for anabolic processes, such as the synthesis of protein during the build-up of muscle.

The total breakdown of muscle protein depends not only on the speed of breakdown but also on the mechanical work done (the number of repetitions using a certain workload). The highest total breakdown of muscle protein occurs during average exercise (65–75% of the maximum strength) and an average number (6–12) of repetitions. Other combinations always result in less breakdown of muscle protein and therefore in less hypertrophy in stressed muscle fiber (Table 6.1).

Workload (number of repetitions)	Speed of breakdown	Mechanical work (number of repetitions)	Total breakdown of muscle protein
1	High	Few	Low
6–12	Average	Average	High
>25	Low	Many	Low

Table 6.1 Breakdown of protein in muscle and power training

Hypertrophy can result from two physiological adaptations:

- an increase in the number of muscle fibers (hyperplasia)
- an enlargement of the cross-section of an individual muscle fiber (hypertrophy).

Hyperplasia

In animal experiments, an increase in the number of muscle fibers has been demonstrated using a program of strength training consisting of a very strenuous workload with few repetitions (Giddings & Gonyea 1992). Until now, there has been a lot of uncertainty about whether human muscle fibers also split as a result of strength training. It appears that the number of muscle fibers remains unchanged during an individual's lifetime (Taylor & Wilkinson 1986).

Myofibrillar hypertrophy

The increase in muscle mass in myofibrillar hypertrophy can be explained by the additional number of myofibrils, which coincides with an increase in the number of actin and myosin filaments. In this manner, more cross-bridges can be formed and the number of sarcomeres connected in parallel will increase. Both these factors will increase the maximum force that a muscle fiber can provide.

Hypertrophy can occur in either slow-twitch (ST; type-I) or fast-twitch (FT; type-II) muscle fibers. The greatest change can be found in FT muscle fibers that have undergone different types of strength training using a limited number of repetitions and almost maximum resistance. Of these two types of fibers, the most hypertrophy is found in oxidative FT fibers when resistance is submaximal. Using an almost maximum resistance and one or two repetitions will give rise only to hypertrophy in glycolytic FT muscle fibers. Hypertrophy in FT muscle fibers affected by endurance training has been verified scientifically (Friden et al 1983, Goldspink 1992). The intensity of the endurance workload is generally too low to bring about such adaptation in ST muscle fibers. During long-distance running, the force of contraction in the groups of muscles involved amounts to only 20–30% of the maximum contractile force. Moreover, because ST muscle fibers are resistant to fatigue, they are quite difficult to exhaust.

Figure 6.5 illustrates the recruitment and exhaustion of various types of motor unit during a single repetition using a maximum workload, and during 12 repetitions using a submaximum load. The motor units of the muscle group under study were composed of type-I, type-IIa, and type-IIb muscle fibers, which have an endurance of 1–100 s. Twelve repetitions were carried out at a speed of one repetition per second. During the first repetition, motor units with type-I muscle fibers were recruited. After six repetitions, these motor units, which have an endurance of <6 s, had become exhausted. As fatigue set in, new motor units must be called upon to generate the necessary force. Such newly recruited motor units are generally type-II muscle fibers, which were exhausted after the preceding repetition. In this way, it becomes clear that hypertrophy in type-I muscle fibers is difficult to bring about because of their apparent indefatigability. Motor units consisting of type-II muscle fibers can be recruited and exhausted by using a single repetition with maximum resistance. This form of strength training causes hypertrophy only in type-II muscle fibers (Zatsiorsky 1995).

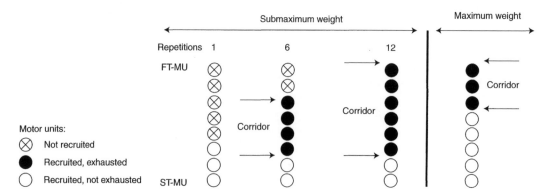

Figure 6.5 The mobilization of different types of motor units using submaximum and maximum workloads
The mobilization of different motor units (MU) using submaximum and maximum weights is illustrated. For a submaximum weight, the recruitment and degree of exhaustion of motor units consisting of slow-twitch (ST-MU) or fast-twitch (FT-MU) muscle fibers is determined after 1, 6, or 12 repetitions. The recruited and exhausted motor units are called the 'corridor'.

It is not advisable for long-distance runners to strive for hypertrophy through strength training. If hypertrophy occurs, the weight of the body will inevitably increase, and this is less favorable from the perspective of energy efficiency. When there is hypertrophy, and so an increase in muscle mass in the legs, much more energy has to be generated in order to speed up and slow down the legs as they move. It is extremely unfavorable from the viewpoint of energy expenditure to have more muscle mass located far from the center of rotation. For these reasons, one must be advised most emphatically against using strength training to cause hypertrophy in the calf muscles.

Another disadvantage of hypertrophy in the leg muscles of long-distance runners is the decline in capillary and mitochondrial accessibility. The exchange between oxygen and carbon dioxide gases will take place with more difficulty, because the distance across which diffusion must take place is greater.

It has already been stated that neural factors play a decisive role in the development of a higher level of strength, certainly when this strength must be converted into functional movement. During hypertrophy training, the ways in which muscle fibers or the neural system are affected are more or less independent processes. Hypertrophy training, therefore, will certainly not contribute to helping a runner improve muscle control. In practice, it appears that hypertrophy training itself has a very negative effect on coordination. This is certainly true for forms of movement such as the sprint, in which extremely high demands are made on the mechanisms of neuromuscular control. First using hypertrophy training and then trying to improve intra- and intermuscular coordination (see also maximum strength, below) is a roundabout path which one should perhaps not travel when training.

Strength endurance training

The definition of strength endurance (see p. 335) indicates the gulf that exists between maximum strength and fast-power, on the one hand, and stamina, on the other hand. Strength endurance is, therefore, a parameter that is impossible to apply in practice. Because the boundaries defining the concept of strength endurance are restricted, the term has become a catchall for performance-determining variables, and is too opaque to be used when planning a goal-oriented training scheme.

No well-delineated boundary can be drawn between the concept of strength endurance and the concepts of stamina and fast-power (Kibele 1995). Quantifying strength endurance by using the intensity and endurance of a workload will always lead to a large number of descriptions, depending on the running distance for which an athlete is training. The training program aimed at strength endurance will be quite different for a marathon runner and a 400-m runner. Thus new concepts, such as endurance in maximum strength and cyclic fast-power endurance, have been introduced (Harre & Leopold 1986). These concepts can be differentiated according to the duration, intensity, and energy-generating processes used. The common denominator lies in one's ability to withstand fatigue. Better strength endurance guarantees that an athlete can show stamina over a longer period at a certain output. This makes the definition of strength endurance too broad, and in practice it is thus an unworkable concept for training.

Maximum strength

The increase in muscle strength through training that cannot be explained directly by hypertrophy is caused by neural adaptation. In particular, during the first 12 weeks of a program composed of strength-training sessions an increase in strength will be observed, and this must be attributed to improvement in coordination. This improvement in coordination can be subdivided further into two aspects:

- intramuscular coordination
- intermuscular coordination.

Intramuscular coordination takes place within an isolated muscle, while intermuscular coordination refers to cooperation between agonists, synergists, and antagonists. Chronologically, adaptation must first be differentiated within intermuscular coordination. Only thereafter will one's intramuscular coordination improve (Huijbregts & Clarijs 1995).

There are three possibilities for improving intramuscular coordination through training. First, more motor units can be recruited. 'Sleeping' motor units, which do not take part in generating force at the beginning of exercise, can become activated. As already stated, the pattern for recruitment is determined by the size principle: small motor units with the lowest stimulus threshold are recruited first; and large motor units, consisting of FT muscle fibers, which are much more difficult to recruit, are called into action only when a higher level of force is needed.

The size principle is a greatly simplified view of the real situation. The degree to which a motor unit is stimulated depends on whether there is stimulation or inhibition. The hypothesis is that, in addition to a stimulus being stronger, at the same time any stimulus that inhibits will be suppressed so that the stimulation threshold can be exceeded in more motor units. For example, the Golgi-tendon organ works as an inhibitor. This receptor is located on the boundary between muscle and tendon and can detect tension in the muscle–tendon complex. The protective action of the Golgi-tendon organ when there is too much tension causes the agonist (autogenic inhibition) to slow down and the antagonist to become activated. In order to suppress the actions of the Golgi-tendon organ more force must be generated. Moreover, in addition to its conservative function, the Golgi-tendon organ also has an important sensory function (see Section 1.7).

For a cyclic motion such as running, there is a stereotypical pattern of recruitment within the muscle involved in the movement. Any small change in this pattern (e.g. in the type of strength exercise used) can cause a different pattern of recruitment. Motor units that have a low stimulus threshold during running may actually have a higher stimulus threshold when the pattern of movement deviates even slightly, as just mentioned, and can therefore become difficult if not impossible to recruit. This underlines the importance of the specificity of strength training. Furthermore, when one is striving to improve intramuscular coordination by increasing the recruitment of motor units, the force loaded must be nearly maximum.

A second way to improve intramuscular coordination through strength training is to increase the frequency of the stimulus. In addition, strength training will also increase the length of time for which a maximum stimulus frequency can be maintained.

A third way to improve intramuscular coordination through strength training is to improve the synchronization of motor-unit activity. Under normal conditions, motor units actually work asynchronously to bring about a flowing motion. When a great deal of force is applied, trained individuals will be better able to activate the motor units synchronously, which can lead to a more rapid build-up of strength.

There are two factors that will affect any improvement in intermuscular coordination. First, strength training will lead to a decrease in co-contractions (Huijbregts

& Clarijs 1995). A co-contraction is the simultaneous tightening of both an agonist and antagonist muscle when a joint moves. Obviously, the agonist will generate a greater contractile force. The advantage gained is heightened stability in the joint. The net (force of the antagonist subtracted from that of the agonist) joint moment, however, is less because of the counter-force generated by the antagonist. Second, power training improves the coordination between the various agonists during a certain pattern of movement. Similar to the improvement in the pattern of intra-muscular recruitment, specific strength training is also required to facilitate the actions between agonists.

Power training/maximum power

The underlying idea behind maximum power training has been discussed in Section 1.8. A number of practical problems that arise during implementation, such as how to actually recognize a limiting factor within a muscle group being trained and how the costs of energy expenditure (exercise) can be weighed against its benefits (effect), are introduced in Section 6.3.

Power training/fast-power becomes reflex-power

A central question that must be answered is: How can one achieve transfer of strength training to the intended movement? In practice, training with light weights (fast-power and explosive power) is often described as the conversion of strenuous strength training to an intended movement. The goal when training fast-power is to bring about a transfer between power training with heavy weights and training speed for a movement used in sports. Furthermore, it is often assumed that a muscle works in the same way when moving rapidly and when lifting heavy weights during training. However, this is not the case. Maximum power training serves to generate the most power possible by way of concentric muscle action. In contrast, when moving rapidly with light weights, reactivity will almost always play a dominant role. From the perspective of coordination, there are different properties for reactive and explosive muscle action. These two forms of action are, therefore, quite different. In addition to the fact that the muscles work differently in the two actions, the emphasis is on different groups of muscles. During maximum power training the monoarticular muscles, such as the gluteus maximus and the quadriceps femoris, are the limiting factor. When training with light weights, the muscles that work concentrically and those that work reactively always function together, although the latter are the limiting factor. A training session must therefore emphasize muscle groups such as the hamstrings and abdominal and dorsal muscles. It is essential for a successful transfer of training, however, that coordination be similar for the different forms of training. Similarities do not simply occur spontaneously; for example, one must search for a long time to find any similarity between extending the body forcefully from a squatting position using bar-bells and coordination during running. One may therefore question the traditional way of thinking.

Training to move rapidly using light weights has almost no function in the transfer of maximum power training to the rapid movements observed in the world of sports. One can ask whether such transfer is actually necessary: muscles working concentrically are easy to coordinate, and this can be fairly easily integrated into movements used in sports. The reason to train with light weights is to learn how to use reactivity when the force is greater than in the intended movement. During the so-called strength of impact using bar-bells, there is greater force in both the pre-stretch and discharge phases. The technique used for reactivity is more difficult for

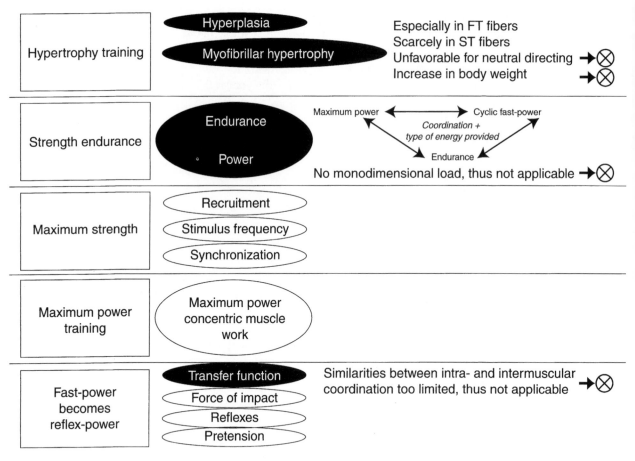

Figure 6.6 Forms of strength training for runners in scheme 1
Black ovals show aspects of strength training that cannot be used in practice by runners. White ovals show aspects of strength training that can be significantly integrated into strength training for runners.

a high than a low peak force and can be compared with the technique used for a service return during a game of tennis. When the service is soft (compared to reactivity, there is a slight prestretch when the external force is small), it is easier to time the return of the ball, but more difficult to do this forcefully (reactivity: discharge is easy, but does not take place forcefully). When the service is hard (a lot of prestretch when the external force is large), it is difficult to time the return of the ball, but easier to give the ball more speed (compared to reactivity, the discharge is difficult to coordinate, but takes place with a large peak force). Learning to handle strength of impact when there is an overload of force is, therefore, a primary concern in coordination training. This aspect of training with light weights is important because reactivity plays such a central role during running.

As a rule, exercising with lighter weight bar-bells and training for strength of impact will prove advantageous when combining reactivity and fixed reflex-response patterns. A much higher peak force can be achieved for patterns of movement supported by fixed reflex responses (e.g. the stumble and inverse-extension reflexes, both of which are important for running) than for patterns of movement in which major reflex patterns do not play a primary role. The overload that can be achieved for movements supported by a reflex action is therefore greater than for

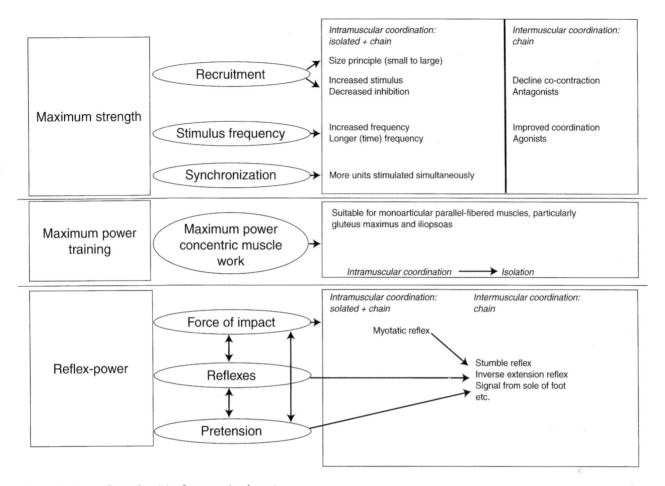

Figure 6.7 Forms of strength training for runners in scheme 2
Aspects of strength training that can prove useful for runners and how they influence inter- and intra-muscular coordination.

movements not supported by reflexes. Types of training in which movements supported by reflexes can be incorporated (i.e. those that work to boost the movement) are therefore extremely effective. Because the motion of running is composed of a series of movements controlled by reflex actions, such forms of training will provide increased specificity with regard to an intended movement, in addition to permitting extra overload. Because a large overload can be combined with a large specificity, the training will be particularly efficient.

A suitable term for such training is 'reflex power': moreover, the quality of how well movement can be implemented will be determined primarily by the quality of the reflex patterns involved. Movements should be carried out as rapidly as possible, and are not isolated, but rather are more or less functional. How well the muscles can be used reactively will be the limiting factor. Between 5 and 10 repetitions will be used in each training session and fatigue will be chiefly neuromuscular (extreme fatigue, but with rapid recovery). In fact, this form of training is tantamount to complex coordination training using a force overload.

In practice, little or almost no attention is given to the role played by reflexes when training reactivity. Nevertheless, because large peak forces can be combined with relevant muscle action, such forms of training offer a wide range of possibilities for runners who want to improve their performance.

6.2 STRENGTH TRAINING AND FUNCTIONAL ANATOMY

6.2.1 Biomechanical aspects

Strength and coordination are closely related. It is therefore obvious that the same basic mechanisms for motion will play a role in both strength and coordination training. These mechanisms (the study of which is termed biomechanics) are dictated to a large extent by the blueprint for the locomotor apparatus.

In Section 3.1 we showed (using a kernel to illustrate movement) how coordination can be organized as three shells (intra- and intermuscular coordination and moving segments) surrounding a central core. The three-layered structure for coordination can also be visualized in other ways. When training coordination, one can imagine a three-story 'house of biomechanics'. Stairways have been built between the floors so that what is constructed on one floor can be transported to another level. The blueprint for movement is designed at ground level. On the first floor, a layout is constructed to show how individual muscles function. On the second floor, models are made to demonstrate how muscles work together according to an established set of patterns. At the top of the house, these patterns are combined to create functional movement.

Training of coordination usually takes place on the second and third floors of the house of biomechanics. Coordination training for individual muscles (constructions made on the first floor of the building) is of little use from the perspective of methodology. If one wants to train an individual muscle, its function must first be isolated. By implementing these exercises in a particular manner, it will be impossible to use other muscle groups to perform the movement. By isolating the muscle, there will no longer be a relationship between muscle function and the total pattern of movement. Moreover, there will almost always be an essential difference in the way in which a muscle contracts in isolation and during functional movement.

This has always been a generally accepted idea when instructing an individual how to run. In contrast, many exercises are still used for strength training that aim to train individual muscles separately. Because strength and coordination are strongly interrelated, however, the question of why training isolated muscles might prove beneficial requires an answer.

The reasons trainers work with isolated muscle are that it is assumed that a single muscle can be stressed better in this way and that the body can be better protected against injury when one muscle is not trained with other muscles. One might well question both suppositions (i.e. that a single muscle can be worked under a larger load and that this method will be safer). Training of the abdominal muscles can serve as an example.

Training the abdominal muscles in isolation has become standard practice. Exercising isolated abdominal muscles is thought to bring about the greatest effect while carrying the lowest risk of injury. In particular, the way in which the iliopsoas works to increase lordosis is thought to be dangerous. Therefore, many ways have been devised to eliminate the action of this muscle so that the abdominal muscles will work only concentrically during practice. However, the spinal column is not well protected until all the surrounding muscles are able to function together as a 'corset', and thus counteract any untoward shifting and rotating movements between the vertebrae as well as pressure on the intravertebral discs in a dangerous

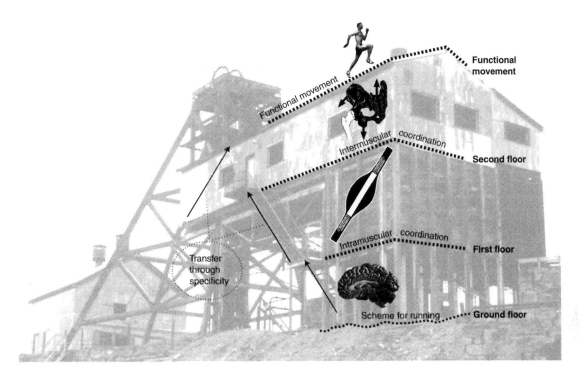

Figure 6.8   *House of coordination*

direction. In fact, when the abdominal muscles actually work alone the spinal column will not be protected, and so untoward movements can occur. It is therefore better to design abdominal exercises in such a way that all the muscles (including the iliopsoas) that work to stabilize the spinal column can be strengthened.

In addition, the idea that exercising abdominal muscles in isolation will prove more effective than when training larger muscle complexes is incorrect. Exercising individual abdominal muscles will always take place concentrically. When movement is rapid, such as during running, the abdominal muscles chiefly work 'reactively' (reactively). When one wants to improve functional movement, it is useless to choose a form of training from the 'ground floor' of biomechanics, which cannot be integrated one level higher. Concentric and reactive muscle actions are two separate processes, and transfer of training (up the stairway between floors) will therefore be minimal using such exercises. Moreover, concentric abdominal exercises can never be performed with the large workload peaks used for a well-coordinated series of reactivity exercises. Although a well-trained athlete can often do 100 concentric sit-ups, he will almost never be able to perform more than 20 reactive abdominal exercises with large strength peaks.

All the muscles that work together to maintain the corset mechanism in the trunk must be well regulated. In this way it is easier to transfer what has been learned to the third floor of the 'house' of biomechanics, and incorporate this information into functional movement. When training the abdominal muscles it may be preferable to use a light workload first in order to study how the other muscles work together. When muscles in the trunk can be coordinated sufficiently, the

347

workload can be intensified. Without much further risk of injury, the abdominal muscles can be stressed in a manner relevant for the movement targeted. This approach will prove much more efficient than when the abdominal muscles are trained separately.

The question of whether muscles should be trained in isolation during strength training or whether it would be better to focus on the basic mechanisms of cooperative muscles must be asked with regard to the training of all muscles. The rule of thumb is that isolated training is only applicable to muscles (concentrically working monoarticular muscles) that can be coordinated easily. All other muscles should be trained on the second floor (in combination with other muscles). However, for other reasons, muscle groups such as the hamstrings are not well suited for isolated training. In particular, the popular leg-curl exercise should not be used for the hamstrings during strength training. Because of its drastic concentric shortening effect, this exercise runs completely counter to the structure and function of these muscles and will more likely result in injury than in improved performance. The exercise is non-functional and will disrupt the state of equilibrium between active and passive muscle segments. The reason why this exercise is nevertheless still included so frequently in training programs is probably that injury generally does not occur while actually performing the exercise, but rather develops later, so that its cause cannot be pinpointed exactly.

On the second floor of the 'house' of biomechanics, muscles that function in line with their own characteristics are required to work together according to fixed mechanisms. For example, the gluteus maximus is responsible for generating the force of contraction, while the rectus femoris and the hamstrings divide this force between the knee and hip joints. Such a fixed interrelationship also exists between the corset function of the abdominal and dorsal muscles when the iliopsoas works, and between the hamstrings and dorsal muscles. During strength training, one generally works with larger systems or chains, thus quickly arriving on the second floor of biomechanics. When working with bar-bells, one will quickly need to adjust how the muscles work together.

On the third floor of biomechanics, one can study the specific function of muscles and the established mechanisms for coordinating their actions during functional movement, which can be defined as motion with a goal, whereby the movements must be adjusted to the conditions in which they will take place (running, jumping, doing a somersault, etc.). High specificity will work effectively for both strength and coordination training. In strength training, however, it is not always possible or effective to carry out an entire pattern of movements that resembles the movement intended. For example, when the entire movement is made using a bar-bell that is too heavy, it will often no longer be possible to work the muscle correctly and as required on the first and second floors of coordination. Movements that closely resemble running must therefore not be made using a large external workload (bar-bell). Prestretch, which takes place quickly with an eccentric moment in the active muscle segments, will have little effect and will easily result in injury. Therefore, during strength training, total patterns of movement are always practiced using lightweight workloads. Speed of implementation is possible if the way in which the muscles work is reactive and technically correct. Regardless of the fact that the weight used is relatively light, the workload ('urged on' by the support of the reflex action) can nevertheless be quite high.

In order to work effectively on all levels in the 'house' of coordination, and in particular to avoid worthless exercises, it is necessary to analyze in detail (on the upper floor) the targeted movement. We have already seen (see Section 3.1) that it is difficult to determine how muscles work together during movement. We also know that muscles do not all have the same structure, and these differences in their anatomy make them more or less suited to certain work. Because a muscle is able to perform a certain type of contraction, this does not automatically imply that it can work only this way. The abdominal muscles of a gymnast, who is hanging in the rings and trying to raise his legs slowly toward the bracket, will work concentrically rather than reactively, although the abdominal muscles are not built to contract over a long trajectory. Thus a question relevant to sports is: When will a muscle group do specialized work suited to its structure and when will it perform other types of work?

The answer to this question can be illustrated by considering a centrifuge. If the muscles are located in the center of the centrifuge, they can be mobilized for different types of work, even performing hybrid forms of muscle activity. For example, they can work at different lengths, simultaneously absorb (limited) external forces while contracting concentrically (i.e. in Hill's model, showing partly contractile element (CE) and partly series-linked elastic component (SEC) behavior), or do positive work while transferring energy (e.g. the hamstrings). When muscles are located near the outer mantle of the centrifuge, they will only function well when working according to their specialized structure; for example, they will only work well at one length or either elastic/isometrically or positive/concentrically. When the centrifuge turns slowly (i.e. slow movements in sports), the muscles will be located in the center. As the centrifuge begins to spin faster, the muscles will be slung toward the

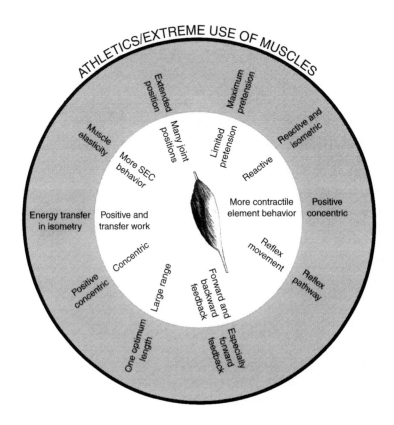

Figure 6.9   Centrifuge of muscle activity

outer mantle. When the spin velocity is high (i.e. movements using maximum speed, such as high-speed running), the muscles will be pressed against the mantle and only contribute significantly to the total movement through their own specializations.

Applying this model to running, it can be seen that a sprinter needs to use his muscles in a more specialized manner than someone running at an easy endurance tempo. In addition, in contrast to an average runner, a top sprinter can expect to use his specialized muscles for more extreme work. An interesting problem is how to estimate the spin velocity when running at, for example, an 800-m tempo. If the muscles have already moved quite a distance toward the mantle of the centrifuge (i.e. the ground contact time is already short), then one can rightly assume that training the muscles according to their own specialized function during strength and technique training may prove worthwhile. It is also useful for long-distance trainers to make a similar analysis.

6.2.2 Strength training, muscle structure, and function

As already stated, there is a strong relationship between muscle structure, the type of work for which a muscle is suited, and the manner in which a muscle functions during running. Furthermore, one must divide muscles into two groups. The first group consists of muscles that are suitable for concentric explosive (i.e. mainly positive) work. These muscles are monoarticular and chiefly parallel-fibered in structure. The second group consists of muscles that are able to work reactively. These muscles generally function to absorb and process external forces. They often have a pennate structure and important passive structures, as well as being biarticular. Naturally, this is a rough division. In reality, muscles are flexible and can have properties of both groups. However, this division into two groups is useful in practice, particularly when organizing a training program. During strength training, a specific approach should be used to train muscles from both groups.

Reactive muscle action

Muscles working reactively will demonstrate a number of characteristics that will have a direct consequence on the way in which a strength training session is implemented.

- The muscle works more or less in isometry. Rapid lengthening and shortening of the active segments is not compatible with reactivity. However, after working reactively, there might be a concentric movement, but it will be of no great importance for running.
- A muscle cannot work reactively equally well over any length range. For functional movements in which reactivity plays an important role, one should attempt to make a muscle work over the length range that is optimal for reactivity. For the lower extremities, the length is optimal when the body is nearly upright.
- The cycle for prestretch and discharge is short, if the muscle fibers have first been tightened.

From the perspective of these muscle characteristics, the following types of workload can be considered for use during strength training:

- *Training for maximum power in isometry with an optimum working range (length at which the muscle is strongest)*. This means that exercises using heavy weights must be done very slowly. Any movement made should not aim to change the range of the muscle (in biarticular muscles, movement by one joint will compensate for movement by another joint, so there will be little or almost no change in length), but rather should try to increase stress in the muscle being trained (i.e. changes in the lever arms). Recruitment and synchronization are quite important and are closely related to one's ability to build up sufficient pretension before the muscle works reactively.

- *Training reactivity by means of the strength of impact (eventually as reflex-power).* Movement is made rapidly, with prestretch using lightweight bar-bells. From the perspective of coordination, these movements are mainly located on the first floor of the biomechanical system. Where possible, they should resemble elements in the pattern of running (second floor) and preferably progress according to a pattern supported by reflex actions. Fatigue is neuromuscular and demonstrates a typical pattern, having a very large peak followed by rapid recovery.
- The most important muscle groups that work reactively during running are the following:
  - the erector spinae group
  - the hamstrings
  - the triceps surae group (the soleus and the gastrocnemius)
  - the rectus femoris
  - small, lower-leg muscles
  - abdominal muscles.

Explosive concentric muscle action

Two statements can be made regarding this type of muscle activity:

- the contractions are concentric over a certain range that is determined by the movement
- the power generated by the muscle is a measure of how much the muscle has been stressed.

During strength training, the ideal situation is to provide the workload appropriate for maximum power (force times acceleration). The power is greatest when using a particular external load (see Section 1.8). If the weight to be moved is lower than the ideal training load, then, although the acceleration may be faster, the product of acceleration times weight will be less than for the ideal weight. Too heavy a weight will result in too little acceleration and less power compared to when using an optimum weight. Such data can be plotted to give a graph showing a minimum–maximum power curve. One must then carry out the extremely difficult task of finding an optimum weight with which to train. First, the specificity of the workload must be considered; one must take into account the muscle's working range where stress will occur (this length must closely match the length actually anticipated during running). Second, the exercise must be set up so that the limiting factor during implementation is actually located within the muscles that will provide maximum power.

The most important muscles for generating power are the gluteus maximus, the iliopsoas, and the vastus segments of the quadriceps. In almost all exercises (even those using equipment), 'power muscles' work together with other muscles (e.g. the hamstrings and the rectus femoris, which distribute energy generated by the gluteus maximus across the knee and hip). Therefore, during a particular exercise, the limiting factor may not be located in the muscles being trained, but rather may be a problem occurring elsewhere.

The most frequently used power exercise is to straighten the body rapidly upward on both legs from a squatting position, while holding a heavy bar-bell at neck level. One must question whether the limiting factor for performance will be the muscles generating power (the gluteus maximus and the vastus heads of the quadriceps femoris). During this exercise, the dorsal muscles are required to exert an enormous amount of force and the strong inhibiting signals sent from the spinal column must be overridden. It is more likely that the limiting factor will be found here than in the concentric force of the gluteus maximus and the quadriceps femoris. Furthermore, from the perspective of coordination, it is probably easier to generate maximum power in one leg rather than twice as much power in two legs. These factors taken together make it doubtful whether the two-leg squat with maximum power output from the muscles being trained will be possible. A single-leg load using a light-weight bar-bell will probably be much more effective. Here the dorsal muscles will need to bear less load, and thus one can concentrate directly on one leg.

In addition to the fact that the correct muscles must be the limiting factor during power training, one should also take into account the relevance of the range over which a muscle will work. During running, muscles usually work over a much narrower range than first assumed. Using other movements as compensation, the degree of movement in a joint can be restricted (see Section 3.2), and consequently the range over which the muscle can be worked will be narrower.

Add up all the problems that maximum power training presents, and the questions that can still be asked about its theory, and one is left with the pressing question of whether maximum power training has any value at all. Whatever the answer, it is advisable to substitute part of the maximum power training of monoarticular muscles by training for maximum strength. In this way the range over which muscles can function can be better regulated and it is easier to control important structures such as the spinal column.

Once an individual is able to maneuver around the obstacles on the road to maximum power training, the only problem remaining is how to measure power output. Good instrumentation for this purpose is difficult to find and expensive to purchase.

The question can now be asked in which relationship should the various muscle groups be trained. How much training is needed for power-generating muscles or for those muscles that work reactively? What emphasis should be used for which type of runner (sprinter, endurance runner, etc.)? Such questions are difficult, if not impossible, to answer. So many factors play a role when deciding which combination will be the best when training an individual that almost no generally applicable principles can be found. In practice, athletes appear to integrate strength training into their total training program, even though they practice the same disciplines in quite different ways but with equal success. One athlete might require a great deal of strength training, while another will need less. Individualization is therefore a key concept. In any case, for sprinters, the explosive power of the quadriceps and the gluteus maximus is important during the start. Once running at speed, reactivity in the hamstrings, dorsal muscles, soleus, etc., will be the most important factor for the sprint. For middle- and long-distance runners, while the start is not important, the most important factor determining performance is also reactivity. For these runners, training for maximum strength in combination with reactive force using lightweight bar-bells is sufficient. In practice, one can easily find distance runners whose lack of skill in the area of reactivity will limit their performance, but hardly any runners sufficiently skilled in reactivity whose lack of power in the monoarticular muscles will limit their performance.

6.3 STRENGTH TRAINING INDIVIDUAL MUSCLE GROUPS

6.3.1 Erector spinae

The erector spinae muscle works across a relatively small range. Its action is switched off when the spinal column is bent. Moreover, the spinal column is vulnerable when flexed. Therefore, strength training of the dorsal muscles must always be done with the spine extended. When the spine is straight, the dorsal muscles can be trained for maximum strength in a number of ways. Having strong dorsal muscles is very important for all runners, but especially for sprinters. During running, the muscles will only work reactively. The degree of movement is so small when these muscles are working reactively that it can only be imitated with difficulty during strength training. Therefore, prestretch and release of power cannot be experienced well enough using isolated exercises. Thus it is better to train dorsal muscles reactively in sequence in cooperation with other muscles. The patterns of movement will be more worthwhile and will dictate reactivity of the dorsal muscles when strictly and correctly implemented.

The so-called hyperextension exercises are controversial. Even when using little ballast, the dorsal muscles will shorten as far as possible, by which the spinal column will be pushed far into a position of lordosis. Although this exercise is considered to be harmful for the spinal column, it is still quite often applied when training (foreign) athletes. The reason for using such forms of exercise cannot lie in their relevance for the range across which the muscle must work, because strong lordosis does not occur during running. These exercises can only be aimed at improving coordination between the muscles that function with regard to the spinal column. The exercise can only be done without causing problems if all the muscles work optimally to protect the spine. In particular, the abdominal muscles must be tightened well. When using hyperextension exercises, such teamwork between the muscles becomes very difficult , and so this form of training must only be used for very good athletes who are well skilled and coordinated.

Many types of training used to exercise the dorsal muscles are carried out while the individual is standing and holding a bar-bell at neck level. As a rule of thumb, when the athlete is standing on two legs, the dorsal muscles are the limiting factor. If one wants to make the leg muscles the limiting factor, the bar-bell exercise must be done while standing on one leg.

How the reactive action of the dorsal muscles is applied within the sequence of exercises is very important. One should pay extra attention to holding the back in an extended position during these exercises.

Figure 6.10   Exercise 1: maximum strength

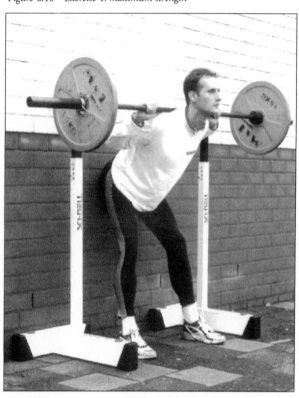

Exercise 1   Maximum strength

Start by standing upright, with the buttocks touching a wall and the feet about 40–50 cm from the wall, placed side by side at shoulder level. A bar-bell is held at neck level, with the weight adjusted accordingly. The back is well extended. The knees are slightly bent so that the hamstrings will not become passive and work insufficiently during the exercise. The trunk then moves forward. The motion must not be made by bending the spine, but rather by tilting the pelvis forward. The lever arm of the trunk with regard to the bar-bell increases and the dorsal muscles must exert more force. The weight of the bar-bell should be heavy enough that the athlete just fails to achieve maximum pelvic tilt. After the maximum degree of movement has been achieved, the trunk will again assume an upright posture. The bar-bell weights used must be heavy. However, the resulting strain on the dorsal muscles depends not only on the weight of the bar-bell, but also on how far the athlete bends forward. When the weight is heavy, the point at which the athlete can no longer lean forward will be reached earlier and more abruptly than when using a lighter weight. Varying the weight used will, therefore, prove useful.

Figure 6.11   Exercise 2: maximum strength using the back-extension bench

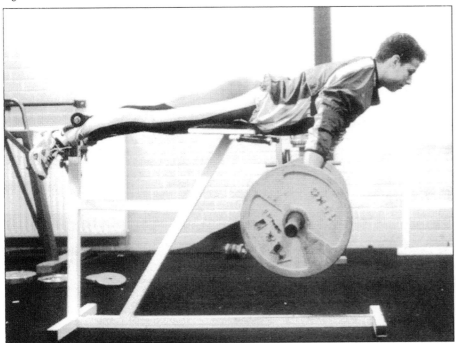

Exercise 2   Maximum strength using the back-extension bench

Start by lying on the stomach with the legs held stationary, the hips supported, and the trunk free. From this position, with the upper body pointing diagonally downward, the trunk will be lifted until the body is completely extended. This position is held momentarily before the trunk is lowered again. It is important that the abdominal muscles remain taut during the entire exercise. The corset action of the muscles works best when the athlete tries to make himself as long as possible while his body is extended. The exercise can be made more strenuous in a number of ways:

- The arms, which were first held in front of the chest in the starting position, can now be clasped in the neck (eventually using an extra weight).
- With the body extended, a helper exerts downward pressure on the shoulder blades. The athlete must try to keep his body extended. Subsequently, this pressure is removed and the upper body drops down again.
- Well-trained athletes can also do this exercise using a bar-bell, which is lifted from and returned to the ground with the arms extended. The range of movement towards the extended position should be small. In this way, good athletes can lift loads that exceed their own body weight.

Figure 6.12   Exercise 3: hyperextension

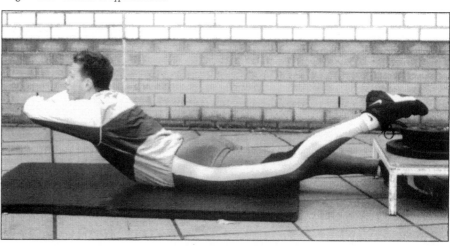

Exercise 3   Hyperextension

Start by lying on the stomach, with the arms extended along the body. One leg is held stationary. The trunk and free leg are lifted simultaneously, while the abdominal muscles tighten. This position is held for several seconds.

Figure 6.13   Exercise 4: reactivity

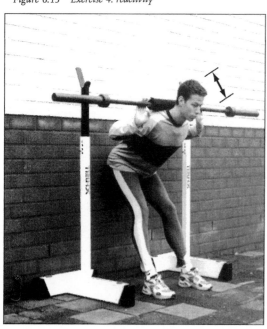

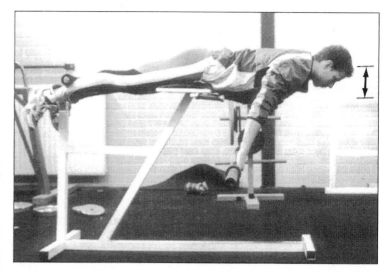

Exercise 4   Reactivity

The body is positioned and the exercise carried out as for Exercise 1 or 2. The bar-bell is now light. The exercise is performed rapidly and with force. The transition from leaning forward to moving back again should be as rapid as possible. The back must remain completely extended and the abdominal muscles must be kept taut.

6.3.2 Hamstrings

One would be wise to approach strength training for the hamstrings as if one were training only for coordination. This means that implementation of the exercise must be technically correct and be of foremost concern at all times (i.e. the magnitude of the workload and number of repetitions should be of secondary concern during the training). The workload may only be intensified once all aspects of coordination (i.e. maintaining correct tension, control over the speed of reactive work, directing other muscles) can be well regulated. Strength training the hamstrings must adhere to exactly the same requirements specified for coordination training (see Section 5.2). The only difference is that the workload can be heavier because bar-bells are being used.

When exercising for maximum strength, it is important that the hamstrings work within the correct range. The angles of the knee and hip must therefore be well coordinated. The exercises should be practiced slowly and with concentration.

Just as when training coordination, with regard to the hamstrings, it is quite worthwhile to train for reactivity in as many ways possible. This can be achieved by varying the position of the body and by training with many different weights. When the weight is heavy, the process of storing and discharging energy takes a relatively long time. Exercises in which body posture and speed deviate from the norm are less specific for running but, considering the major role played by the hamstrings during running, the use of somewhat non-specific exercises will contribute enough to affect the level of performance.

The most important way to train the hamstrings to work reactively is to exercise while standing with a bar-bell. The emphasis of this exercise can frequently be directed toward the hamstrings by bending the knees slightly and allowing the movement to take place, especially by extending the hips powerfully. For example, when this action of moving the bar-bell occurs when the knees are nearly extended, the hamstrings are stressed well.

Figure 6.14   Exercise 1: maximum strength

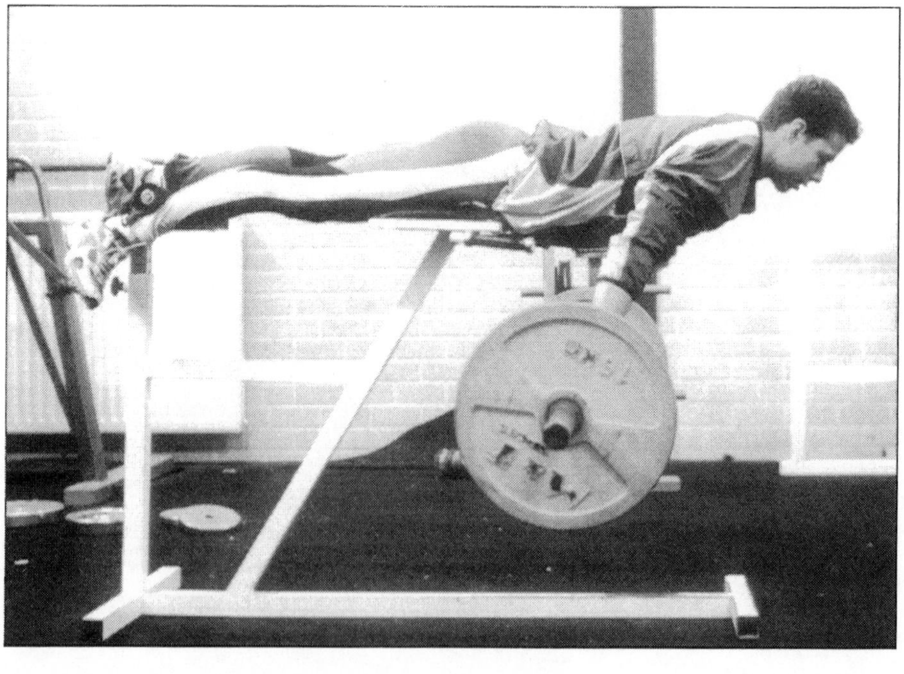

Exercise 1   Maximum strength

Exercising on the back-extension bench to obtain maximum power from the dorsal muscles can also be done with one leg held stationary and one leg free. The free leg must not be lifted to act as a counterweight. Because the weight must now be absorbed by one rather than two hamstring groups, the strength of the hamstrings will be the limiting factor.

Figure 6.15   Exercise 2: maximum strength body snap

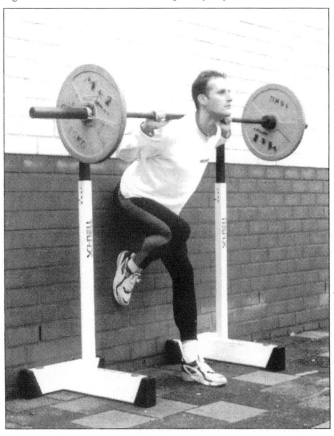

Exercise 2   Maximum strength body snap
This exercise, which is used to train the dorsal muscles, can also be carried out while standing on one leg. The other leg is either placed on an elevation or against the wall at the level of the supporting knee, and will serve only to maintain balance. In this variation also, the strength of the hamstrings will be the limiting factor.

Figure 6.16   Exercise 3: maximum strength by bending one knee

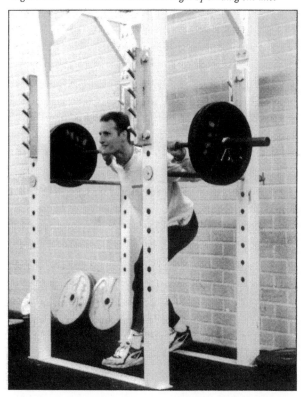

Exercise 3   Maximum strength by bending one knee

Start by standing with the feet slightly apart (60 cm) while holding a bar-bell at neck level. For a good athlete, the weight of the bar-bell will be equal to or heavier than his own body weight. The athlete stoops down until the thighs are nearly horizontal. Subsequently, the trunk and bar-bell are moved forward until the weight is approximately above the front knee. This movement causes the weight to have a larger lever arm with regard to the hip joint, while the lever arm with regard to the knee becomes smaller. Therefore, only very little force will be needed to keep the knee from bending further, but more force will be needed to keep the hip from bending. In such a situation, the hamstrings work together with the gluteus maximus to keep the hip extended. The force moment that the hamstrings still exert to bend the knee will be compensated for by the action of the vastus segment of the quadriceps femoris. The amount of force demanded of the hamstrings therefore depends on the weight and magnitude of the lever arm with regard to the hip. One must find a weight that is heavy enough to work the muscle at the limit where it can still function when the shoulders are moved to the front. A still heavier weight will be useless (now the shoulders cannot be moved as far to the front).

Figure 6.17   Exercise 4: maximum strength in the hamstrings

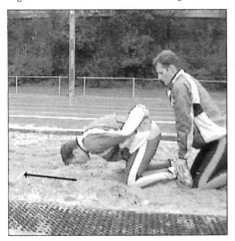 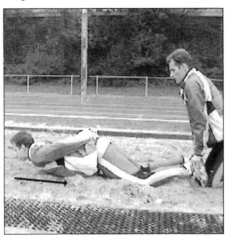

Exercise 4   Maximum strength in the hamstrings
Kneel on a very soft surface (preferably sand). Bend the trunk forward until the face is just above the ground. The lower legs are held stationary by a helper. Subsequently, the trunk is moved forward so that the hips and knees are slowly extended. The face remains just above the ground surface. The hamstrings are increasingly stressed up to the maximum, before returning the trunk to its original position.

Figure 6.18   Exercise 5: reactivity due to strength of impact

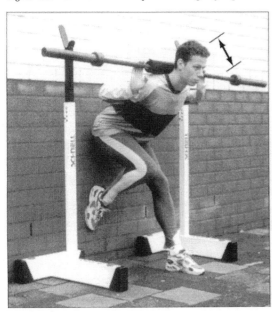 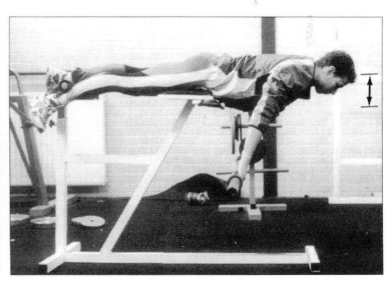

Exercise 5   Reactivity due to strength of impact
This exercise is performed as for the variation described in Exercise 1 or 2 using a bar-bell which, however, is now lighter. Start by holding the body extended, with the bar-bell raised off the ground. Slight bouncing motions are made while maintaining tension in the body. If tension drops as the downward motion is absorbed, the load is too heavy and the exercise should be done either with no weight or with a lighter bar-bell.

Figure 6.19   Exercise 6: reactivity due to reflex-power

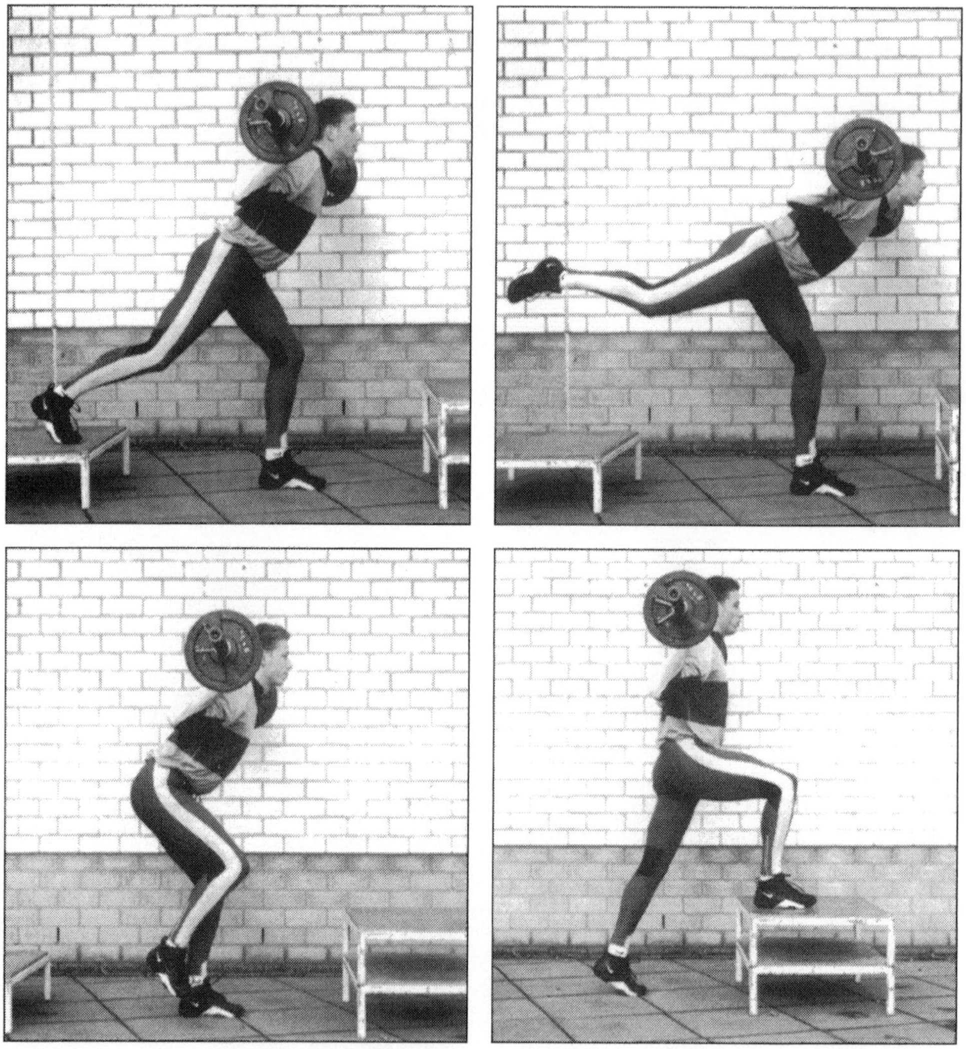

Exercise 6   Reactivity due to reflex-power

Start by standing on one leg with a bar-bell held at neck level. The free leg is extended to the rear, with the foot on an elevation (to maintain balance). The trunk is bent forward, with the back kept extended. The knee of the stance leg is slightly bent. Next, the back leg is lifted quickly before being swung forward and placed on an elevation with the knee bent. At the same time, the trunk is brought upright forcefully. The stance leg extends outward here, but the motion is not emphasized and only takes place after the trunk has been brought upright. During the course of these movements, the hamstrings are of major importance during the transfer of energy (from the knee to the hip). When the exercise is performed using a light bar-bell, one can work using short but powerful forward movements. The trunk first drops forward before snapping back briskly. Here the motion of the swing leg resembles the way in which it moves during running, making a useful running pattern together with other muscles (the gluteus maximus, dorsal muscles, gastrocnemius, etc.).

Figure 6.20   Exercise 7: jumping back and forth

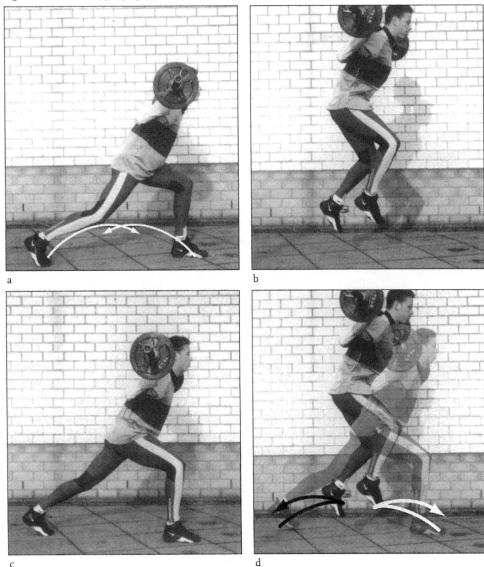

a

b

c

d

Exercise 7   Jumping back and forth
Start with the feet spread apart while holding a bar-bell (about 40 kg for a trained athlete) at neck level.
The upper body must be held forward during the entire exercise so that the weight remains positioned
above the front foot (a). Subsequently, jump back and forth briskly while keeping the hips stable (no
vertical tilt) and the ground contact time short. In (b) the runner's hips are too high. Instead of placing
the other foot forward while jumping (c), the exercise can be varied by landing with the same foot in
front. During the floating phase, the feet are first moved closer together and then further apart, with
the body again landing in the starting position (d).

6.3.3 Triceps surae group (soleus and gastrocnemius) and small lower-leg muscles

The muscles of the lower leg are particularly important during running, and the logical conclusion is that they should be frequently exercised during strength training. Corresponding to their function, these muscles and their reactive properties should be trained for maximum strength. They are not suited for concentric work.

However, a large problem arises when one tries to strength train these muscles. During running and jumping, the forces that these muscles must absorb is extremely large (see Section 1.6). The forces working on the muscles, particularly during running, are so great that it will be difficult if not impossible to create an overload during an individual strength training session. Therefore, training the small muscles in the lower leg should mainly be directed at learning how to regulate their function better (coordination training). Exercises carried out on teeter-boards serve to help maintain greater pretension in the lower-leg muscles, without actually making the muscles stronger (certainly in trained runners).

Considering the enormous load that would be necessary when using bar-bells to create an overload with regard to jumping and running, using strength training for the triceps surae group would prove hopeless, and is therefore best forgotten. Instead, it is more useful during other types of training to place higher demands on how these muscles function (see Section 5.2.1).

This problem of how difficult it is to create an overload is frequently acknowledged by athletes and trainers, who sometimes attempt to create overload by means of vertical rebounding jumps holding a bar-bell at neck level. However, when an individual jumps while holding a bar-bell, the drop will be less than when not using a weight. For the lower-leg muscles, there will be hardly any overload, if any. However, the muscles in the area of the trunk will be heavily (and sometimes dangerously) stressed. Reactive jumping while holding a bar-bell weight must therefore be carried out using very light weights (an empty bar) or avoided completely.

6.3.4 Abdominal muscles

During running, the abdominal muscles function simultaneously as an elastic band and as a corset. Furthermore, the presence of pretension and coordination between other muscles is important. Coordination is also needed during strength training. When exercising, the spinal column must remain well protected. Good intermuscular coordination ensures that this occurs and is absolutely necessary if one wants to increase a workload without endangering the body. One must first learn how to control the corset function of the muscles; only thereafter will increasing the workload prove worthwhile. In order to learn how to do this, one must practice the exercises slowly. In this manner, the abdominal muscles can work concentrically, eccentrically, and statically. Only after the technique has been mastered can an athlete begin using exercises that will actually contribute to improving the function of the abdominal musculature during running.

Because they work reactively, in principle the abdominal muscles can be considered when training for maximum strength and reactive force. One can object to maximum strength training for two reasons. Trying to use a workload that is too heavy can lead to an imbalance throughout the entire corset area (problems in the back, groin, etc.). In addition, pressure in the abdominal cavity will be increased due to the large amount of tension in the abdominal muscles, and it will prove quite difficult to keep this pressure from reaching an unhealthy level when the workload is extreme. Therefore, maximum strength training is best avoided. However, the abdominal muscles can be exerted reactively using the power of impact. Although the peak forces last only for a short time, they can be very large. Furthermore, breathing can be well regulated in this situation.

The process of learning to control muscle coordination and to work the abdominal muscles reactively shows considerable differences in development between individuals. While one athlete might hardly need any basic training and be able to exercise his abdominal muscles immediately without difficulty, another individual might be unprepared to absorb a rapid power impact even after years of training. The agility in the joints (pelvic tilting and flexibility in the lumbar spinal column) determines whether a movement can be made easily or whether it will be difficult, if not impossible. Because they are not agile enough, some sportsmen cannot even move beyond their point of inertia while doing simple sit-ups. In this case, an athlete is better advised to choose other forms of exercise and spend more time improving agility in the trunk and pelvis. Therefore, when exercising the abdominal muscles, it is necessary to use a custom-designed training program that focuses on individual special needs.

In the series of exercises described below, particular attention is paid to working the abdominal muscles reactively. Many excellent articles can be found in the literature on basic techniques and the cooperation between abdominal and other muscles.

In addition to strength training, jumping can also be used to help the abdominal muscles work better reactively. In particular, a squatting leap on two legs, where there is a large horizontal displacement, will give rise to large peak forces affecting the abdominal muscles.

Figure 6.21a–d Exercise 1: corset function 1

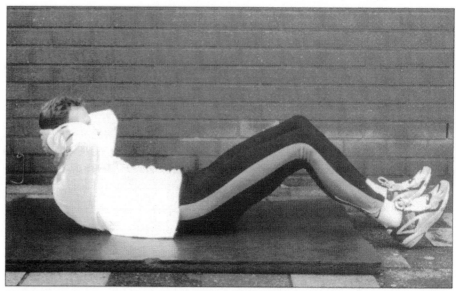

a

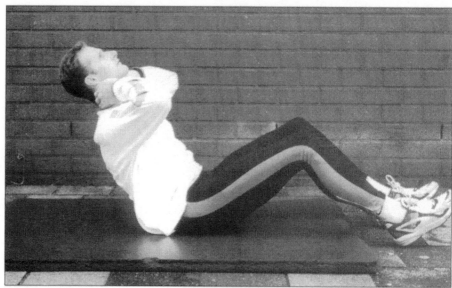

b

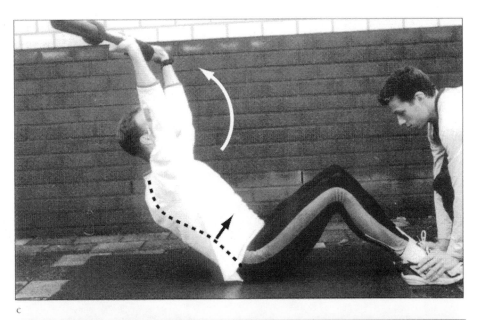

c

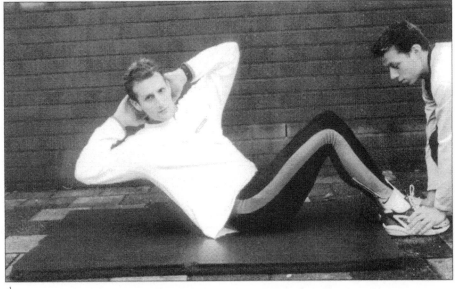

d

Exercise 1   Corset function A

Start by laying on the back with the legs slightly retracted before raising the upper body to a sitting
position. Clasp the hands behind the neck (a). Just before the trunk is erect, the back should be
extended (lower back flat and chest pointed forward). Here the elbows are pressed towards the
rear (b). Thereafter, the back rounds out again as the trunk returns to its starting position. The
entire exercise must be done slowly and be kept well under control. In particular, close attention
must be paid to how the body is returned to its starting position and the motion must be well executed.

- The exercise can be made more difficult by lifting the knees further. Extending the body outward
  will then take place while the trunk is still leaning quite far backward.
- The exercise can be performed while holding a bar-bell. From the starting position, the arms are
  extended and raised vertically. The arms remain extended during the sit-up. At the point where the
  back must be extended (before the trunk is vertical), the arms must be aligned with the trunk (c).
- At the point where the back is extended, torsion will develop as one elbow moves forward and the
  other elbow moves toward the rear (d).

367

Figure 6.22   Exercise 2: corset function 2

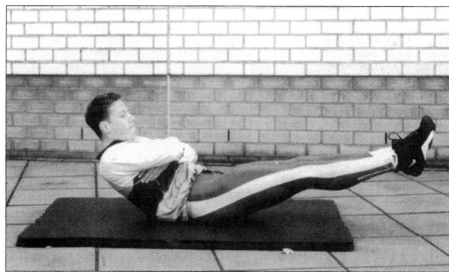

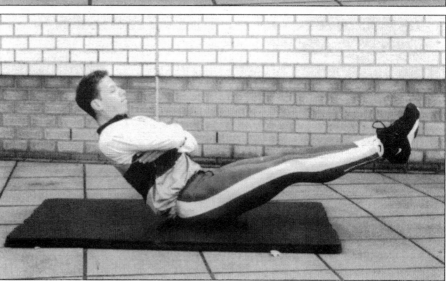

Exercise 2   Corset function 2

Start by reclining on the back with the legs extended. Both the legs and upper body are lifted so that only the buttocks are touching the ground. Both the feet and shoulders are raised 20–30 cm from the ground. The pelvis tilts first backward and then forward. The back is rounded as the pelvis tilts backward. The pelvis is tilted forward while the back is straightened by tightening the dorsal muscles. While first rounding the back before making it hollow, the feet and shoulders must remain stationary. The abdominal and dorsal muscles working together are responsible not only for moving the body but also for maintaining its balance. This exercise should be performed slowly and kept well under control. It can be made more difficult either by weighting down the feet (with ankle weights) or by extending the back while torsion develops in the spinal column.

Figure 6.23   Exercise 3: reactivity arising from a hard stroke 1

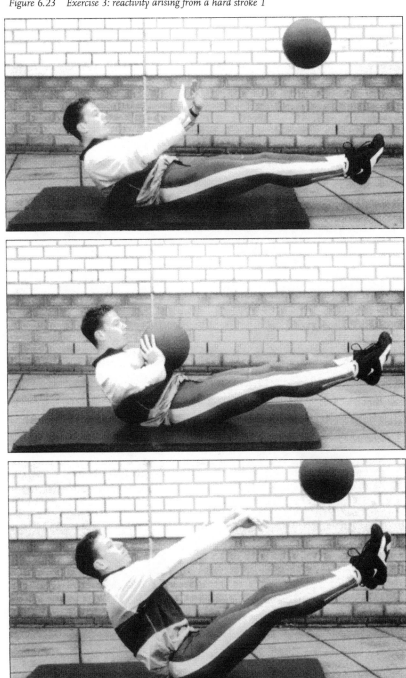

Exercise 3   Reactivity arising from a hard stroke 1

Start as described for Exercise 2: only the buttocks are touching the mat. A helper stands near the feet and throws an exercise ball in the direction of the head/chest. The athlete catches the ball and thrusts (not throws) it back again as hard as possible. The abdominal muscles must repeatedly absorb the shock of impact, which works eccentrically, and then immediately release this energy by thrusting the ball back again. The time between the catch and return must be kept as brief as possible. As a variation, this exercise can be performed sideways, in which case the weight of the load will be more on the oblique abdominal muscles.

Figure 6.24   Exercise 4: reactivity arising from a hard stroke 2

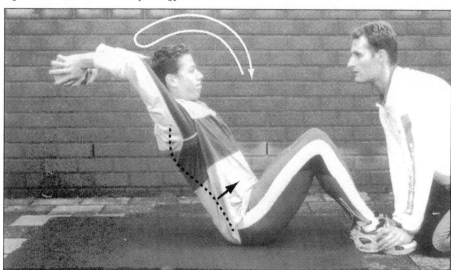

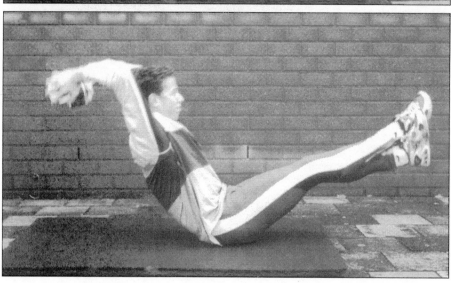

Exercise 4   Reactivity arising from a hard stroke 2

Start by reclining on the back with the knees bent (90°). The feet are kept stationary and a weight is held in front of the chest with both hands. A half sit-up is made while moving the weight directly upward and then behind the head. Subsequently, the weight is returned as rapidly as possible in front of the chest before the body returns to its starting position. The weight can also be lifted upwards and to the side. The movement must be carried out with increasing speed and more force each time, placing emphasis on the way in which the weight is pulled back in front of the chest. This exercise can also be performed without keeping the legs stationary. In the starting position, only the buttocks touch the ground and the knees are pulled up against the chest. At the same time that the weight is pushed backwards, the legs are extended in the opposite direction. After extending, the body returns to its starting position. The body should be extended so far that the exercise can still be performed without the back and feet touching the ground. When the feet are kept stationary, this exercise can be intensified by working on a slanting surface so that the feet are higher than the hips.

Figure 6.25   Exercise 5: reactivity arising from a hard stroke 3

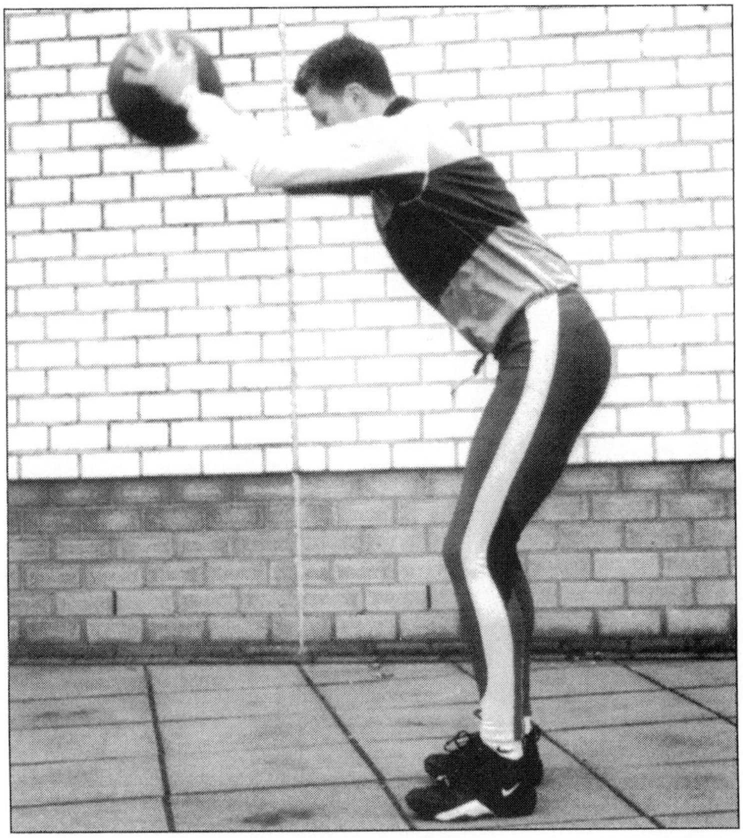

Exercise 5   Reactivity arising from a hard stroke 3
Stand upright holding a ball between the hands. The ball is bounced from above the head as hard as possible onto the ground just in front of the feet. As the ball rebounds, it is caught for the next throw. The exercise is carried out rapidly and with as much force as possible. During the throw, the abdominal muscles will be stressed eccentrically. Prestretch is converted reactively, and the upper body snaps forward to increase the downward velocity of the ball. This exercise trains the arms as well as the abdominal muscles and is very suitable for middle- and long-distance runners because of the conditional moment that makes this implementation intensive.

Figure 6.26 Exercise 6: reactivity arising from a hard stroke 4

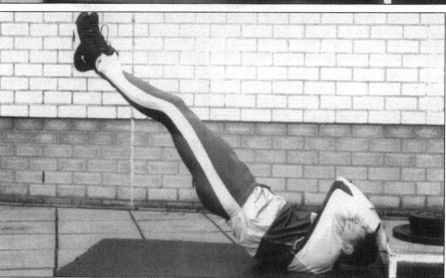

Exercise 6 Reactivity arising from a hard stroke 4

Start by laying on the back with the knees pulled toward the chest. The hips are off the ground and the hands grip a rigid support above the head. The entire lower body extends diagonally upward, making an angle of about 45° with the ground, so that only the shoulders remain on the floor. Subsequently, the knees are briskly pulled back to the starting position. The hips must not be allowed to touch the floor here. The smaller the angle between the extended body and the floor, the greater will be the forces working on the abdominal muscles. Movement of the legs must therefore be as even as possible.

6.3.5   Quadriceps femoris

In principle, the three vastus segments of the quadriceps femoris can be strengthened by means of maximum power training. In addition, training for maximum strength is also useful. Furthermore, exercises on one leg, rather than two, are always preferred. Strong vastus muscles are particularly important for sprinters. These muscles can be trained without having to pay much attention to the transfer (for 'dumb' muscles, transfer is easy). This means that the angles of the knee and hip with which one is working do not have to correspond too closely to those angles found when carrying out the running movement targeted.

For the biarticular segment of the quadriceps, the rectus femoris, the opposite is true. The structure of this muscle is even more specific (more pennate) than that of the hamstrings. Because biarticular muscle works isometrically and reactively, it requires maximum strength and impact training. The function of the muscle is embedded in how it will function in coordination with other muscles, and so it is not useful to attempt to train it alone. In most exercises, the rectus femoris works together with other muscles: in sit-ups, when the feet are held stationary it works together with the iliopsoas and the abdominal muscles, and in squatting exercises it works with the gluteus maximus.

6.3.6   Gluteus maximus

The major motor at work during running is the gluteus maximus. This muscle (especially its lower section) is suited for concentric work, and therefore for maximum power training. Because it is almost impossible to work the gluteus maximus in isolation during strength training, one cannot determine which ballast will be optimal. Therefore, one is best advised to seek only exercises that actually emphasize the gluteus maximus itself. Once such an exercise has been found and it can be implemented easily close to isometry, then one can put aside the issue of speed and train the muscle for maximum strength.

In practice, it appears to be both easy and useful to train the gluteus maximus and the quadriceps femoris together. Because they work together as a team, the total movement will be much greater than if either muscle were trained in an extreme situation of isolation. Because the movement is more all-round, it will be somewhat easier to reach an extreme degree of effort than if the movement was restricted to a single joint. Exercising on one leg, rather than two, is always preferred during such intermuscular teamwork.

Figure 6.27   Exercise 1: maximum strength while bending one knee

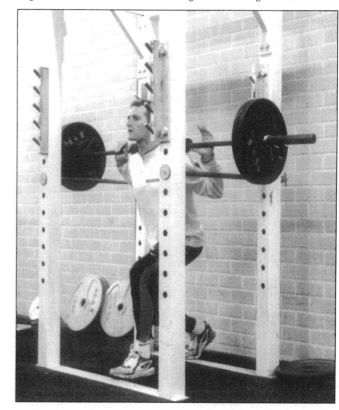

Exercise 1   Maximum strength while bending one knee
When training for maximum force in the hamstrings, the shoulders are brought forward as the knees bend. In this exercise, emphasis is placed on the quadriceps (together with the gluteus maximus), instead of the hamstrings, by holding the shoulders and bar-bell directly above the hips. In this way, the back leg can absorb more weight, and the weight of the bar-bell can thus be heavier than when training the hamstrings. The lever arm acting on the knee is now large and the load on the quadriceps femoris (including the rectus femoris) and gluteus maximus is large. This exercise is not suited for training for maximum power because it is somewhat difficult to maintain balance.

Exercise 2   Hack squat
When using leg-press or hack-squat equipment to train, a weight is pushed either horizontally or diagonally upward by the feet. When using hack-squat equipment, the load is placed on the shoulders and the weight glides up and down along guidelines. It is preferable to position the feet so that, when squatting, the angles of both the hip and the knee measure 90°. When the feet are placed in alignment with the body, the angle of the knee will be more acute when squatting. Not only will the lever arm be less favorable, but the hip cannot be bent very much either, because the angle of the knee is less than 90° and must be avoided. The best position for exerting the most force will differ substantially according to the type of training equipment used. The machine will dictate the movement. Therefore, an athlete must first become accustomed to the apparatus with which he will be training before using heavier workloads successfully. Exercising on one leg is preferable. Concentrating on one leg will make it possible to generate more force. Furthermore, the safety of the equipment should not be overestimated. The athlete must remain well in control of the corset function of the muscles around the spinal column. Because of the compulsory nature of the movement, oblique forces and torsion develop that are perhaps greater than when working with a bar-bell. To prevent the load from becoming too heavy, power exercises (rapid extension) should always be performed standing on one leg.

Figure 6.28   Exercise 3: hack squat using a bar-bell

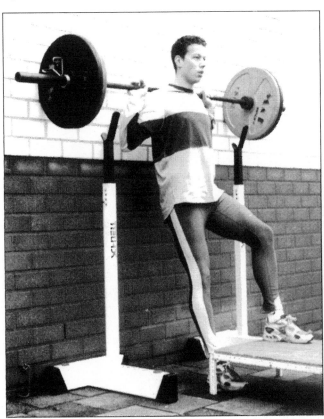 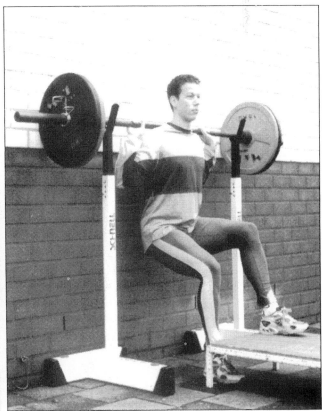

Exercise 3   Hack squat using a bar-bell

When training with bar-bells, one can also work in a squatting position in which the angles of both the knee and the hip are 90° and the load remains positioned directly above the hips. Stand with the back against a wall, holding a bar-bell at neck level with its discs touching the wall (this exercise must be performed using an 'Olympic' bar-bell). The hips are placed directly beneath the shoulders and near the wall. One foot is on the ground about 2–3 foot lengths from the wall. The other foot is placed on a low elevation and serves only to maintain balance. The upper body slides downward while the bar-bell discs roll along the wall until the thigh is directly horizontal. The angle of the knee should be 90°. If this is not the case then the foot must be repositioned. The exercise must be carried out while wearing a weightlifter's belt because it is an important that the trunk be kept well under control. This exercise can be used to train for maximum strength and power.

Figure 6.29   Exercise 4: reactivity arising from rapid loading

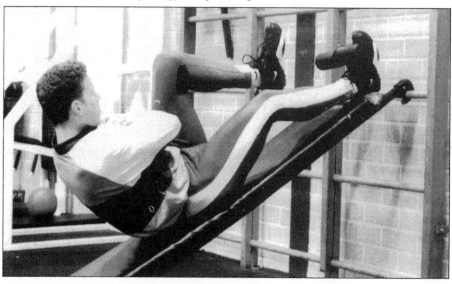

Exercise 4   Reactivity arising from rapid loading

This exercise is for the rectus femoris. Start in a sitting position. One leg is held stationary with the knee bent and the foot on the ground, while the other leg is free, with the hip and knee bent quite far. The upper body swings rapidly forward and backward. The degree of movement is slight and the load can be increased by holding the upper body farther backward, on average. The dorsal muscles must be tightened quite well so that the degree of movement developed will be caused as much as possible by tilting the pelvis. This exercise can be performed on a hard surface or one that slants downward as illustrated.

6.3.7 Iliopsoas

Electromyograms (EMGs) have not been recorded for the iliopsoas during running or at impractical lower speeds. Therefore, we have no insight regarding the range over which this muscle can function during running. With respect to training, it is best to work the muscle across a relatively large trajectory in which it contracts. It is more difficult to find an exercise for the range of the muscle when the hip is extended. When training the iliopsoas, it is impossible to determine an exact load for obtaining maximum power. It is therefore not very important which workload or speed is used during the exercise. When this muscle is worked rapidly, the muscles responsible for protecting the spinal column must be tightened adequately. If this becomes impossible due to the speed used, it is better to exercise more slowly while using a heavier workload.

Exercise 1 Concentric hip bending 1
The starting position is identical to that for exercising the rectus femoris reactively. If possible, the leg should only be held secure above the knee. There is now a lot of room for movement while the tempo is slow. The rectus femoris is not actually suited to shorten very far, so the movement is chiefly carried out by the iliopoas. The back must remain as extended as possible so that movement can be generated particularly when the pelvis is tilted.

Figure 6.30   Exercise 2: concentric hip bending 2

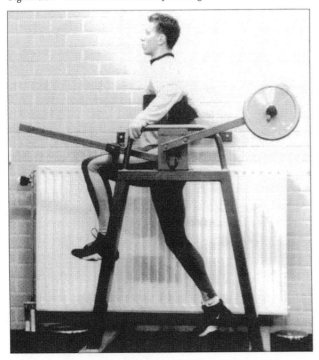

Exercise 2 Concentric hip bending 2
The 'Schnell trainer' is frequently used and particularly effective for exercising the iliopsoas. A bar exiting the apparatus and running parallel to the thigh holds a roller, which rests on the thigh. This roller can be pressed upward with a great deal of force. It is important that close control is maintained over the upper body during the exercise, because the iliopsoas will exert a great deal of force on the spinal column.

6.3.8   Small gluteal muscles

The small gluteal muscles and the uppermost section of the gluteus maximus are responsible for lifting the free half of the pelvis during the stance phase of running. This movement is preceded by a downward movement in the opposite direction. The speed with which these movements occur in sequence is quite fast. These muscles work reactively during running. One can train for maximum force by means of abduction in the leg. Running and jumping exercises can be used to train the muscles to work well reactively. It will be nearly impossible to exceed the power peaks generated in this way by using bar-bells.

Figure 6.31   Exercise 1: abduction on the Schnell trainer

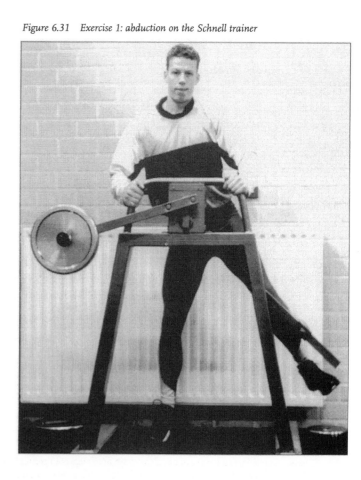

Exercise 1   Abduction on the Schnell trainer
The small gluteal muscles can also be trained on the Schnell trainer. Here the roller is placed on the outer side of the ankle and the athlete abducts his hip.

Figure 6.32   Exercise 2: abduction with resistance

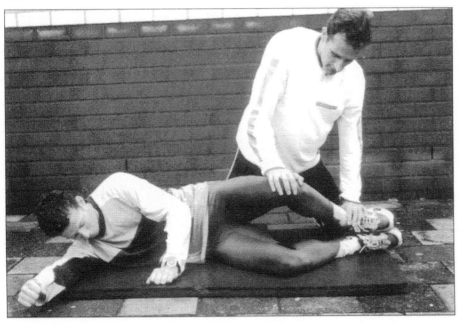

Exercise 2   Abduction with resistance

Start by laying on one side with the hip bent 45° and the knees bent 90°. An assistant provides resistance to the outer side of the top knee while the athlete tries to push his knees as far apart as possible. The exercise can be performed well when the top foot is held securely by the assistant. The pelvis must not be allowed to rotate toward the back. This exercise is suitable for training maximum strength. It can also be started with the knees held far apart. The assistant tries to press the athlete's knees together while the athlete resists.

6.4   STRENGTH TRAINING FOR MUSCLE CHAINS WORKING TOGETHER

Many exercises can be carried out for which the quality of implementation will depend to a large extent on the manner in which the muscles work as a team. Such mutual cooperation forms the second floor (coordination) in the biomechanical 'house' and precedes functional movement. It is also useful to train coordination using relatively heavy bar-bells. One must be careful to observe which groups of muscles will limit performance, and also if the various muscles are actually working together correctly (i.e. technique).

Figure 6.33   Exercise 1: dead weight

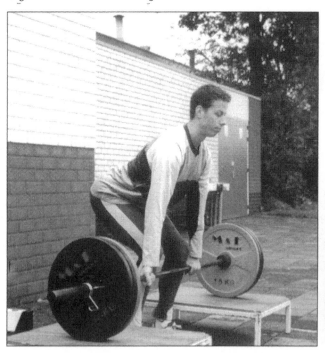 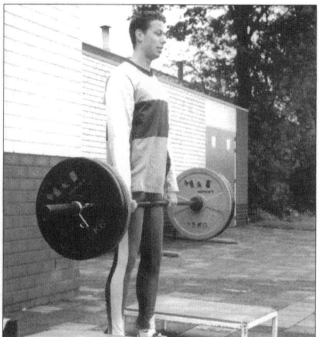

Exercise 1   Dead weight

A bar-bell is placed on two elevations so that the bar is just below the level of the knees. The bar is held in a mixed grip. The knees are near the bar, with the feet placed at shoulder width. The body extends upward as the bar-bell is lifted. While standing erect, the shoulder blades are moved backwards until they reach their final position. Thereafter, the bar-bell is returned to the elevations in a well-controlled manner. The dorsal muscles are the limiting factor and work together with the gluteus maximus and the hamstrings.

Figure 6.34   Exercise 2: classic pumping weights

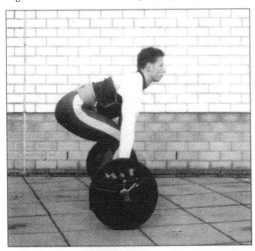

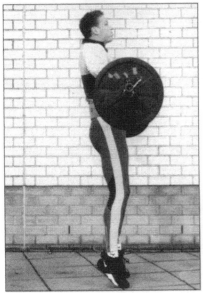

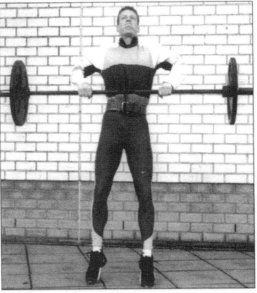

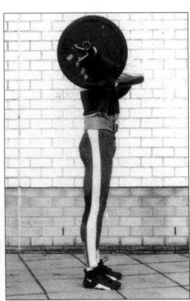

Exercise 2   Classic pumping weights

Start by holding the bar-bell 30–50 cm above the ground. The back is extended, the knees are near the bar, and the buttocks are kept as low as possible. The arms are extended while the hands hold the bar at shoulder width. The bar-bell is lifted off the ground while keeping the arms and back as extended as possible. The knees and hip extend simultaneously. The bar-bell is moved upwards with increasing speed close to the front of the body. When the bar-bell reaches hip level the arms push it on through in an upward motion. Here the elbows are raised high to the side. Next, the athlete twists his wrists so that the elbows are pointing forward. The motion ends with the body upright and the bar-bell held in front of the chest. During the first part of the movement, the bar-bell is quickly lifted upwards so that the elastic muscle segments that are working reactively can be preloaded. As soon as the bar-bell has reached a certain velocity, the stored energy is unloaded, thus causing further acceleration. During this pattern of movement, all the muscles involved in the extension sequence are working together and reactivity plays an important role. This is a very suitable exercise for instructing how to coordinate reactive muscle action with large peak forces.

Figure 6.35a–d   Exercise 3: pumping weights (variation)

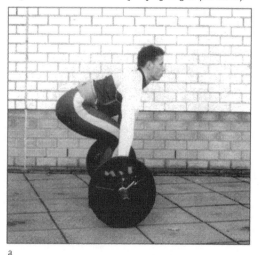

a

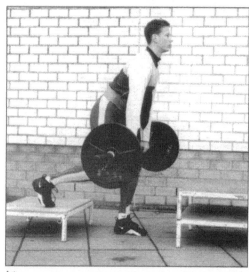

b1

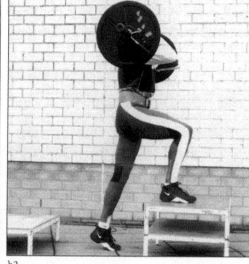

b2

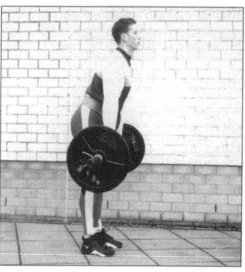

c

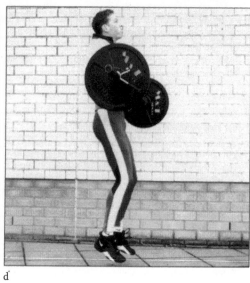

d

Exercise 3 Pumping weights (variation)
This type of exercise is usually only practiced in its basic form. However, some variations are of particular significance for runners.

- Carry out the movement with the knees kept more or less extended (see Section 6.3.2). Now emphasis is placed on the hamstrings. An extended back is required (a).
- Carry out the movement standing on one leg. In the starting position the bar-bell must be held just above the knee. One leg is bent strongly at the knee and rests toward the back with the foot on an elevation. This leg only serves to maintain balance. The other (support) knee is near the bar-bell. Otherwise, the movement is identical to that for the basic exercise. Because the body is supported by one leg, there is strong emphasis on the reactive action of the hamstrings (b1, b2).
- Start with the body nearly extended with a bar-bell held to the front at hip level. The movement is carried out with as little forward motion as possible. Because prestretch cannot be built up during the first acceleration of the bar-bell, it is necessary to create pretension in the body on purpose before movement is initiated (c).
- Building up pretension can be facilitated by first bending the trunk slowly forward from its extended position. The hip bends while the knee remains straight. When the trunk is leaning forward by about 45° there is a great deal of tension in the muscles, especially the hamstrings. Subsequently, the trunk is slowly returned to an erect posture, by which tension in the muscles is consciously maintained as fully as possible. Once a nearly upright posture has been reached, the forward motion of the bar-bell will follow. When pretension is good, the bar-bell will accelerate faster, especially just after the movement has begun, than would have been possible without the extra pretension.
- Classic pattern. As the wrists twist, the feet briefly leave the ground. Therefore, reactivity must be unloaded somewhat faster (d).
- From an extended posture, by which the feet briefly leave the ground.

Figure 6.36   Exercise 4: extension exercise 1

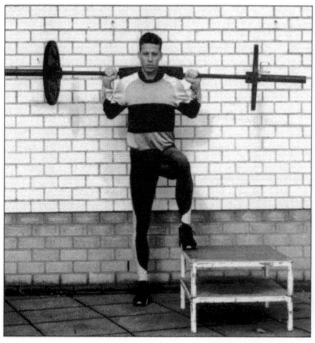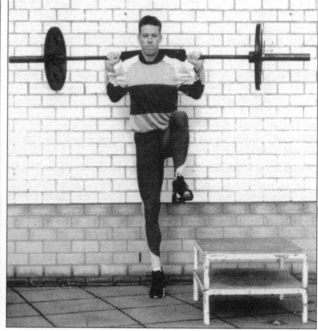

Exercise 4   Extension exercise 1

Stand on one foot while holding a heavy bar-bell at neck level. The other leg is bent at the knee, with the forward foot resting on an elevation. The stance leg is completely extended at the ankle and knee so that the weight of the body is on the forefoot. At the same time, the bent leg is lifted as high as possible without also extending the knee. This position is held for 1 s. This exercise demands a lot of work from the gluteal muscles, hamstrings, and (unilaterally) dorsal muscles. The bar-bell may be heavy.

Figure 6.37a–c   Exercise 5: extension exercise 2

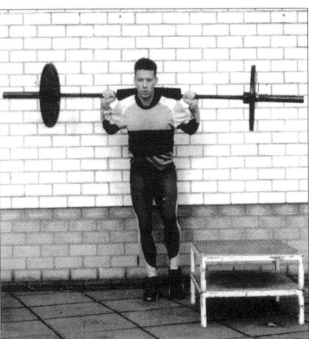
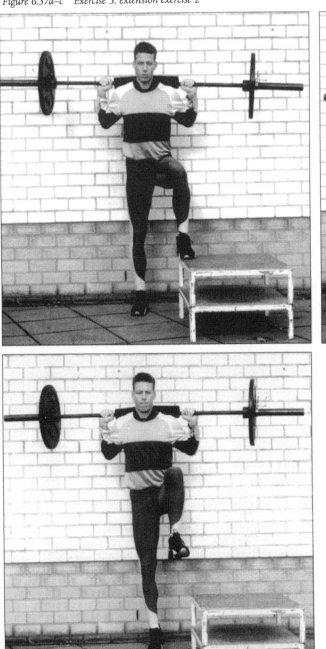
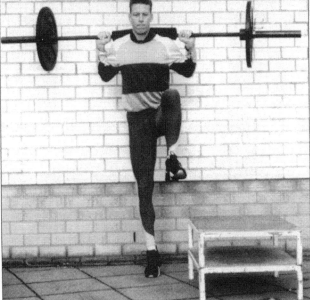

Exercise 5   Extension exercise 2
The starting position is identical to that in Exercise 4. Bend the stance leg slightly at the knee. The other leg is bent and rests on an elevation. This leg is lifted from the elevation in order to tap the ground next to the foot of the stance leg. After tapping, the foot is returned to the elevation as quickly as possible, with the stance leg extending as forcefully as possible. Extension has now been coupled to the upward swing of the stance leg (inverse-extension reflex).

Exercise 6   Hammer throw

Backward hammer throw using heavy weights (see Section 5.2.3). To a certain degree, this exercise can be compared with the classic pattern of movement shown in Figure 6.34 (Exercise 2). Both exercises use extending movements. In the first part of the movement elastic tissues are preloaded, and in the second part stored energy is released.

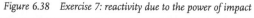

Figure 6.38   Exercise 7: reactivity due to the power of impact

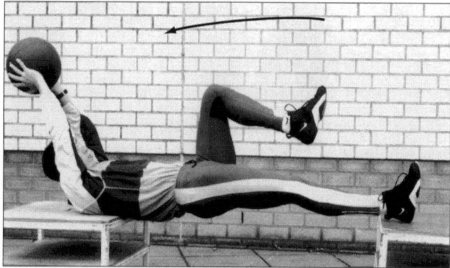

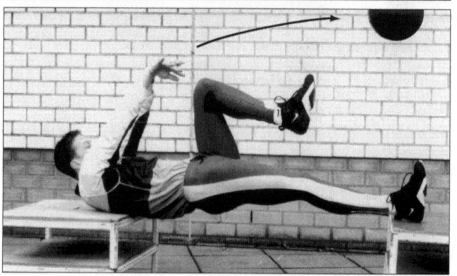

Exercise 7   Reactivity due to the power of impact

Start by reclining on the back with the body extended. The shoulders and one foot are resting on elevations. The remainder of the body is held off the floor. The free leg is bent 90° at the knee and hip. An assistant standing at the foot end throws a training ball into the hands of the athlete, who catches it with arms extended and throws it back as rapidly and with as much force as possible. The motion of tossing the ball reactively stresses, in particular, the hamstrings and the dorsal and abdominal muscles.

6.5 STRENGTH TRAINING FOR PATTERNS OF MOVEMENT RESEMBLING RUNNING

The total pattern of movement is formed by elements of locomotion and is supported by reflexes. The intensity of implementation is always high. Some exercises can be carried out using heavy weights, while others involve the use of only light weights. Coordination always remains an important issue when performing these exercises. Exertion at the neuromuscular level is very high. As an illustration a series of exercises is described, each of which is related to the step-up movement.

Figure 6.39   Exercise 1: step-up

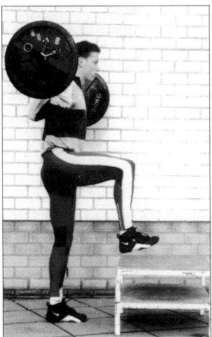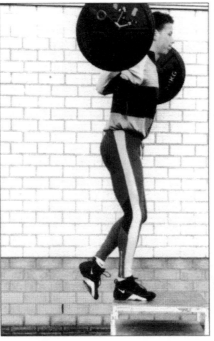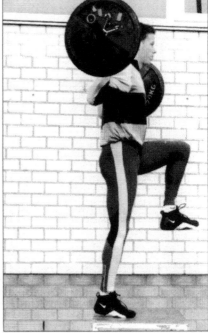

Exercise 1   Step-up
Stand with a bar-bell at neck level in front of an elevation that is lower than the knee. Next, lift the right leg and place it on the elevation. This step-up motion is carried out as forcefully as possible. Just before the right foot is placed on the elevation, the left leg must push off with as much force as possible and then swing upward rapidly. This upward swing ends at the front, with the knee and hip bent 90° and the foot lifted. The powerful push-off and upward swing of the free leg reinforces the extending motion of the step-up leg. Moreover, at the end of push-off, the swinging motion and bent position of the leg help prevent the back from undergoing strong lordosis during step-up. This exercise can be performed using various bar-bell weights. Because a reflex pattern is involved, it is advantageous to use a heavy weight as well as varying the bar-bell load, and therefore the speed of implementation.

Figure 6.40   Exercise 2: body snap before step-up

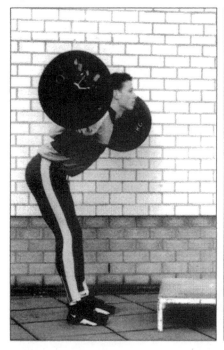
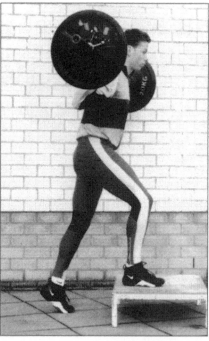
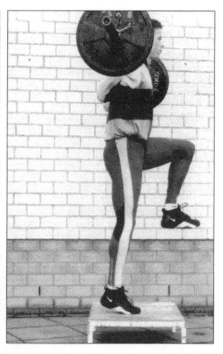

Exercise 2   Body snap before step-up

Stand upright on both feet in front of an elevation while holding a bar-bell at neck level. Next, snap the body forward. The movement must be made by tilting the pelvis forward while keeping the back extended. Next, extend the body upward. As the trunk is raised, one leg is lifted off the floor and makes a step-up movement. The step-up is carried out the same way as in Exercise 1. This exercise can be performed using various bar-bell weights. When the weight is heavy, the degree of movement during the body snap is quite small, so the elevation should be low. Even when using a heavy weight, rapid implementation of, in particular, the step-up movement is important. When the load is lighter, the snapping motion of the trunk can be performed more quickly. Here the degree of movement must not be too large. The elevation upon which the foot must step may be higher with a lighter weight than with a heavier one. For this exercise also, varying the weights and the height of the elevation is useful. The movement should be continuous without pausing, and the athlete should feel that the energy stored during the body snap is being released during the step-up.

Figure 6.41   Exercise 3: body snap and forward leap

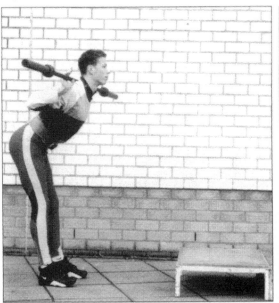
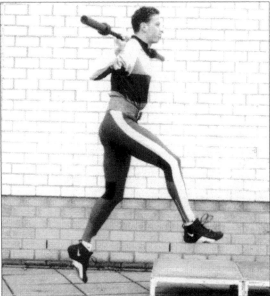
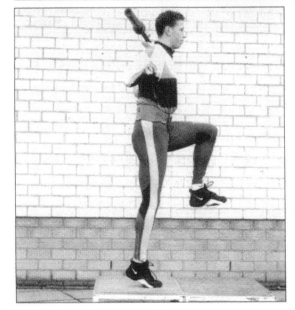

Exercise 3   Body snap and forward leap

This exercise is basically identical to Exercise 2. However, the bar-bell is lighter (eventually the bar may have no weights attached) and the elevation is only 20 cm high. The step-up now has a floating phase and becomes a leaping motion. Push-off from the ground is more powerful, and during the floating phase the leading leg causes backward flexion in the hip. Pulling this leg toward the rear causes the swing leg to accelerate forward. At the moment of foot strike, the stance leg is fully extended at the hip. In this exercise, the peak forces are somewhat lower than those in Exercise 2, but the processes of loading and releasing energy occur more rapidly. One must look for ways to implement this exercise more rapidly during training.

Figure 6.42   Exercise 4: upward push and forward leap

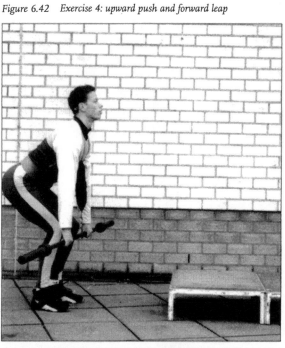
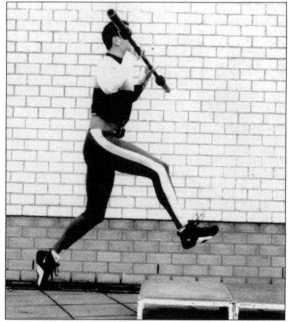
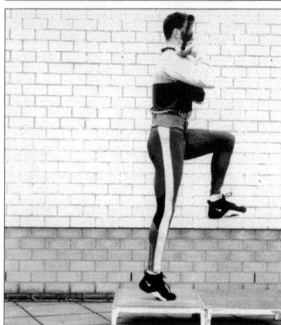

Exercise 4   Upward push and forward leap
Instead of standing upright with the bar-bell at neck level, the starting position is identical to that in Exercise 2 (Figure 6.34), in which the bar is held just below the knee. The weight of the bar-bell is rather light. The leaping motion is begun after pushing the bar-bell upward and ends with the bar-bell held in front of the chest. Here also the speed of implementation is important.

Figure 6.43   Exercise 5: variation while standing on one leg

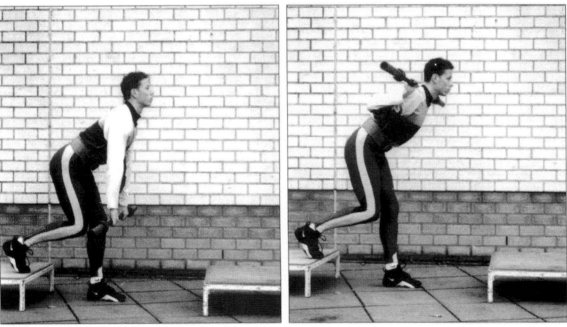

Exercise 5   Variation while standing on one leg
The two previous exercises can also be performed while standing on one leg. During the body snap and push up, the free leg, which is extended toward the back, is lifted before the swing phase is initiated. The free leg is also the leg that will land on the elevation.

FRANS BOSCH (1954) earned his degree (MOP) in 1977 at the Catholic Academy for Physical Education in Tilburg. Thereafter he was employed as a physical education teacher before becoming a self-employed expressive artist, in particular painting, in 1985. His style is considered to belong to the school of realism. Since 1980, he has been a trainer in the field of athletics. Today he works as a trainer of top athletes, namely sprinters and high-jumpers, of whom the Olympic high-jumpers Wilbert Pennings and Tora Harris are the most well-known. He has also worked for the KNAU as a teaching instructor (biomechanics, power-speed-jumping, and running techniques). Furthermore, Bosch has combined his talent as an expressive artist and his knowledge of anatomy by working as a medical–biological illustrator. In 1998, he published the book *Anatomy op het oog* (Elsevier Gezondheidszorg, Maarssen).

E-mail: fmpbosch@xs4all.nl

RONALD KLOMP (1962) earned his degree (MOP) in 1984 at the Catholic Academy for Physical Education in Tilburg. From 1985 to 1996, he was employed as a physical education teacher. During his final years as a teacher, he also studied the science of locomotion, specializing in the physiology of exercise. From 1993 to 2000, he was co-owner of a center that administered professional tests for physical exercise to athletes. Since 1983, Klomp has been a trainer of middle- and long-distance runners. During the past 10 years, he has been particularly involved in coaching top athletes, of whom the most well-known are Ellen van Langen, Marcel Laros, Simon Vroemen, and Jim Svenøy. At present, in addition to being a trainer, he is an instructor for various sports associations and develops applications for the internet.

E-mail: rklomp@mac.com

References

1 Anatomy of the locomotor apparatus and basic principles of motion

Aruin AS, Prilutskii BI. Relationship of biomechanical properties of muscles to their ability to utilize elastic deformation energy. Human Physiol 1985;11:8–12.

Bobbert MF, Huijing PA, Ingen Schenau GJ van. An estimation of power output and work done by the human triceps surae muscle–tendon complex in jumping. J Biomech 1986;18:899–906.

Bobbert MF, Yeadon MR, Nigg BM. Mechanical analysis of the landing phase in heel–toe running. J Biomech 1992;25:223–34.

Bobbert MF, Gerritsen KGM, Litjens MCA, Soest AJ van. Why is countermovement jump height greater than squat jump height? Med Sci Sports Exerc 1996;28(11): 1402–1412.

Bogduk N. Clinical Anatomy of the lumbar spine and sacrum. London: Churchill Livingstone 1997.

Brooks GA, Fahey TD, White TP. Exercise physiology, human bioenergetics and its applications. Mountain View: Mayfield 1996.

Burgerhout WG, Mook GA, Morree JJ de, Zijlstra WG. Fysiologie. Utrecht: Bunge 1995.

Cavagna GA. Storage and utilization of elastic energy in skeletal muscle. Exerc Sports Sci Rev 1977;5:89–129.

Cavagna GA, Kaneko M. Mechanical work and efficiency in level walking and running. J Physiol 1977;268:467–81.

Cavagna GA, Saibene FP, Margaria R. Mechanical work in running. J Appl Physiol 1964;18:1–9.

Chapman AE, Caldwell GE. Kinetic limitations of maximal sprinting speed. J Biomech 1983;16(1):79–83.

Cranenburgh B van. Neurowetenschappen. Maarssen: De Tijdstroom 1997a.

Cranenburgh B van. Schema's Fysiologie. Maarssen: Elsevier/De Tijdstroom 1997b.

Doorenbosch CAM, Welter TG, Ingen Schenau GJ van. Intermuscular co-ordination during fast contact leg task in man. Brain Res 1997;751:239–46.

Fox EL, Bowers RW, Foss ML. Fysiologie voor lichamelijke opvoeding, sport en revalidatie. Maarssen: Elsevier/De Tijdstroom 1996.

Gollnick PD, Piehl K, Saltin B. Selective glycogen depletion pattern in human muscle fibers after exercise of varying intensity and at varying pedal rates. J Physiol 1974;241:45–7.

Henneman E, Clamann HP, Gillies JD, Skinner RD. Rank order of motoneurons within a pool, law of combination. J Neurophysiol 1974;37:1338–49.

Hof AL, Geelen BA, Berg JW van den. Calf muscle moment, work and efficiency in level walking: role of series elasticity. J Biomech 1983;16:523–37.

Huijbregts PA, Clarijs JP. Krachttraining in revalidatie en sport. Utrecht: De Tijdstroom 1995.

Huxley AF, Huxley HE. Muscle structure and theories of contraction. Prog Biophys Biophys Chem 1957;7:255–318.

Ingen Schenau GJ van. Kracht en snelheid 1: het moment-hoeksnelheidsdiagram. Geneeskunde Sport 1983;16:173–6.

Ingen Schenau GJ Van, Tousaint H. Biomechanica. Amsterdam: Vrije Universiteit 1994.

Ingen Schenau GJ van, Boer RW de, Vergoesen I. Kracht en snelheid 3: de counterbeweging. Geneeskunde Sport 1984;17(2):44–8.

Ingen Schenau GJ van, Dorssers WMM, Welter TG, Beelen A, Groot G de, Jacobs R. The control of monoarticular muscles in multijoint leg extensions in man. J Physiol 1995;484(1):247–54.

Jacobs R, Ingen Schenau GJ van. Intermuscular co-ordination in a sprint push-off. J Biomech 1992;25:953–65.

Jacobs R, Bobbert MF, Ingen Schenau GJ van. Function of mono- and biarticular muscles in running. Med Sci Sports Exerc 1993;25:1163–73.

Jacobs R, Bobbert MF, Ingen Schenau GJ van. Mechanical output from individual muscles during explosive leg extensions: the role of biarticular muscles. J Biomech 1996;28: 513–22.

Jones DA, Round JM. Skeletal muscle in health and disease. Manchester: University Press 1990.

Ker RF, Bennet MB, Bibby SR. The spring in the arch of the human foot. Nature 1987;325:147–9.

Kraaijenhof H. Powertraining, een nieuwe ontwikkeling binnen de krachttraining. Richting Sportgericht 1994;48(3):122–4.

Lohman AHM. Vorm en Beweging. Utrecht: Bohn, Scheltema & Holkema 1977.

Loo H van der. Krachttraining? Powertraining! Specialisatie krachttraining 1–7. Nieuwegein: KNAU 1996.

Mann RA, Moran GT, Dougerty SE. Comparative electromyography of the lower extremity in jogging, running and sprinting. Am J Sports Med 1986;8:345–50.

Martin PE, Cavanagh PR. Segment interactions within the swing leg during unloaded and loaded running. J Biomech 1990;23:529–36.

Martini FH. Fundamentals of anatomy and physiology. Upper Saddle River, NJ: Prentice Hall 1998.

McNiell Alexander R. The spring in your step. New Scientist 1987;42–4.

McNiell Alexander R. Elastic mechanisms in animal movement. Cambridge: University Press 1988.

Prilutskii BI, Zatsiorsky VM. Tendon action of two-joint muscles: transfer of mechanical energy between joints during jumping, landing and running. J Biomech 1994;27(1): 25–34.

Poel G van der. De kracht-snelheidsrelatie van een spier. Versus, Ned T Fysiother 1993;5:258–65.

Rozendal RH, Huijing PA. Kinesiologie van de mens. Houten: Robijns 1996.

Snijders CJ, Nordin M, Frankel VH. Biomechanica van het spierskeletstelsel. Utrecht: Lemma 1995.

Tittel K. Beschreibende und funktionelle anatomie des menschen. Jena/Stuttgart: Gustav Fischer Verlag 1990.

Williams KR, Cavanagh PR. Relationship between distance running mechanics, running economy, and performance. Am Physiol Soc 1987;63:1236–46.

Wilmore JH, Costill DL. Physiology of sport and exercise. Champaign, IL: Human Kinetics 1994.

Wingerden BAM van. Voetspieren in revalidatie en preventie. Sportgericht 1999;1:29–34.

Zuurbier CJ, Huijing PA. Influence of muscle geometry on shortening speed of fiber, aponeurosis and muscle. J Biomech 1992;25:1017–23.

2   Generation of energy

Anderson GS, Rhodes EC. A review of blood lactate and ventilatory methods of detecting transition thresholds. Sports Med 1989;8(1):43–55.

Arts FJP, Kuipers H. The relation between power output, oxygen uptake and heart rate in male athletes. Int J Sports Med 1994;15(5):228–31.

Balsom PD, Söderlund K, Ekblom B. Creatine in humans with special reference to creatine supplementation. Sports Med 1994;18(4):268–280.

Basset JR, Howley ET. Limiting factors for maximum oxygen uptake and determination of endurance performance. Med Sci Sports Exerc. 2000;32(1):70–84.

Bernús G, Conzález de Suso JM, Alonso J, Martin PM, Prat JA, Arús C. ^{31}P-MRS of quadriceps reveals quantitative differences between sprinters and long distance runners. Med Sci Sports Exerc 1993;25:479–84.

Billat VL, Flechet B, Petit B, Muriaux G, Koralsztein JP. Interval training at VO_{2max}: effects on aerobic performance and overtraining markers. Med Sci Sports Exerc. 1999; 31(1):156–63.

Billat V, Renoux JC, Pinoteau J, Petit B, Koralsztein JP. Reproducibility of running time to exhaustion at VO_2max in sub-elite runners. Med Sci Sports Exerc 1994;26(2):254–7.

Billeter R, Hoppeler H. Conditions for oxygen and substrate transport in muscles in exercising mammals. J Exp Biol 1991;160:263–83.

Bon M van. Wielrentraining. Haarlem: De Vrieseborch 1998.

Brooks GA. Anaerobic threshold: review of the concept and directions for future research. Med Sci Sports Exerc 1985;17(1):22–34.

Brooks GA, Fahey TD, White TP. Exercise physiology, human bioenergetics and its applications. Mountain View: Mayfield 1996.

Cheethan, ME, Boobis LH, Brooks S, Williams C. Human muscle metabolism during sprint running. J Appl Physiol 1986;61(1):54–60.

Connett RJ, Honig CR, Gayeski TEJ, Brooks GA. Defining hypoxia: a system view of VO_2, glycolysis, energetics, and intracellular PO_2. J Appl Physiol 1990;68(3):833–42.

Costill DL, Wilmore JH. Physiology of Sport and Exercise. Champaign, IL: Human Kinetics 1994.

Costill DL, Winrow, E. Maximal oxygen intake among marathon runners. Arch Phys Med Rehab 1970;51(6):317–20.

Fox EL, Bowers RW en Foss ML. Fysiologie voor lichamelijke opvoeding, sport en revalidatie. Edited and translated by J de Bruijne and HCG Kemper. Maarssen: Elsevier/De Tijdstroom 1997.

Goolberg T van de, Swinkels JM. De basisprincipes van de training. Voorburg: Isidoro 1994.

Greenhaff PL. Creatine and its application as an ergogenic aid. Int J Sport Nutr 1995;5:S100–10.

Greenhaff PL, Casey A, Short AH, Harris R, Söderlund K, Hultman E. Influence of oral creatine supplementation of muscle torque during repeated bouts of maximal voluntary exercise in man. Clin Sci 1993;84:565–71.

Harris R, Söderlund K, Hultman E. Elevation of creatine in resting and exercise muscles of normal subjects by creatine supplementation. Clin Sci 1992;83:367–74.

Hitchcock HC. Recovery of short-term power after dynamic exercise. J Appl Physiol 1989;67(2):677–81.

Hoogeveen AR, Hoogsteen J, Schep G. The maximal lactate steady state in elite endurance athletes. Jpn J Physiol 1997;47(5):481–5.

Howley ET, Bassett JR, Welch DR, Welch HG. Criteria for maximal oxygen uptake: review and commentary. Med Sci Sports Exerc 1995;27(9):1292–301.

Ingen Schenau GJ van, Toussaint H. Biomechanica. Amsterdam: Vrije Universiteit 1994.

Jeukendrup AE, Hesselink MKC, Snyder AC, Kuipers H, Keizer H. Physiological changes in male competitive cyclists after two weeks of intensified training. Int J Sports Med 1992;13(7):534–41.

Kloosterboer T. Elementaire trainingsleer en trainingsmethoden. Haarlem: De Vrieseborch 1996.

Loat CE, Rhodes EC. Relationship between the lactate and ventilatory thresholds during prolonged exercise. Sports Med 1993;15(2):104–15.

Marsh GD, Paterson DH, Potwarka JJ, Thompson RT. Transient changes in muscle high-energy phosphates during moderate exercise. J Appl Physiol 1993;75(2):648–56.

Martini FH. Fundamentals of anatomy and physiology. Upper Saddle River, NJ: Prentice Hall 1998.

Maughan RJ. Creatine supplementation and exercise performance. Int J Sport Nutr 1995;5:94–101.

Meyer RA, Sweeney HL, Kushmerick J. A simple analysis of the 'phosphocreatine shuttle'. Am J Physiol 1984;246:C365–77.

Myers J, Ashley E. Dangerous curves. A perspective on exercise, lactate and the anaerobic threshold. Chest 1997;111(3):787–95.

Newsholme E, Leech T, Duester G. Keep on running. New York: Wiley 1994.

Noakes TD. Implications of exercise testing for prediction of athletic performance: a contemporary perspective. Med Sci Sports Exerc 1988;20(4):319–30.

Noakes T. Lore of running. Champaign, IL: Leisure Press 1991.

Ohira Y, Tabat I. Muscle metabolism during exercise: anaerobic threshold does not exist. Ann Physiol Anthropol 1992;11(3):319–23.

Rehunen S, Näveri H, Kuoppasalmi K, Härkönen M. High-energy phosphate compounds during exercise in human slow-twitch and fast-twitch muscle fiber. Scand J Clin Lab Invest 1982;42:499–506.

Silverthorn DU. Human Physiology: an integrated approach. Upper Saddle River, NJ: Prentice Hall 1998.

Söderlund K, Greenhaff PL, Hultman E. Energy metabolism in type I and type II human muscle fibres during short term electrical stimulation at different frequencies. Acta Physiol Scand 1992;144:15–22.

Spurway NC. Aerobic exercise, anaerobic exercise and the lactate threshold. Br Med Bull 1992;48(3):569–91.

Stryer L. Biochemistry. New York: WH Freeman 1995.

Swinkels JM. Tendensen in de periodisering en hun rol in de blessurepreventie. In: Brouns F, JM Swinkels (eds), Congresverslag blessurepreventie. De Haarlem: Vrieseborch 1980.

Tanaka K. Lactate-related factors as a critical determinant of endurance. Antropol 1990;9(2):192–202.

Tesch PA, Thorsson A, Fujitsuka N. Creatine phosphate in fiber types of skeletal muscle before and after exhaustive exercise. J Appl Physiol 1989;66(4):1756–9.

Thoden JS. Testing aerobic power. In: MacDougall JD, Wenger HA, Green HJ (eds), Physiological testing of the high performance athlete, 2nd edn. Champaign, IL: Human Kinetics 1991.

Vandenberghe K, Gillis N, Leemputte van, Hecke M van, Vanstapel P, Hespel FP. Caffeine counteracts the ergogenic action of muscle creatine loading. J Appl Physiol 1996;80(2):452–7.

Vander AJ, Sherman JH, Luciano DS. Human physiology: the mechanism of body function. New York: McGraw-Hill 1994.

Vrijens J. Basis voor verantwoord trainen. Gent: Publicatiefonds voor lichamelijke opvoeding 1984.

Westra H. Spiervermoeidheid: zijn we dichter bij de oplossing van het raadsel spiervermoeidheid? Richting Sportgericht 1993;47(5):273–6.

Zintl F. Duurtraining. Haarlem: De Vrieseborch 1995.

3 Running techniques

Bhowmick S, Bhattacharyya AK. Kinematic analysis of arm movement in sprint start. J Sports Med Phys Fitness 1998;28:315–23.

Bobbert MF, Yeadon MR, Nigg BM. Mechanical analysis of the landing phase in heel–toe running. J Biomech 1992;25:223–34.

Cappozzo A. Force actions in the human trunk during running. J Sports Med 1983;23:14–22.

Cavagna GA, Saibene FP, Margaria R. Mechanical work in running. J Appl Physiol 1964;18:1–9.

Chapman AE, Caldwell GE. Kinetic limitations of maximal sprinting speed. J Biomech 1983;16(1):79–83.

Hinrichs RN. Upper extremity function in distance running. In: Cavanagh PR (ed), Biomechanics of distance running. Champaign, IL: Human Kinetics 1990.

Jacobs R, Ingen Schenau GJ van. Intermuscular co-ordination in a sprint push-off. J Biomech 1992;25:953–65.

Jacobs R, Bobbert MF, Ingen Schenau GJ van. Function of mono- and biarticular muscles in running. Med Sci Sports Exerc 1993;25:1163–73.

Mann RA, Moran GT, Dougerty SE. Comparative electromyography of the lower extremity in jogging, running and sprinting. Am J Sports Med 1986;8:345–50.

McClay IR, Lake MJ, Cavanagh PR. Muscle activity in running. In: Cavanagh PR (ed), Biomechanics of distance running, p 173. Champaign, IL: Human Kinetics 1990.

McMahon TA, Cheng GC. The mechanics of running: how does stiffness couple with speed? J Biomech 1990;23:65–78.

Miller D. Ground reaction forces in distance running. In: Cavanagh PR (ed), Biomechanics of distance running. Champaign, IL: Human Kinetics 1990.

Ounpuu S. The biomechanics of walking and running. Clin Sports Med 1994;13(4): 843–63.

Pink M, Perry J, Houglum PA, Decine DJ. Lower extremity range of motion in the recreational sport runner. Am J Sports Med 1994;22:541–9.

Simon C, Mendoza L. Effizienz und ökonomie im mittel und langstreckenlauf. Leistungssport 1998;4:35–40.

Williams KR, Cavanagh PR. Relationship between distance running mechanics, running economy, and performance. Am Physiol Soc 1987;63:1236–45.

4 Training and adaptation

Åstrand P-O, Rodahl K. Textbook of work physiology. Singapore: McGraw-Hill 1986.

Bompa TO. Periodization, theory and methodology of training. Champaign, IL: Human Kinetics 1999.

Bon M van. Wielrentraining. Haarlem: De Vrieseborch 1998.

Brooks GA, Fahey TD, White TP. Exercise physiology, human bioenergetics and its applications. Mountain View, CA: Mayfield 1996.

Bunc V, Leso J. Ventilatory threshold and work efficiency during exercise on a cycle and rowing ergometer. J Sports Sci 1993;11:43–8.

Cannon WB. Organization of physiological homeostasis. Physiol Rev 1929;9:398–402.

Costill DL, Wilmore JH. Physiology of sport and exercise. Champaign, IL: Human Kinetics 1994.

Costill DL. Inside running: basics of sports physiology. USA: Benchmark Press 1986.

Daniels J. Running formula. Champaign, IL: Human Kinetics 1998.

Davis JA. Anaerobic threshold: review of the concept and directions for future research. Med Sci Sports Exerc 1985;17(1):6–18.

Fallowfield JL, Wilkinson DM. Improving performance in middle and long distance running. New York: Wiley 1999.

Foster C. Monitoring training in athletes with reference to overtraining syndrome. Med Sci Sports Exerc 1998;30(7):1164–8.

Foster C, Daniels JT, Seiler S. Perspectives on correct approaches to training. In: Lehmann M, Foster C, Gastmann U, Keizer H, Steinacker JM (eds), Overload, performance, incompetence and regeneration in sport. pp. 27–41. New York: Kluwer/Plenum 1999.

Gaesser GA, Poole DC, Lactate and ventilatory thresholds: disparity in time course of adaptations to training. J Appl Physiol 1986; 61(3) 999–1004.

Gaesser GA, Poole DC, Gardner BP. Dissociation between $VO_{2\,max}$ and ventilatory threshold responses to endurance training. Eur J Appl Physiol 1984;53:242–7.

Hettinger T. Isometrisches muskeltraining. Stuttgart: Thieme Verlag 1966.

Holloszy JO, Coyle EF. Adaptations of skeletal muscle to endurance exercise and their metabolic consequences. J Appl Physiol 1984;56(4):831–8.

Hooper SL, Mackinnon LT, Howard A, Gordon RD, Bachmann AW. Markers for monitoring overtraining and recovery. Med Sci Sports Exerc 1995;27:106–12.

Lehmann M, Dickhuth HH, Gendrisch G, Lazar W, Thum M, Kuminski R, Aramendi JF, Peterke E, Wieland W, Keul J. Training-overtraining: a prospective, experimental study with experienced middle and long distance runners. Int J Sports Med 1991;12:444–52.

Matveyev LP. Periodisierung des sportlichen trainings. Berlin: Bartels & Wernitz 1972.

Morgan WP, Brown DR, Raglin JS. Psychological monitoring of overtraining and staleness. Br J Sports Med 1987;21:107–14.

Myers JN. Essentials of cardiopulmonary exercise testing. Champaign, IL: Human Kinetics 1996.

Noakes TD. Implications of exercise testing for prediction of athletic performance: a contemporary perspective. Med Sci Sports Exerc 1988;20(4):319–30.

Noakes T. Lore of running. Kaapstad: Oxford University Press 1992.

Os AG van. Men wordt niet als marathontopper geboren. Arnhem: NOC*NSF-publication BOK, January 1999.

Roovers M. Voorwaarden voor supercompensatie, deel 1. Richting Sportgericht 1999;1:25–7.

Silverthorn DU. Human physiology: an integrated approach. Upper Saddle River, NJ: Prentice Hall 1998.

Simon J, Young JL, Blood DK, Segal KR, Case RB, Gutin B. Plasma lactate and ventilation thresholds in trained and untrained cyclists. J Appl Physiol 1986;60(3):777–81.

Swinkels J. Tendensen in de periodisering en hun rol in de blessurepreventie. In: Brouns F, JM Swinkels JM (eds), Congresverslag blessurepreventie. Haarlem: De Vrieseborch 1980.

Swinkels JM, Goolberg T van de. De basisprincipes van de training. Voorburg: Isidoro 1994.

Tschiene P. Die neue 'theorie des trainings' und ihre interpretation für das nachwuchstraining. Leistungssport 1989;23(6):4–6.

Urhausen A, Kindermann W. One and two-dimensional echocardiography in body builders and endurance-trained subjects. Int J Sports Med 1989;10:139–44.

Verchoshansky J. Das ende der 'periodisierung' des sportlichen trainings im spitzensport. leistungssport 1998;(5):14–19.

Verchoshansky J. Effektiv trainieren. Berlijn: Sportverlag 1987.

Verchoshansky J. Ein neues trainingssystem für zyklischen sportarten. Münster: Philippha Verlag 1992.

Viru A. The mechanism of training effects: an hypothesis. Int J Sports Med 1984;5:219–27.

Viru A. Adaptation in sports training. Boca Raton, FL: CRC Press 1995.

Wasserman K, McElroy MB. Detecting the threshold of anaerobic metabolism. Am J Cardiol 1964;14:844–52.

Wasserman K, Hansen JE, Sue DY, Whipp BJ, Casaburi R. Principles of exercise testing and interpretation, 2nd edn. Philadelphia, PA: Williams & Wilkins 1997.

Young K. The theory of collapse. Runners World, September 1973.

Zatsiorsky VM. Science and practice of strength training. Champaign, IL: Human Kinetics 1995.

Zintl F (trans. Jeukendrup AE, Kuipers H) Duurtraining. Haarlem: De Vieeseborch 1995.

5 Running techniques in practice

Bobbert MF, Yeadon MR, Nigg BM. Mechanical analysis of the landing phase in heel–toe running. J Biomech 1992;25:223–34.

Cranenburgh B van. Neurowetenschappen. Maarssen: De Tijdstroom 1997.

Doorenbosch CAM, Welter TG, Ingen Schenau GJ van. Intermuscular co-ordination during fast contact leg task in man. Brain Res 1997;751:239–46.

Jacobs R, Ingen Schenau GJ van. Intermuscular co-ordination in a sprint push-off. J Biomech 1992;25:953–65.

Jacobs R, Bobbert MF, Ingen Schenau GJ van. Function of mono- and biarticular muscles in running. Med Sci Sports Exerc 1993;25:1163–73.

Pink M, Perry J, Houglum PA, Decine DJ. Lower extremity range of motion in the recreational sport runner. Am J Sports Med 1994;22:541–9.

6 Strength training for runners

Costill DL, Wilmore JH. Physiology of sport and exercise. Champaign, IL: Human Kinetics 1994.

Friden J, Seger J, Sjoestroem M, Ekblom B. Adaptive response in human skeletal muscle subjected to prolonged eccentric training. Int J Sports Med 1983;4:177–83.

Giddings CJ, Gonyea WJ. Morphological observations supporting muscle fiber hyperplasia following weight-lifting exercise in cats. Anat Record 1992;233:178–95.

Goldspink G. Cellular and molecular aspects of adaptation in skeletal muscle. In: Komi PV (ed), Strength and power in sport, pp. 211–29. Oxford: Blackwell Scientific 1992.

Häkkinen K, Alén M, Komi PV. Changes in isometric force and relaxation-time, electromyographic and muscle fiber characteristics of human skeletal muscle during strength training en detraining. Acta Physiol Scand 1985;125:573–85.

Harre D, Leopold W. Kraftausdauer und kraftausdauertraining. Theor Prax Körperkult 1986;35:335–59.

Hollmann W, Hettinger TH. Arbeits- und Trainingsgrundlagen. Stuttgart: Sportmedizin 1980.

Huijbregts PA, Clarijs JP. Krachttraining in revalidatie en sport. Utrecht: De Tijdstroom 1995.

Ingen Schenau GJ van, Toussaint H. Biomechanica. Amsterdam: Vrije Universiteit 1994.

Kibele A. Bedingungsfaktoren von kraftausdauerleistungen. Frankfurt am Main: Verlag Harri Deutsch 1995.

Nett T. Zum begriff 'schnellkrafttraining'. Lehre der Leichtathletik 1968;25:743–6.

Scholich M. Die Bewegungseigenschaften und ihre komplexität. Theor Prax Körperkultur 1965;14:481–95.

Schröder W. Die erscheinungsformen der kraft und ihre ausbildung. Theor Prax Körperkultur 1969;18:1076–85.

Taylor NAS, Wilkinson JG. Exercise-induced skeletal muscle growth: hypertrophy or hyperplasia. Sports Med 1986;3:190–200.

Zatsiorsky VM. Science and practice of strength training. Champaign, IL: Human Kinetics 1995.

INDEX

abdominal muscles 5, 6, 7, 40–2, 124, 346–8
    strength training 347, 364–5
abduction 3, 4, 378–9
acceleration 321–9
acceleration phase 172–6
accent period 194
acetone 98
acetyl-CoA 97, 100, 101
Achilles tendon 31, 35, 47
actin 12–14, 15–16
    filamentous (f-actin) 13
    globular protein (g-actin) 13
actomyosin complex 16
adaptation 189, 207–8
    cardiovascular 208–12
    metabolic 213–21
    respiratory 212–13
adduction 3, 4
adenosine monophosphate *see* AMP
adenosinediphosphate *see* ADP
adenosinetriphosphate *see* ATP
adenylate kinase (myokinase) 84, 85, 86–8
adenylate phosphokinase 85–6
ADP 15, 83, 86, 87, 88, 219
aerobic pathway 84, 85, 86, 95–9
afferent bundles 62
afferent innervation 62–4
all-or-none principle 20
all or nothing principle *see* all-or-none principle
alternating-tempo endurance running 227
alveolus 108
AMP 86, 87
anabolism 191
anaerobic threshold 93, 94, 214–18
ankle 8–11
    function of 243–62
    position in start and acceleration 321–2
    rigidity and reactive running 316
    sensory information 243
    storage and release of energy 249
aponeurosis plantaris 10
arch, foot 9, 10
arm
    in acceleration 327
    during start 147–50, 177, 327
    for endurance tempo 187
arteriovenous oxygen difference ($_{a-v}VO_2$) 115, 208, 212
asynchrony of recovery processes 192